Complete **Callanetics**

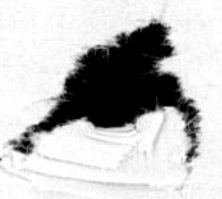

Complete Callanetics

The Bestselling Collection of Callan Pinckney's Exercises

INCLUDING
CALLANETICS

SUPER
CALLANETICS

Callan Pinckney

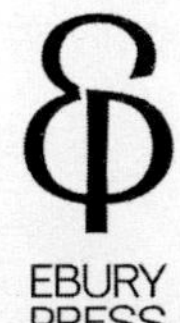

EBURY
PRESS

WARNING:
There are risks inherent in any exercise programme. The advice of a doctor should be obtained prior to embarking on any exercise regimen. This programme is intended for persons in good health.

TO PREGNANT WOMEN:
Under no circumstances should any woman in the first trimester of her pregnancy do any of the exercises which also use the stomach muscles featured in this book. During the second and third trimester do not attempt to do the exercises unless your doctor has actually done them to feel how deep the contractions are.

Do not just show your doctor the book. These exercises appear to be very easy, but looks in this case are extremely deceiving.

This edition published in 1993
by BCA by arrangement with Ebury Press,
an imprint of Random House UK Ltd,
20 Vauxhall Bridge Road, London SW1V 2SA

CN 8673

Callanetics first published in Great Britain in 1989 by Arrow Books Ltd
Copyright © 1984 Callan Pinckney

Super Callanetics first published in Great Britain in 1991 by Arrow Books Ltd in association with Ebury Press
Copyright © 1991 Callan Production Corp.

The Random House Group Limited supports The Forest Stewardship Council® (FSC®), the leading international forest-certification organisation. Our books carrying the FSC label are printed on FSC®-certified paper. FSC is the only forest-certification scheme supported by the leading environmental organisations, including Greenpeace. Our paper procurement policy can be found at www.randomhouse.co.uk/environment

Printed and bound in Great Britain by Clays Ltd, St Ives plc

Contents

Also by Callan Pinckney

Callanetics for Your Back
Callanetics Countdown
Quick Callanetics: Legs
Quick Callanetics: Stomach
Quick Callanetics: Hips and Behind
am/pm Callanetics

Callanetics: 10 Years Younger in 10 Hours

CALLAN PINCKNEY
with Sallie Batson

Photographs by Gary Moody

SPECIAL CREDITS

Travel photos by whoever could aim the camera and push the button.

Medical Researcher: Michelle Dellapenta, R.N., C.N. II
Special Researcher: Valerie S. Brown

Sculptures by Edwina Sandys
Hair and Makeup by Lillian Cortez

Consultants: Mary Ann Castro, R.N.; New York City Police Sgt. John P. Codiglia, Mr. New York's Finest, State Body Building Champion in 1982 and 1983; Ellen M. Godowitz, M.Th.; Hiromichi Hayashi, M.C., P.C.; Kim Johnson; Dr. Laurie Langer; Dr. Pasquale A. Luongo; Dr. Patrick M. Luongo; Charles McCarroll; M.S.C., C.S.W.; Carl Bruno Menkel; Norman Miller Associates; Jacqueline I. Ross, R.P.T.; and Leonard Russell of the Sheridan Square Health Club.

Special Thanks to: Peggy Batson, Helen Mary Breen, Dianne Brooks, Lulu Buras, Irene Cara, Dara Cohen, Susan Croft, Mark Dixon, Valdev Duggal, Mitch Douglas, Louise Duncan, Paula Fierman, Larry Finley, Barbara Friedlander, Pat Golbitz, Tina Jorgenson-Rubbo, Charles and Suzanne Lecht, Marie McGrath, Lynne Meena, Tanya Mendoza, Jane Pinckney Middleton, Lane Middleton, Page Middleton, Janet Milazzo, Alan Peseri, Joan Poole, Karl S. Sabo, Ray Steinberg, Elba Tanburino, Arlene Tarte, Tara Terrell, Neal Thompson, Anna Tipton, Lynn Tuttle, Jennifer Williams, to Jane Angus, who wrote the initial proposal, and, especially, to Ebba Olsen Thomson, my ballet teacher.

Contents

THIS BOOK IS DEDICATED:

—to my precious, darling mother, who faithfully massaged my legs three hours a day for five years;
—to all the people around the world who were so concerned for my safety, for without their kindnesses I probably would have never made it home;
—and to my students who have taught me so much and eased my readjustment into the American way of life.

CHAPTER ONE

Who Is Callan Pinckney and Why Is She Writing This Book?

Callan Pinckney is not a celebrity, model, or movie star, nor is she a medical doctor with a string of degrees. She is a teacher, albeit unorthodox, of one of the most innovative exercise programs today. How she became a teacher is not so simple to explain. How she devised the program began somewhere between Savannah, Georgia, and Southeast Asia, sometime in the 1960s.

On paper, Callan's life looks like the figment of a fertile imagination, a scenario for a movie script:

A ninth-generation American Southern debutante, Callan hopped a freighter bound for Germany in 1961 and hitch-hiked around the world for the better part of ten years, completely missing the turbulent sixties in this country.

She shoveled snow in London, tracked migrating herds in Central Africa, painted the decks of a freighter as a member of its crew, sold peanuts table to table in a fashionable Tokyo rooftop restaurant, and taught British pronunciation to four hundred Chinese children in Hong Kong. These are but a few of her survival jobs.

Born with spinal curvatures (scoliosis and swayback), one hip higher than the other, and feet turned inward so severely that she wore leg braces to her waist for seven years of her childhood, Callan went on to study classical ballet for twelve years with a protégé of the legendary Michel Fokine.

Today she teaches exercise to diplomats and ambassadors, recording stars, actors and actresses, housewives, doctors, as well as to business and professional people of all sizes, shapes, and ages.

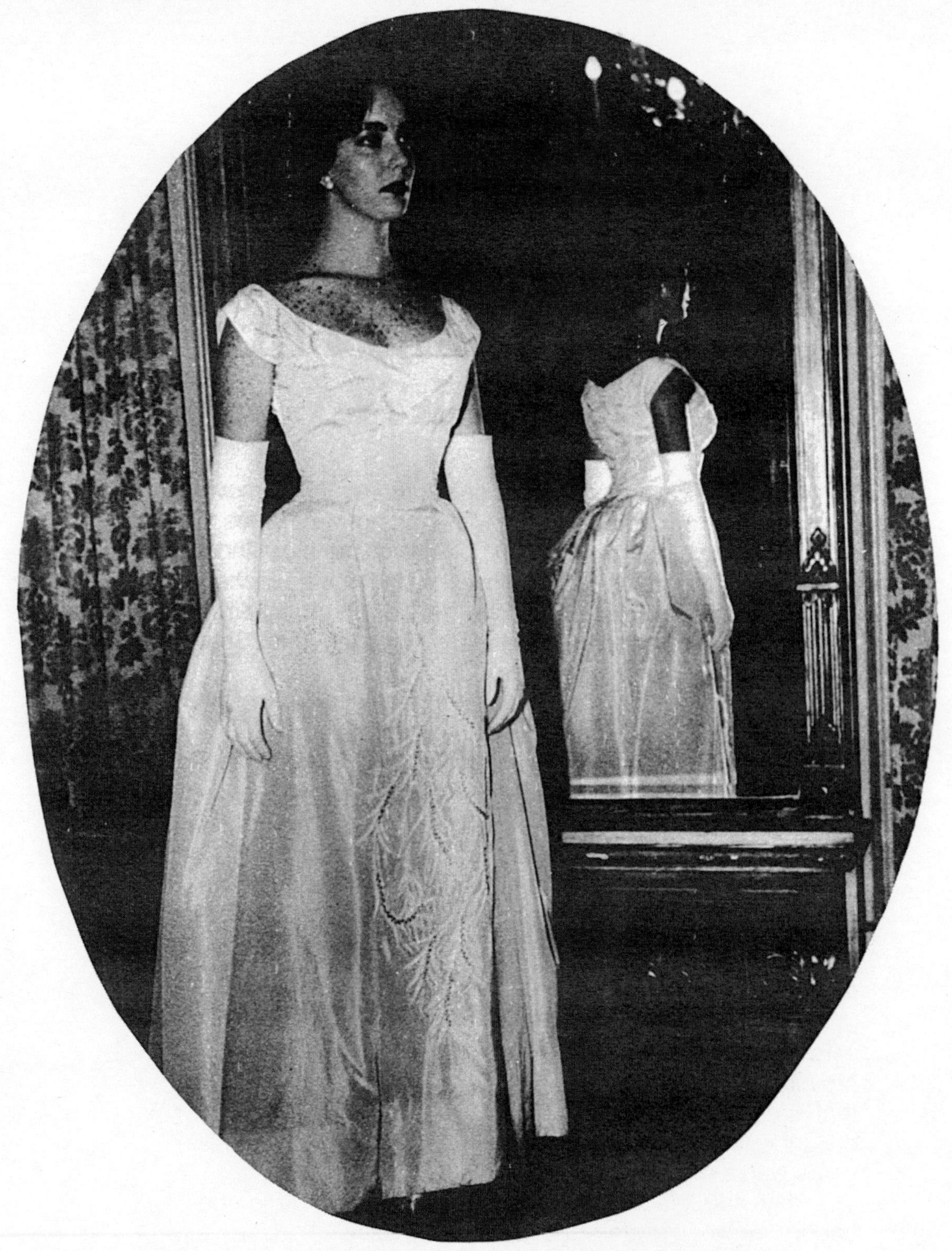

Callan was presented to Savannah society at the 1959 Debutante Cotillion. Her formal portrait shows her in an intricately beaded gown before a massive antique mirror. Within two years, she stepped through a looking glass of another sort and this traditional southern lifestyle was, for her, gone forever. ▲

Descended from the same Pinckney family that was instrumental in the founding of this country, especially South Carolina, even helping to draft the Constitution of the United States, Callan comes from a long line of special achievers. At the age of seventeen, Eliza Lucas Pinckney was singlehandedly responsible for finding the process that made indigo the most profitable export crop of the colonies for more than thirty years until the American Revolution severed our relationship with the primary consumer, Great Britain. George Washington was a pallbearer at her funeral. Charles Cotesworth Pinckney, her son, negotiated the Pinckney Treaty of 1795 with France, laying the groundwork for the purchase, less than a decade later, of the entire Louisiana Territory.

The United States of America was not the first country that the Pinckneys helped to settle. They were with William the Conqueror at the Norman Invasion in 1066. A British noblewoman quipped to a contemporary Pinckney family historian: "My God, you Pinckneys cover the world!"

Callan's maternal ancestry contributes further to this colorful woman's spirit of adventure. These hearty souls—the Pfeiffers—trekked from the heart of the Pennsylvania Dutch territory, across the Oregon Trail, to settle in the Pacific Northwest.

Growing up in and around Savannah, Georgia, Callan was taught to be a proper Southern Lady, with all the trimmings, rebelling all the way. "I was suspended by almost every school I attended," she confesses. "I didn't want to be there. I was busy dreaming of being in foreign lands. I wanted to experience life and people, not read about them in books."

Despite her aversion to academic ventures, Callan completed two years of college. The final straw was when she spotted her hosts at a fraternity party spying through a peephole into the ladies' room. "If those boys were to be the future of our country, I didn't want any part of them," she recounts. "I sold my books and went back to Savannah."

Callan worked as a clerk in a department store, saving every penny and plotting her "getaway." This was a bit scandalous, considering her family's background, but she was not thinking of appearances: The sales job paid more than anything else she could find, and money was what she was after, keeping expenses to a minimum, saving the balance for her travels.

Her father had adamantly prohibited her going abroad until she completed her college education. Callan was equally adamant about going. "My father's telling me I couldn't live three months without his support was the first major challenge in my life."

Her Great Escape came when she threw her suitcase from a second-story window and climbed out after it, leaving her parents' home behind. Friends drove her to the depot where she caught a bus for Wilmington, North Carolina. There she boarded a freighter bound for Germany.

The year was 1961. There was little indication of what lay ahead for this country during the decade to follow. Kennedy was President. Everyone was singing about Camelot. Women wore skirts to go shopping and dressed up when they traveled by plane. Men had weekly haircuts, wore socks that matched their Madras sportscoats and oxford-cloth shirts, and opened doors and tipped their hats for ladies. The Love Generation and the antiwar movement were yet go to public.

Armed with little more than her passport, Callan Pinckney was off to see the world.

Arriving in Bremerhaven, West Germany, the petite brunette had no particular itinerary, just an insatiable curiosity that led her through Europe for almost a year. In Germany, she acquired a Volkswagen for a friend. This was to become her home to cut expenses.

Without work permits, Callan took odd jobs to supplement her savings. Her first winter in London, she shoveled snow and coal for what amounted to $3.36 for an eight-hour day. There was no central heating and Callan was not accustomed to the frigid temperatures. She lived on biscuits and jam, cookies, and quantities of starchy foods to insulate her body in fat. Before long, she weighed 129 pounds—quite a jump for someone who is only an inch over five-feet tall and whose previous top weight had been 105.

Hearing about Africa from people she met in London, Callan explored the possibilities of going there. She was unable to get the necessary travel permits in England, so she hitchhiked to Hamburg and secured papers there, returning briefly to London to tie up loose ends and to purchase the rucksack that was to be her "mobile home" for the next eight or nine years.

For a while Callan worked in Capetown for an advertising agency by day and as a waitress by night. She talked her way into most of the jobs she held during her travels, determined to learn whatever skills were necessary once she secured the position.

Her soft, cultured Southern accent was foreign to Callan's British and Afrikaans employers and co-workers. Consequently, she was asked to come to the office a half hour early every morning to be tutored in "proper English pronunciation." "I was quite insulted. I told them I spoke *modern* English, not Elizabethan," she laughs. Today, her accent is part American, part British, and all Callan. She is a verbal chameleon, reflecting the accents of those around her.

She spent almost a year in the bush of Central Africa. Part of this time she helped track animal migrations from place to place, leaving Zimbabwe, then Rhodesia, Zaire, then the Congo, and Kenya, when trouble began to brew.

Her survival instincts kept her body alive, but did not keep her fit and healthy. Her rapid weight gain in England had caused stretch marks on her hips. Her erratic, often inadequate, diet lead to malnutrition and three debilitating bouts of amoebic dysentery. ("I had diarrhea for eight years.") She dropped from a pudgy 129 to 78 pounds during the worst of these attacks. She was on Cyprus and had to be evacuated from the RAF Hospital there to make room for the wounded soldiers brought in from battle daily.

Callan further abused her body by doing menial labor to earn money and by carrying her backpack. Weighing almost as much as she did, it pulled her collar bones and strained her back and knees mercilessly.

For most of her odyssey, Callan lived among peasants, without any of the conveniences she had taken for granted all of her life. To this day she brushes her teeth without water. She usually wears a sweater or has one handy even in summer, remembering her fear of freezing for lack of clothing. "When I first returned to the States, I identified with the street people, the shopping bag ladies," she confides. "I wanted to know what they carried in their bags, if the contents resembled what I had carried."

In most of the countries where she lived or traveled, there was nothing written in English, not even signs on buildings. Callan tells that she had been living in New York for several years, following her travels abroad, wondering how people always knew the names of stores and streets. She had spent so much time in places where signs were unreadable that she had forgotten to look at them.

Callan maintained a detailed diary throughout her travels. As she left a country, she mailed a diary to her parents, making sure she could not be traced. "I never knew where I would be going next," she explains. "I went where the roads and rides took me. I didn't care where they went." As for her diaries: "To this day I haven't read them. I don't think I ever shall."

Much of this time she was alone, although sometimes she traveled with a Canadian girl whom she met early in her trip.

Callan planned to hitchhike from Johannesburg to Japan. She expected the trip to take about six months. It took seven years.

In Bombay, India, she was in an air raid. "I was walking down a street when a plane flew over and began shooting. I froze. Two men grabbed me and threw me into a doorway for cover. I hid my face in my arms and waited for the shooting to stop. When I looked up, I saw a hand with only three fingers next to me. I was lying next to a leper. One of my greatest fears while traveling the world was contracting that disease."

This prompted Callan to travel south to Ceylon. She and her Canadian companion, joined by an American girl who had been staying in the same place in Bombay, rode third class on the train to the border. Callan slept on luggage racks because the compartments, which had comfortable space for fifteen people, contained as many as sixty.

The trio missed the boat from India to Ceylon (now Sri Lanka) and had to wait a week for passage. To occupy their time, Callan introduced her American cohort to basic ballet. "That was the first time I noticed I could not do movements I had once been able to do so beautifully. I had no flexibility or extension. My muscles had no tone."

She did not understand why it hurt whenever she sat. Her behind had fallen so much that it was now on her hips. Sitting on her sweater to cushion her tailbone had become second nature. Sleeping with a rag between her knees to keep them from rubbing together was a necessity.

Newspapers and current events were no longer a part of Callan's life. Her day-to-day considerations were personal safety, drinkable water, clean food for survival, and finding a safe place to sleep.

Once Callan reached Japan, she recorded British voice-over tapes for advertising, wrote about her travels for a Japanese magazine, and modeled miniskirts. She also managed a bar and was responsible for hiring Western waitresses.

At that time, Callan was becoming increasingly aware of her body's need for care. Back in London, she began to work seriously on her body. This was a slow, painful process for someone who had become so run-down. Doctors advised her to have surgery on her travel-damaged knees and cautioned that her back would never recover. "I looked terrible and was in constant pain. I thought that if I had to hurt all the time, I might as well look good. I had no other choice."

When Callan returned to the United States, she appeared so emaciated and old that her mother fainted upon seeing her emerge from the plane.

Callan's first job upon returning to the United States in 1972 was at a New York City exercise salon. "I left there because I didn't approve of the way clients' bodies were being treated. I was told to change the way I had been instructed to teach the exercises, supposedly so we could handle more clients in the salon. The owner of the franchise prohibited my asking the women I worked with if they had back problems, yet my back hurt when I did some of the exercises. Other people might have been hurting as well. This was extremely upsetting for me. The salon's owner and I had studied this program from a woman who is a master in this field. I believed in my teacher's program, and, in all fairness to her and to myself, I could not continue the way things were going."

After leaving the salon, Callan experimented with other techniques, and the movements learned while studying ballet. "I found that if I felt back pain, I could simply shift my position as little as a fraction of an inch until my back no longer hurt. I got incredible results. I was determined not to do anything to start the back spasms again. I was amazed to see how strong and tight my body had become. My back had stopped hurting. I felt and looked as though I had been exercising for three hours a day for five years after only a few hours of these movements. I concluded that these delicate, precise movements are the key to successful exercising. I was so excited that I couldn't wait to share the results with other people. I felt absolutely magnificent, as if I could spring like a majestic gazelle."

When Callan began teaching on her own, she instructed students privately in their homes. "I carried a metal pole with me from place to place to hang in doorways as a *barre*. We exercised on their living-room floors." Soon, she offered classes in her own studio apartment.

"It was a circus. I had a *barre* across my closet door. Students looked at my pitiful wardrobe while they exercised. I rearranged it every week so they wouldn't get bored at my interpretation of American clothes."

For the past seven years, Callan has been teaching in her penthouse that overlooks New York's East River.

There is no pulsating music, no shrill cadence called by an instructor. There is no grotesque machinery to make the place look like a modern-day torture chamber. Students, men and women of all ages, sizes, and shapes, work at their own speed under Callan's careful scrutiny. She moves about the room, attending to each individual's needs.

Callan's classes are a far cry from the usual fitness center environment: indoor-outdoor carpeting; wall-to-wall people blinding in fluorescent lighting; overly chlorinated pools; and a sea of humanity, everyone doing the same things at the same time, whether or not their bodies are capable of it.

A new student observed, "Coming to Callan's at seven o'clock in the morning is a terrific way to start the day. Someone wanders in at seven ten, someone else at seven twenty. Callan may be having breakfast or putting cream on her face, teaching while still in her nightgown. Despite this chaotic appearance, Callan has her hawkeye on everyone in the room. The way the mirrors are set up, she doesn't miss a trick.

"The sun comes through the greenhouse glass and literally bathes the room in warm light, exposing every roll and bump in your body. You see *exactly* what you look like on the beach and it scares the daylights out of you."

The natural light, reflected in the thirteen-foot mirrored walls, and the clear panorama of the city—the sky, rivers and skyscrapers—are magnificent inducements to exercise.

"One student told me that she had always thought her body was flawless . . . until she came here and saw it in bright light," Callan laughs. "I believe people need this kind of objectivity so that they will be able to *work* on their bodies."

There is a magnetic energy between Callan and her students. It's a powerful combination.

Callan Pinckney is a one-of-a-kind woman, and this is a one-of-a-kind book. Through it you will embark on a true adventure into body awareness . . . for obtaining your new, true shape of things to come.

—*Sallie Batson*

CHAPTER TWO

Excuses! Excuses! Excuses!

If your personal exercise program never gets beyond the thinking stage, you must take a close look—a *very* close look—at what is keeping you from fitness. Read through this list of excuses and check off the ones you have used, and the ones you have thought of using, to explain why you are carrying around all that extra flab.

- ☐ I have big bones.
- ☐ It's my thyroid. My glands are really out of whack.
- ☐ I retain water.
- ☐ I might throw my back out.
- ☐ I hate to get all sweaty.
- ☐ My husband/wife/boyfriend/girlfriend likes me the way I am.
- ☐ I want to lose a little weight first. Then I'll start exercising.
- ☐ If I exercise now, all this fat will turn into muscle, and muscle is harder to lose than fat.
- ☐ I don't have time.
- ☐ My diet makes me too weak to exercise.
- ☐ If I had the kind of money he/she does, I'd look good too.
- ☐ Anybody can look great when they're sixteen.
- ☐ My whole family is big (fat).
- ☐ Exercise is boring.
- ☐ I've been sick.
- ☐ I have arthritis.

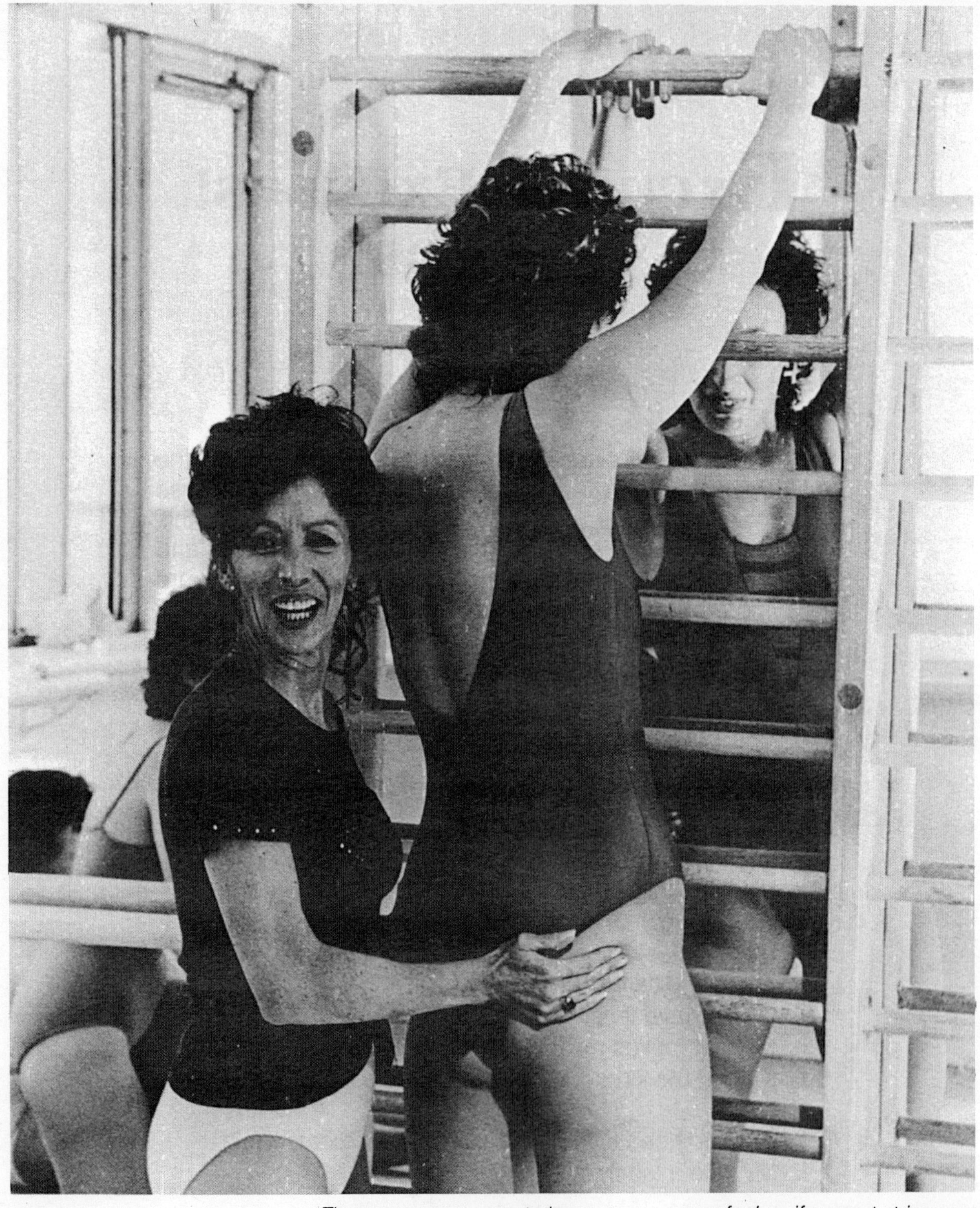

There are no excuses to keep anyone from tightening their thighs and lifting their behind for that wonderful, youthful feeling of childhood. Remember what that was like? If you can't, I'll remind you: When you walk, you feel as if puppet strings are pulling your buttocks into the air. If you never had that experience, it can be yours within hours, no matter your age, sex, or size. ▲

- ☐ I get enough exercise cleaning my house.
- ☐ I'm too tired to exercise when I come home from work.
- ☐ Once you've had a baby, your stomach goes to pot anyway.
- ☐ Saddle bags are a fact of life for women as we get older.
- ☐ I have to close this business deal first.
- ☐ Why should I lose? Men secretly like big women.
- ☐ I'm afraid I'll hurt myself.
- ☐ I just had my hair done.

Got the picture? I've heard them all, and so have you.

Quit whining. Put on some comfortable clothes and get to work on your body.

CHAPTER THREE

Chasing the Impossible Dream

Things are not always what they seem, especially when you look at pictures of gorgeous bodies in magazines and, sadly, even in exercise books.

Every day, women around the world give up on their bodies because they can't transform themselves into the images of beauty created by the media. Who can compete with those incredibly young beauties in the fashion magazines? Real people like you and me could not possibly look like that!

No wonder we mere mortals suffer with low self-images. We buy every cosmetic on the market, try the latest hairstyles and fashions, use hip wraps and reducing creams, go on the latest diets, drink the right mineral waters, and we still fail to come close to Ideal Beauty.

My own lack of confidence in my body was due to conditioning. I had false expectations about how I should look. Despite years of compliments, I remained insecure about my appearance. New students, meeting me for the first time, often exclaimed, "You have the tightest, most beautiful body I've ever seen." I thought they were trying to flatter me so that I would go easy on them. It was impossible for me to consider. After all, I saw my body in the mirror every day. I knew what I looked like. How could they put *me* in the same league as those tall, exquisite young creatures in bathing suits cut up to their waists to show their perfect hips and legs?

I never suspected that the goddesses we see in the magazines don't always look that perfect either. I would have

Most weight loss by artistic means, be it airbrushing, cut-and-paste, or photography, is subtle: a bustline is raised, a hipline trimmed, a behind lifted and rounded, a waist cinched, and thighs slimmed and smoothed. These touches, as insignificant as they may seem, have monumental impact on the egos of unknowing women who think that what they see is real. To illustrate this point I have taken rather drastic steps, reducing a 230-pound woman to "normal" size. Were these photos used to advertise a diet or exercise plan, wouldn't you believe it worked? This is the only photograph in this book to receive any type of artistic editing. Every other body you see in the book or on the jacket is as it is in real life. ►

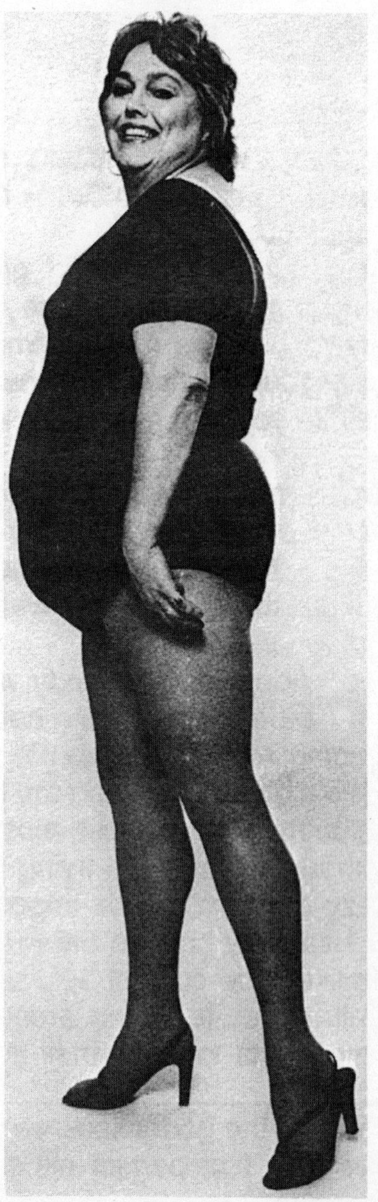

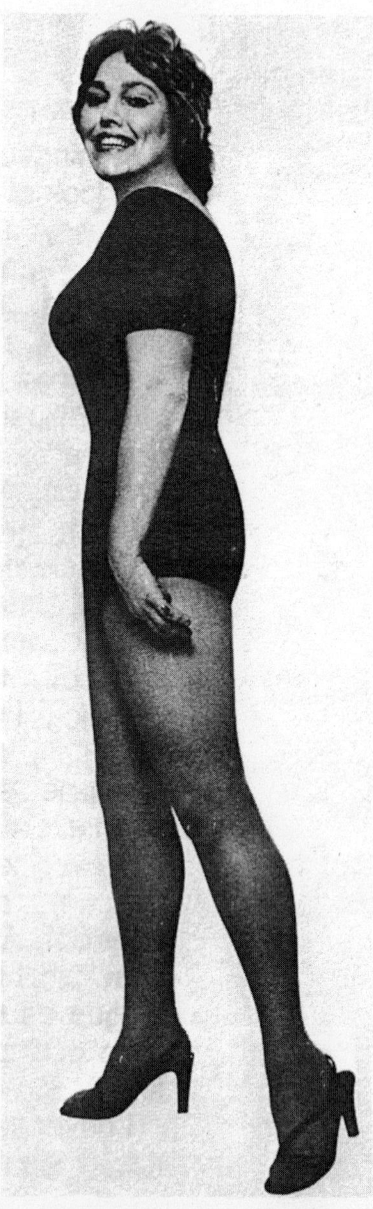

This, and only this, photograph is airbrushed. ▲

sold my soul to have the body of one particular swimsuit model, until I saw her in person. I recognized her in a store where she was trying on high heels. As I watched her prance back and forth before the mirrors, I became more and more bewildered. She wore shorts. Her buttocks sagged and globs of cellulite sat on her hips. Her legs jiggled like tofu in a blender. I could not believe that the woman I had seen trying on shoes was the *real* person and the one in the magazines was the creation of a team of art directors, photographers, stylists, makeup artists, and airbrushers—The Army Corps of Image Engineers. You and I could look like the most beautiful women in the world too if we had this professional team to back us up.

Here's how they work:

The stylists—one for hair, one for makeup, and another for clothes—coif, curl, lift, paint, and primp you until there are no visible flaws.

You would then be directed to sit or stand about a perfectly appointed set, either in a photographer's studio or a real room, striking poses and moving in ways that show off your body to ultimate advantage.

Now, another sleight of hand begins. Lights are adjusted to create the desired (translate that "artificial") image, and a high-powered wind machine gives your hair and clothes that perfect billowy look. How many of us can lug around a four-foot fan to give us that perfect windblown look without a strand out of place?

Then, the photographer, using the appropriate cameras, lenses, films, filters, and angles, fires away, immortalizing your beauty in hundreds, if not thousands, of shots to obtain the *one* shining example of physical perfection.

If these techniques fail, have no fear: The cosmetic surgeons (known as the Art Department) can remedy anything else that may be considered wrong. They even correct any mistakes there might be in Mother Nature's handiwork. They operate on photographs, not living bodies.

Hips too wide? No problem. Able artists can use their scissors to cut off anything in the way, "amputating" bones if necessary, to give you a perfectly straight hipline.

Feet too big: again, no problem. They can chop off yours with scissors and glue on a prettier, younger, smoother, and yes, even smaller, pair in less time than it takes for *you* to slip into your stockings.

Flabby body but fabulous face? You can acquire a new figure, custom-made. Artists can superimpose your head and face onto the body of their choice. Or they can brush away any offending parts, such as thunder thighs, whale tails, droopy bosoms, tree-stump ankles, bulging bellies, and cellulite (or whatever you care to call those hideous ripply pockets of fat that so many women have). Gone, in an instant! Scissors, glue, and an airbrush machine—that's all an artist needs to create the most beautiful body in the world.

Airbrushing is one of the best kept secrets in this universe, outside of the advertising business. It is the final touch. This is a precision artistic technique, akin to spray painting, used to subtract or add parts of a picture. It can lighten or even remove shadows, iron out wrinkles in clothing *and* bodies, and take away any hair out of place. It can turn the *real* into the *perfectly unreal.*

No wonder we give up all hope of looking like the paper dolls in our favorite magazines. Our self-images are destroyed before we leave home!

Most women view their bodies as flawed. When someone comes to me for her first class, I ask her to stand in front of the mirrors and look objectively at her body. (I ask students not to wear tights—black tights hide multitudes of sins—or chic, belted leotards. I want them to wear something comfortable, yet revealing.) I ask her, "What would you like to change? What is it that you do not like about your body?" With nine out of ten of my students, the flaw they *think* they see is not a flaw at all.

Don't be tricked into thinking that everyone else you see is "perfect" and you are not. Work with what you have. There is always room for improvement. No one has a so-called perfect body.

I am writing about the methods of artistic deception because these techniques have damaged a lot of people. Every day I meet women and men who are depressed about their bodies. Many can't see how lovely, or potentially lovely, their bodies are.

It is harder for me to get a student to give up a negative self-image than it is for me to teach her how to exercise. I help my students to erase those false images that have been with them since their teens. I teach them how to see their bodies realistically and to stop chasing the impossible, retouched dream.

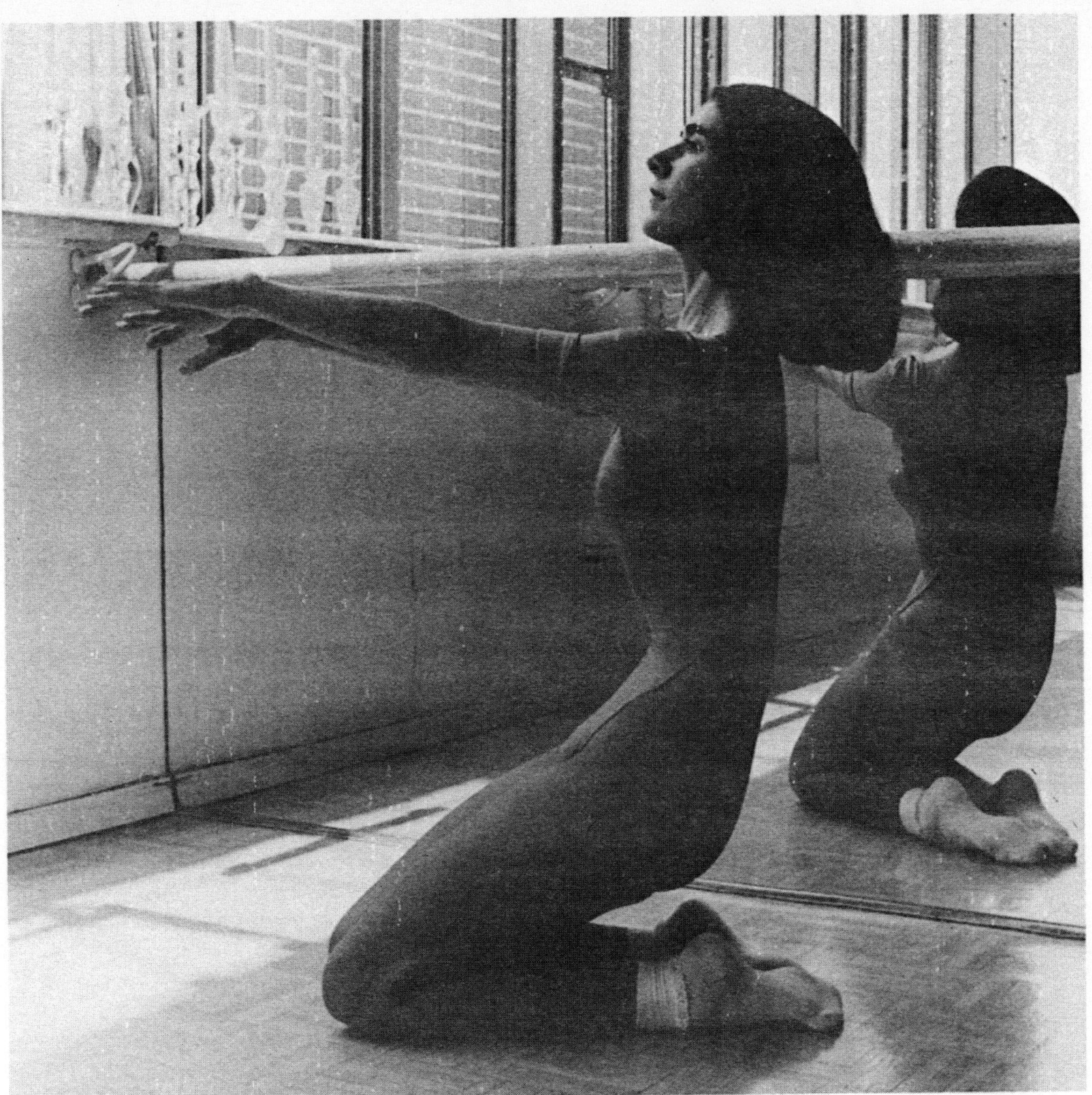

My student Page was an active, athletic teenager. However, when she went to college, she ate the typical cafeteria and junk foods that kept the average student alive. She ballooned before she took charge of her body and began a sensible routine of a nutritionally sound diet and my exercise program. Today her body is amazingly beautiful. It's better than airbrushing any day. ▲

CHAPTER FOUR

Portfolio of Proof

The exercises you are about to learn produce fast results.

I could tell you that this is a complete, comprehensive program that will restore your body to its lithe, firm, young form and protect your back at the same time. And I could explain that if you follow the basic program outlined here, you can have a round, firm, peach-shaped behind, just like the little suntanned girl in the Coppertone suntan oil ads, in what seems like days. That is because an hour of these exercises equals approximately seven hours of conventional exercise and twenty hours of aerobic dancing, as far as firming the body and pulling it up is concerned.

Knowing your considerations, I have prepared a portfolio of pictures proving that these exercises work. By comparing the pictures of my students, you will be able to see for yourself that a flat, taut tummy and a high, round behind are possible for anyone who wants them.

To demonstrate the validity of my claim that these exercises work in a matter of hours, several of my students—all but one were beginners at the time—agreed to have their progress photographed for documentation. Some of these sequences were taken by a professional photographer. I took the others myself with a Polaroid camera. You will recognize the ones I took immediately! They were taken in the midst of dressing-room madness, hardly the best conditions for photography. On the pictures I took, you will see a line around the left-hand side of each body, thanks to less than perfect lighting. The darkroom technicians could have removed this photographic flaw, but I was committed to my promise that no pictures in this book would be altered.

For purposes of comparison, each student was photographed from the rear and in profile, immediately after class. The exact classes in each sequence are listed under each set of pictures. Samples of the progress made by participants in the project are included in this portfolio. One student, Jeanne,* was selected to show her hourly progress. Most of her photos are shown.

Joyce, my advanced student pictured here, became involved in the project when she told me that her body was "tight enough." She did not plan to continue classes because she did not see how her body could pull in any more than it already had. I picked up the challenge and said, "Let's take pictures and see." Joyce was surprised at the results. She had already pulled in dramatically and her continued progress was quite encouraging. I wasn't surprised. I see it happen every day. Unlike some other programs of exercise, this one continues to work as long as you do it.

Study the pictures. You can see a number of dramatic changes in each photo series. Hips become smaller and develop smoother lines. Behinds become higher, tighter, and rounder. Locate an identifying mark—a scar, birthmark, mole, stretchmarks, wrinkly fat deposits—and notice how they move higher and higher as the body becomes tighter.

If you see pouches of cellulite appear after you have worked to get your figure in shape, don't panic. The tightening from the exercises has only revealed what was there all along. My experience is that, if you change your diet, you can get rid of the unsightly, pebbly fat. For me, I eliminated coffee, red meats, dairy products, sugars, and processed foods from my diet. I ate a lot of vegetables and fish and drank at least eight glasses of water daily. I also took calcium supplements. My cellulite disappeared in six weeks.

Though their changes are not so radical, even men experience remarkable tightening and change. Women start out gooshier than men, so improvement is more visible from the start.

You can also see how students' postures improve. Remember what your mother said about standing up straight? Well, she had a point. Compare the first side views and subsequent side views of everyone in the portfolio. Notice how the bodies begin to change and how they become more and more erect. That's because the exercises tighten the hips and pull in the behind, which pulls in the inner thighs and, in turn, tips the pelvis up, which stretches the spine. The process reminds me of a Rube Goldberg contraption

*Names have been changed.

where you turn a tiny wheel to Point A, which sets off a sequence of reactions to make the cage fall on the mouse at Point Z.

The entire figure-shaping process is accomplished automatically—the way Nature intended. However, for most of us, Nature needs a boost. That's where these exercises come in. See for yourself how well they work.

LUCY
Age: 40

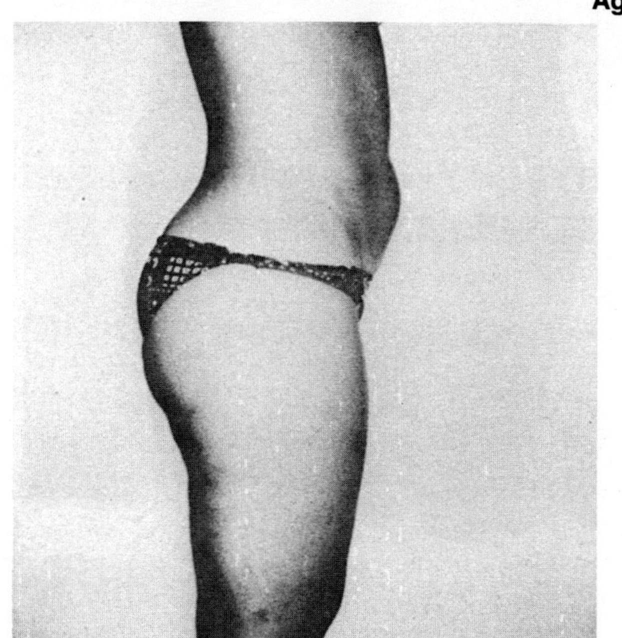

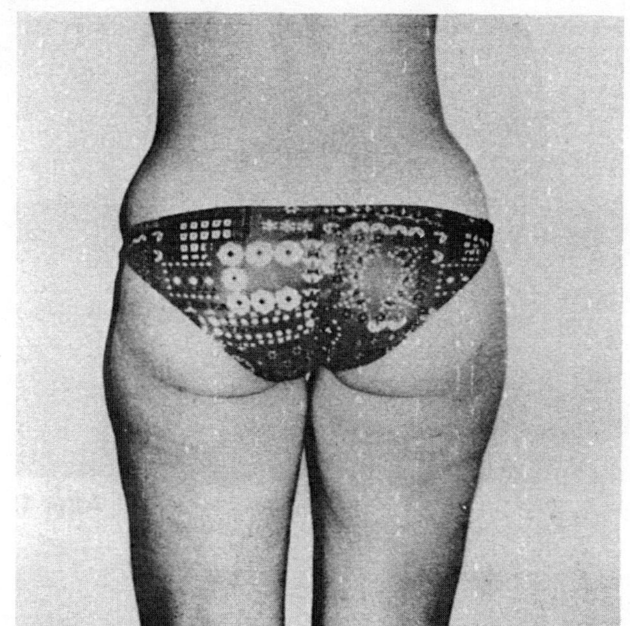

After 1st Class

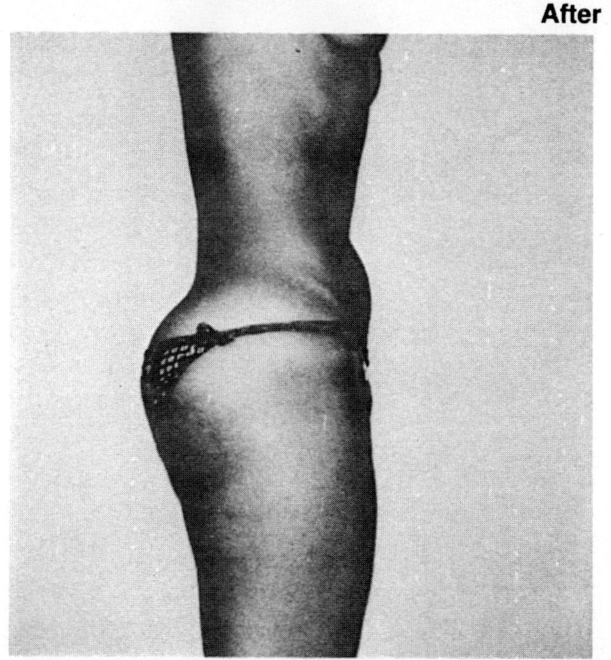

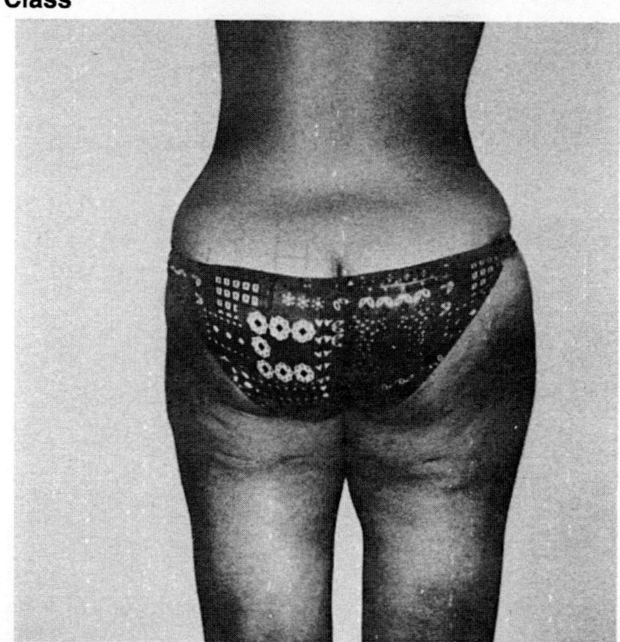

After 4th Class

GERTRUDE

Age: 32

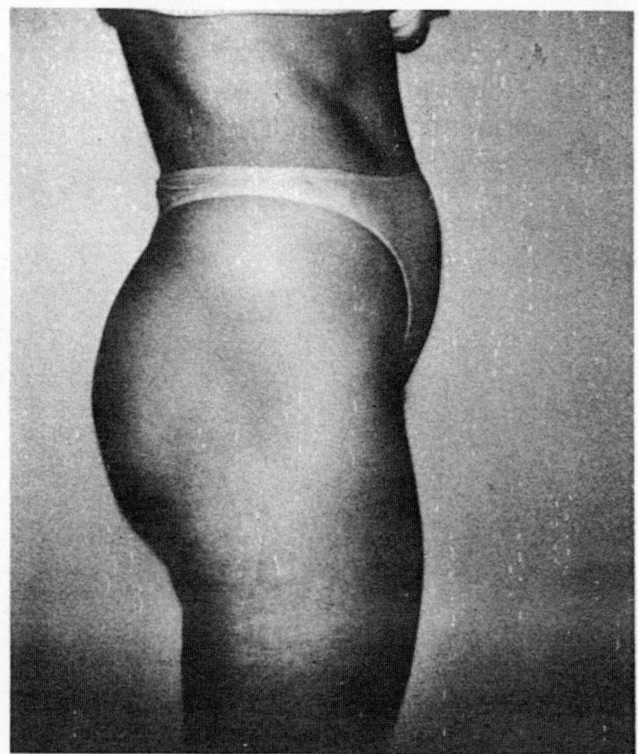

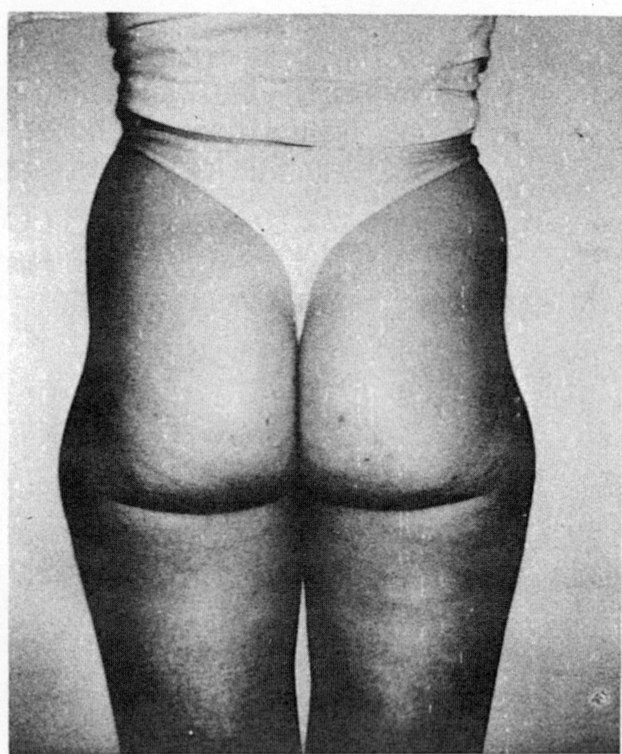

After 1st Class

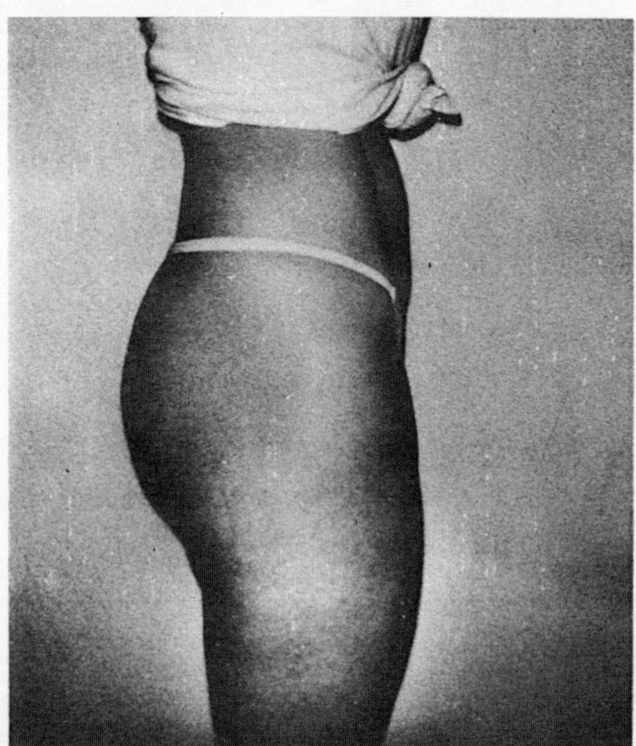

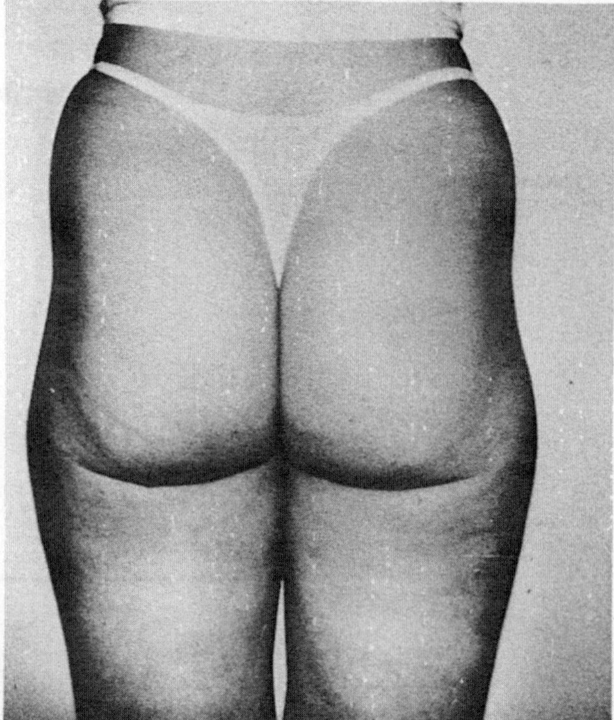

After 3rd Class

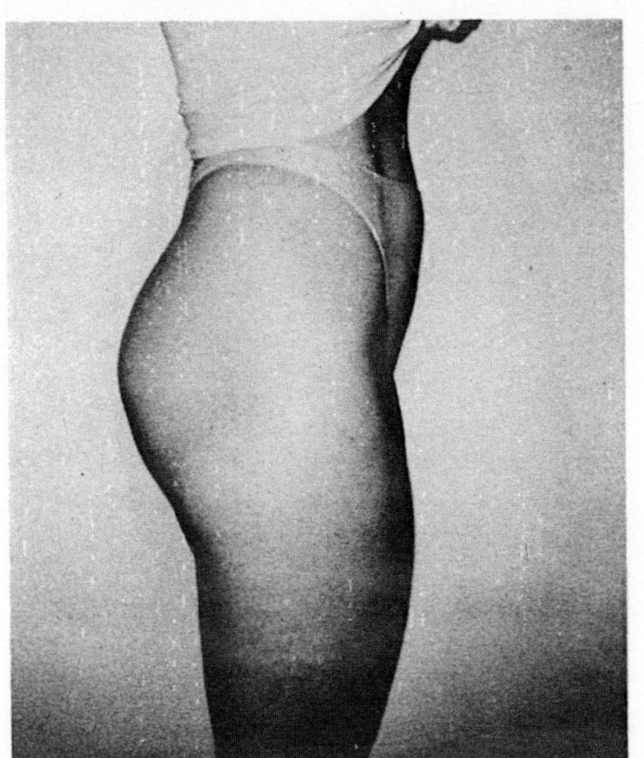

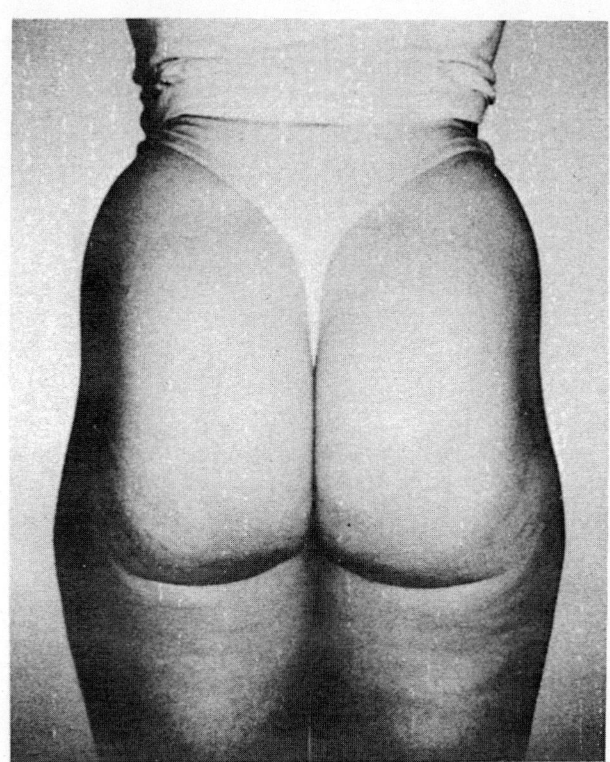

After 4th Class

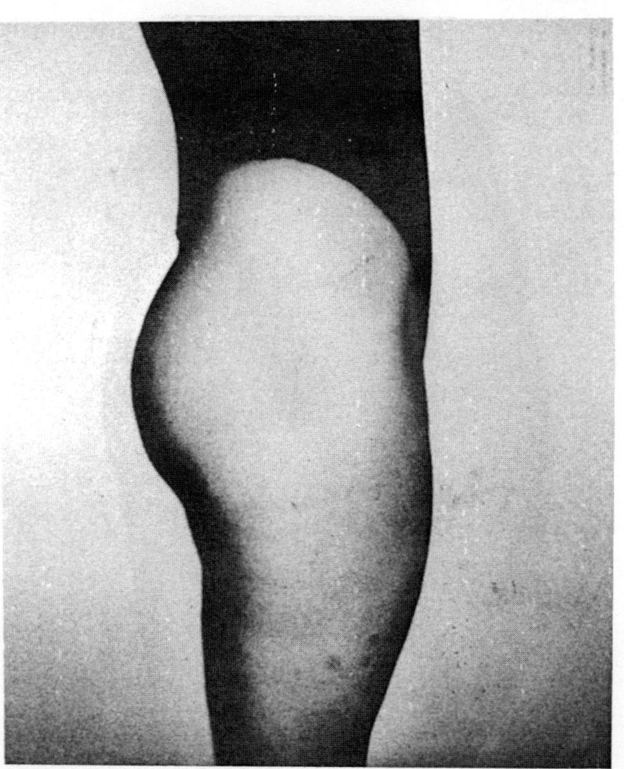

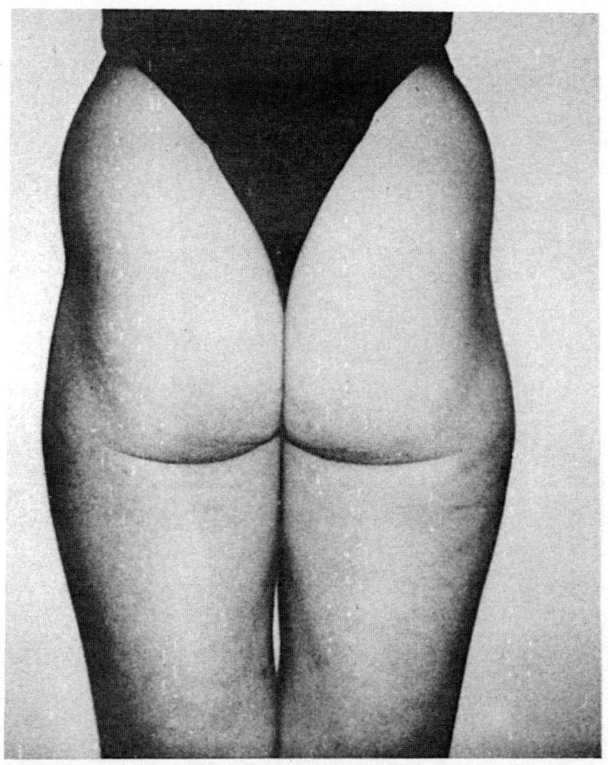

After 5th Class

MARCIE

Age: 37

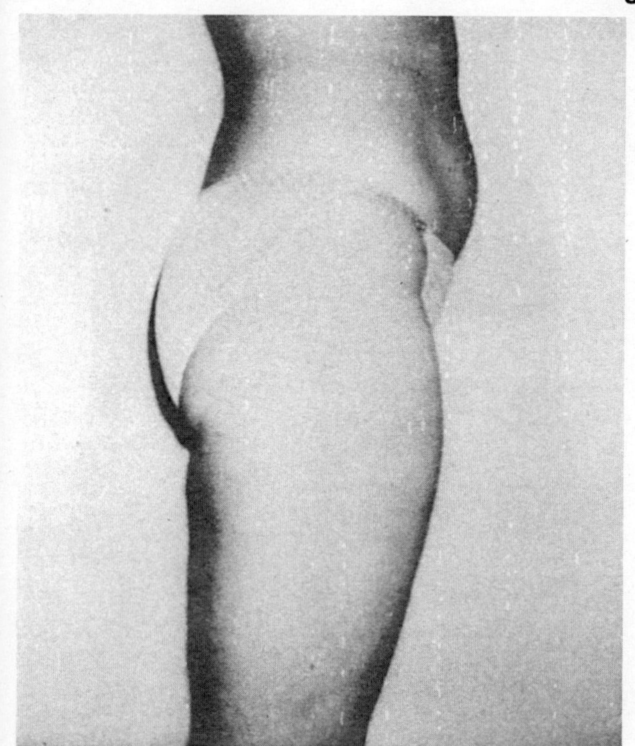

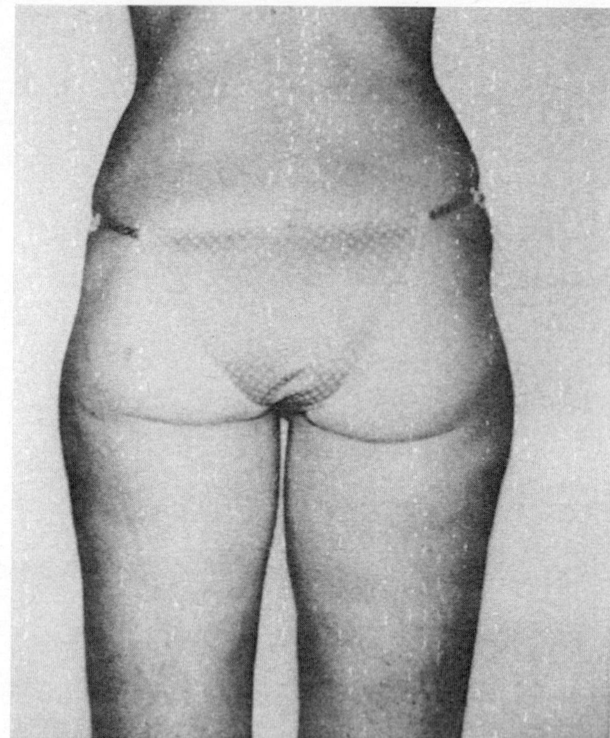

After 1st Class

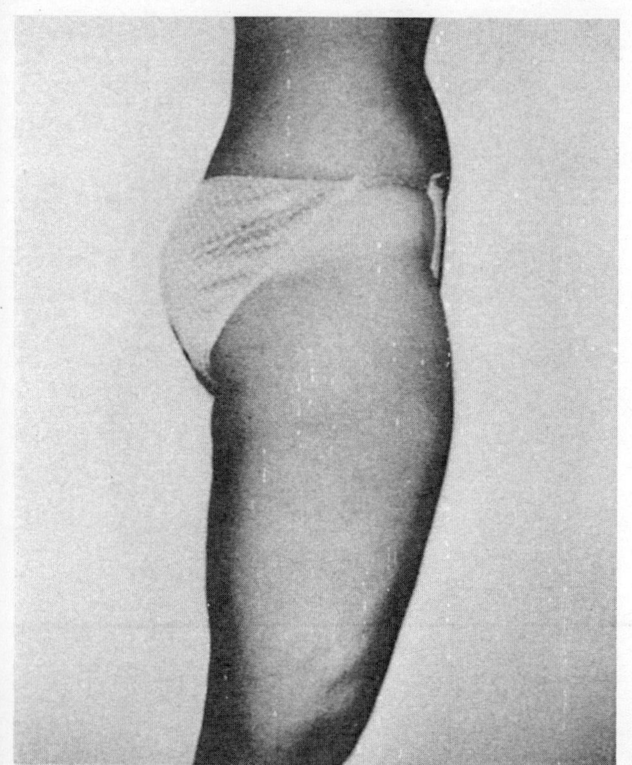

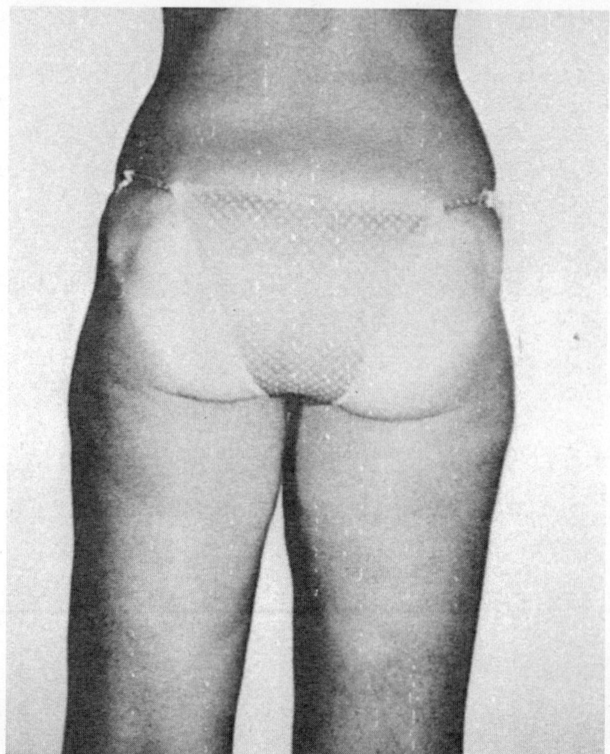

After 7th Class

CHRISTINE

Age: 27

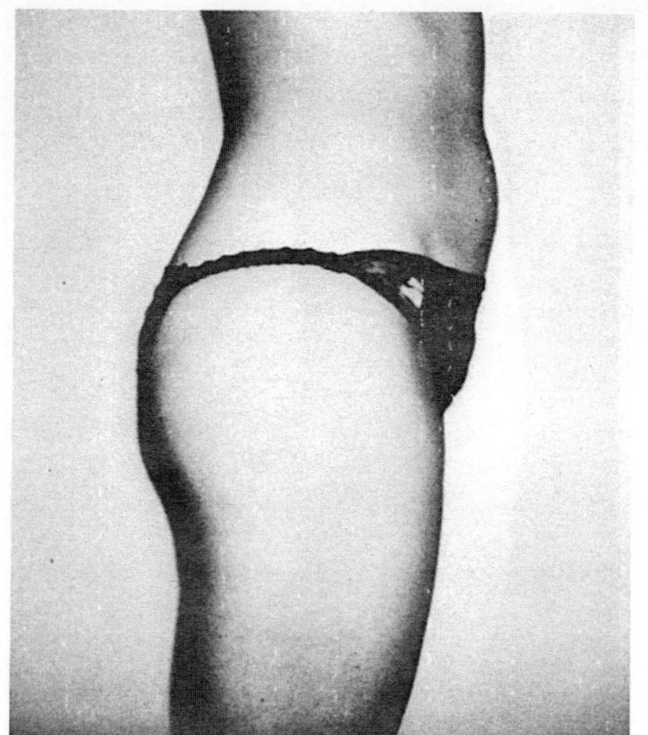

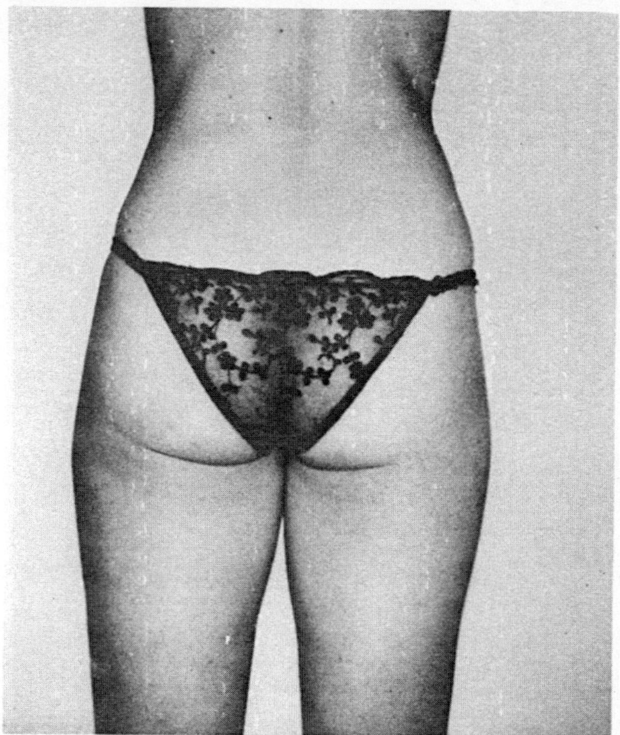

After 1st Class

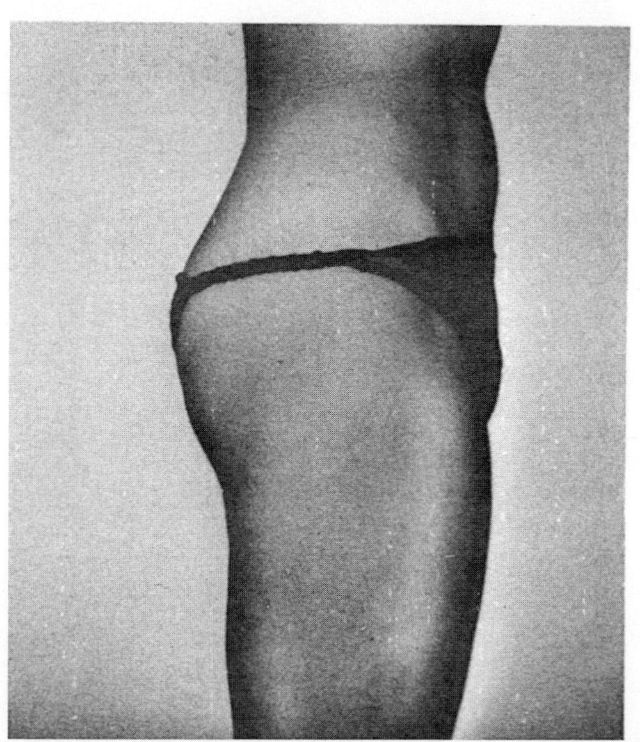

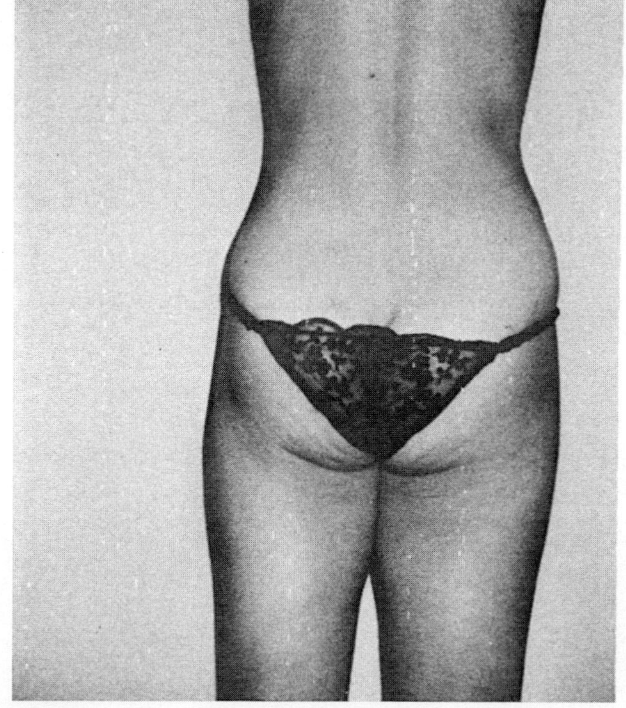

After 5th Class

MARK

Age: 27

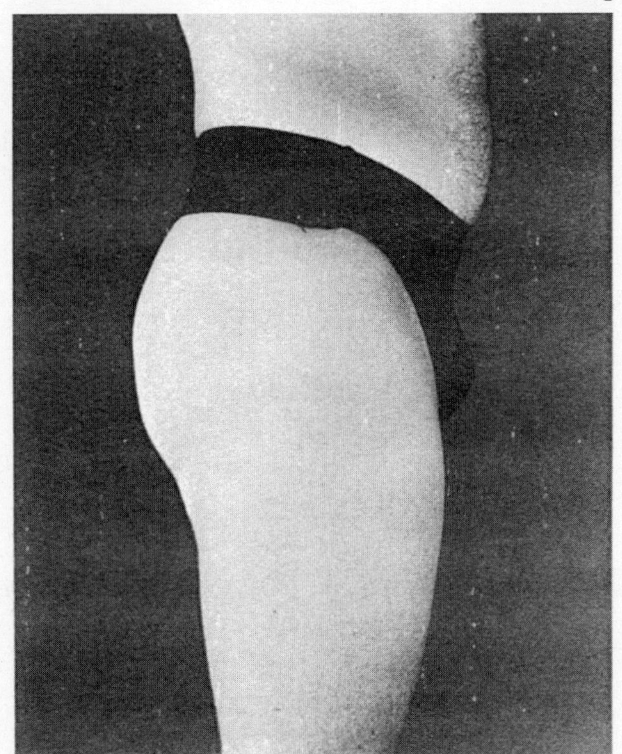

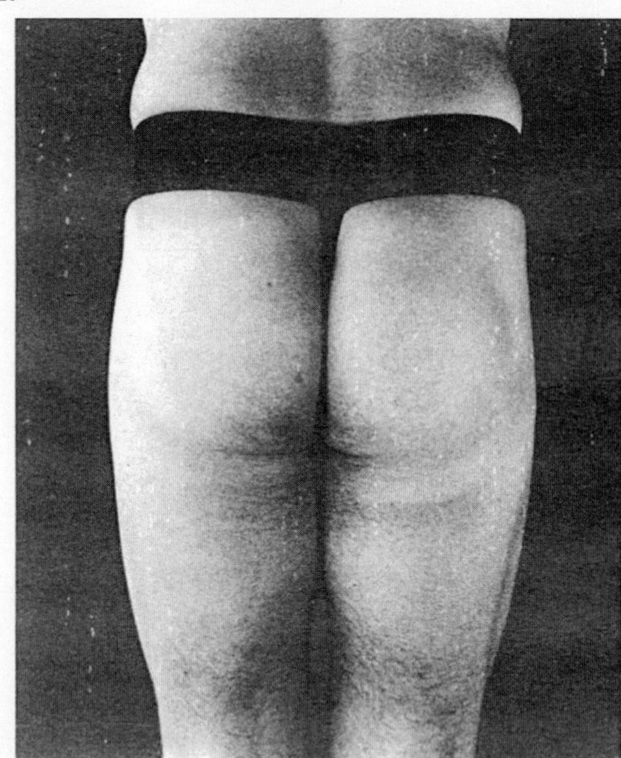

After 1st Class

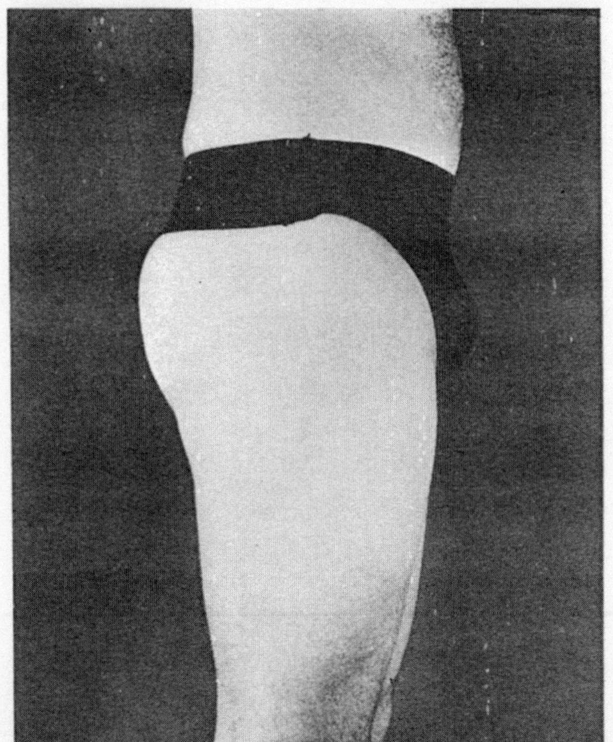

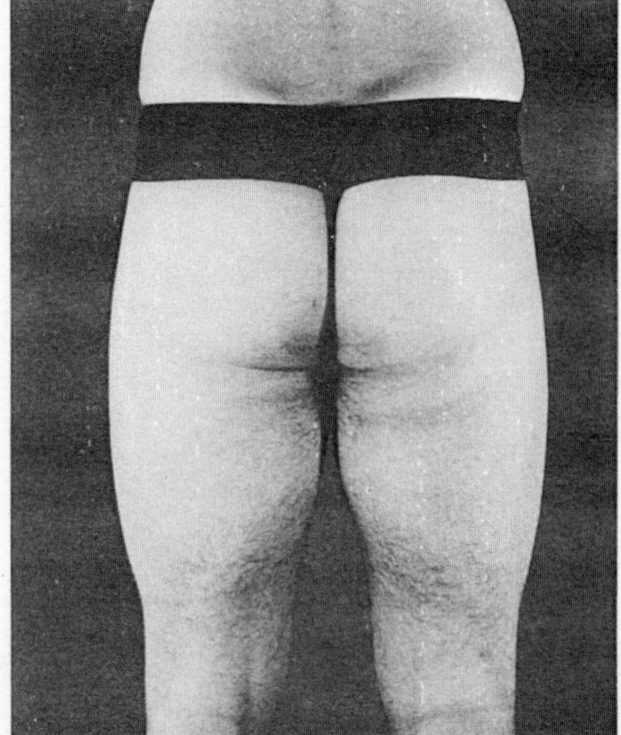

After 4th Class

JOYCE

Age: 28

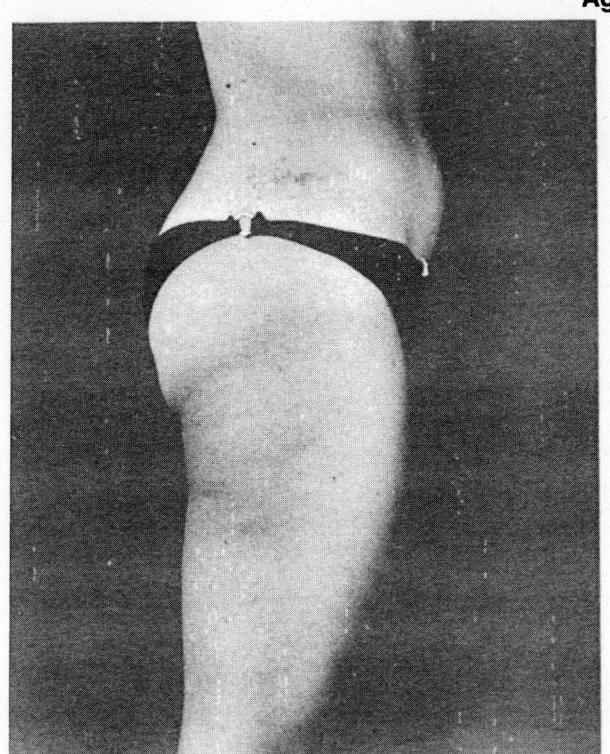

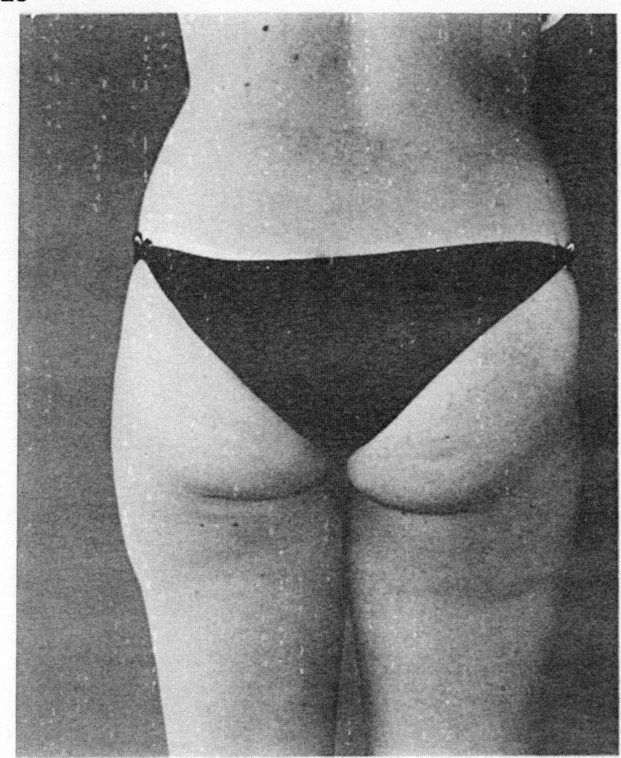

After 14th Class

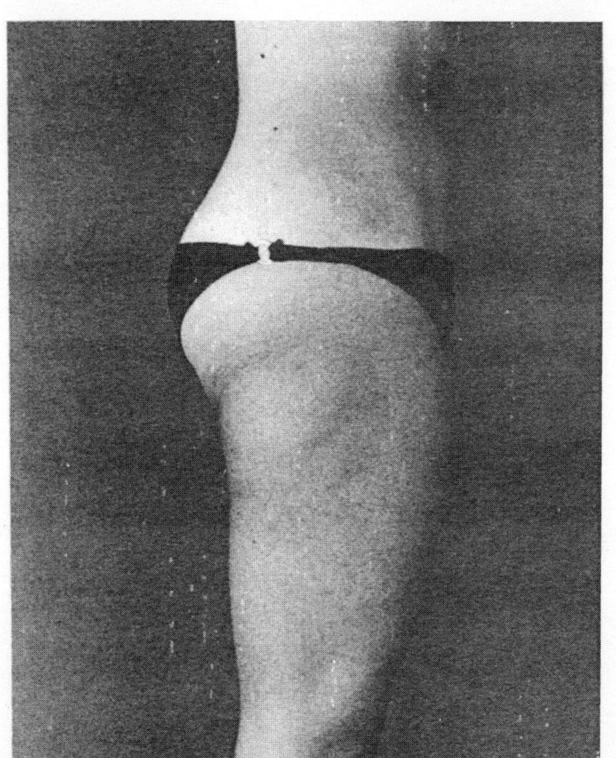

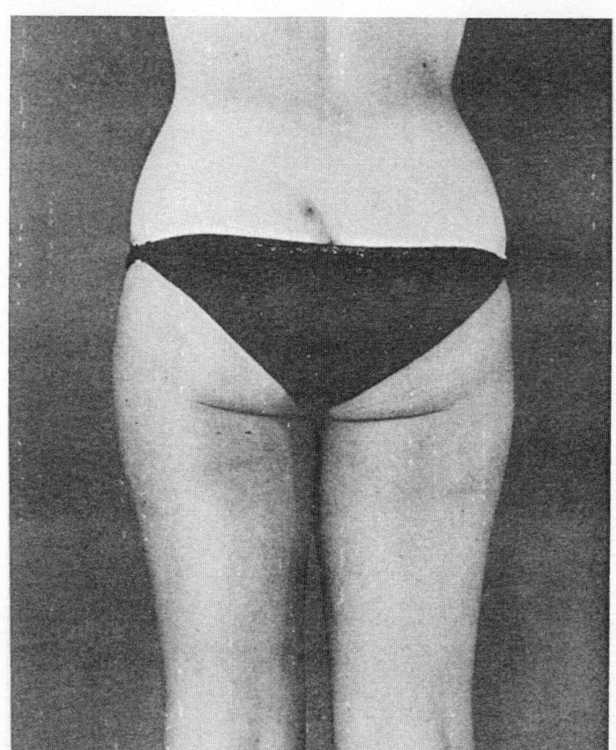

After 24th Class

CHARLES

Age: 41

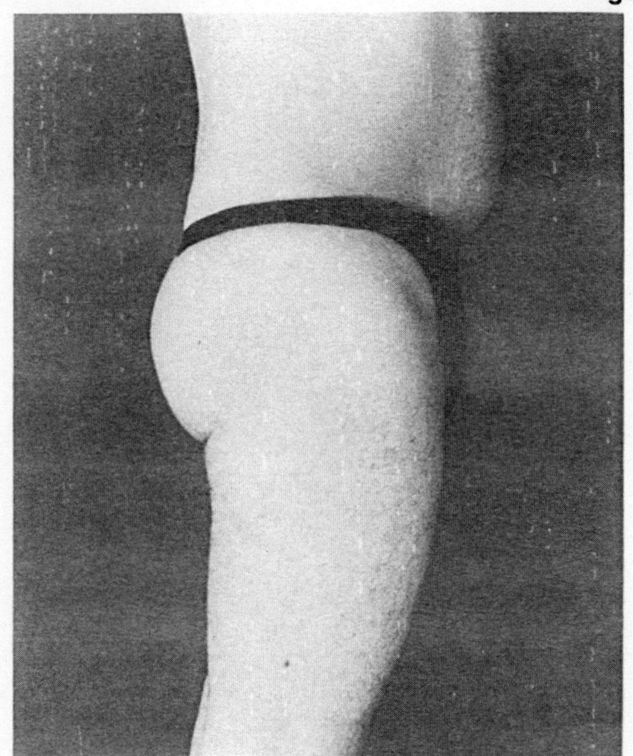

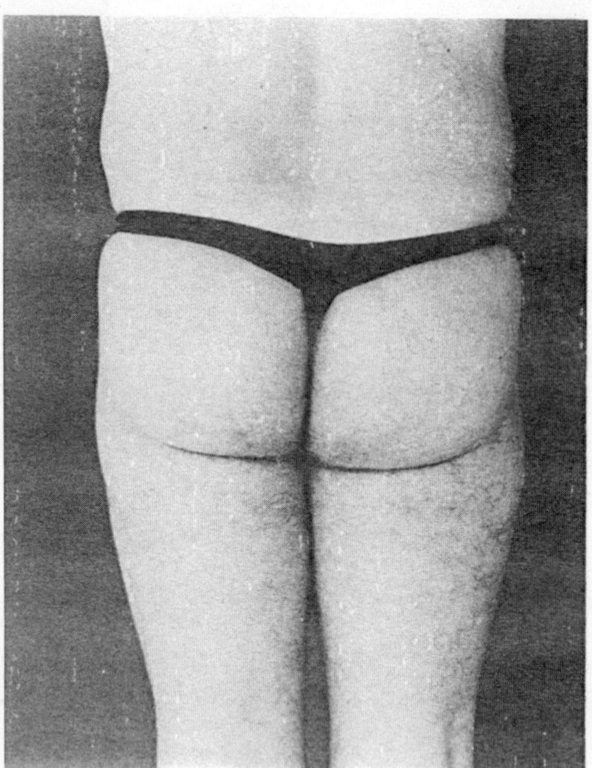

After 2nd Class

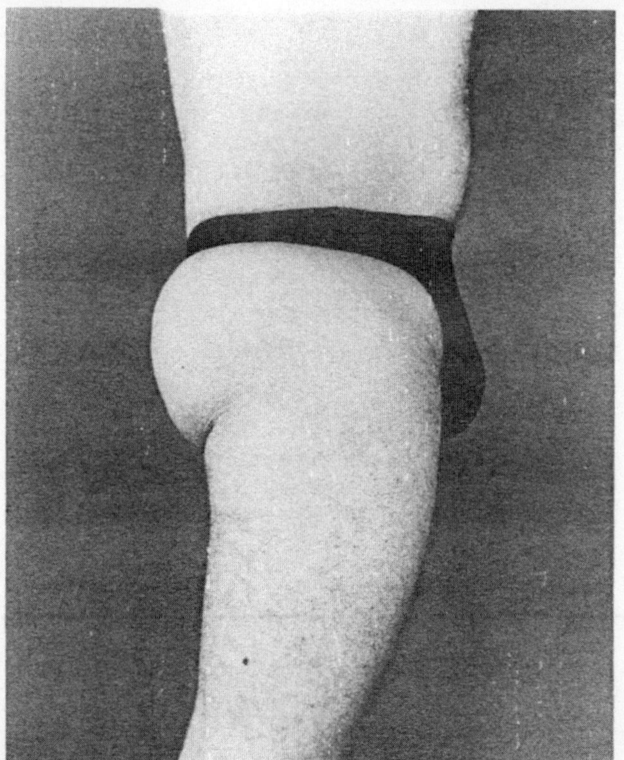

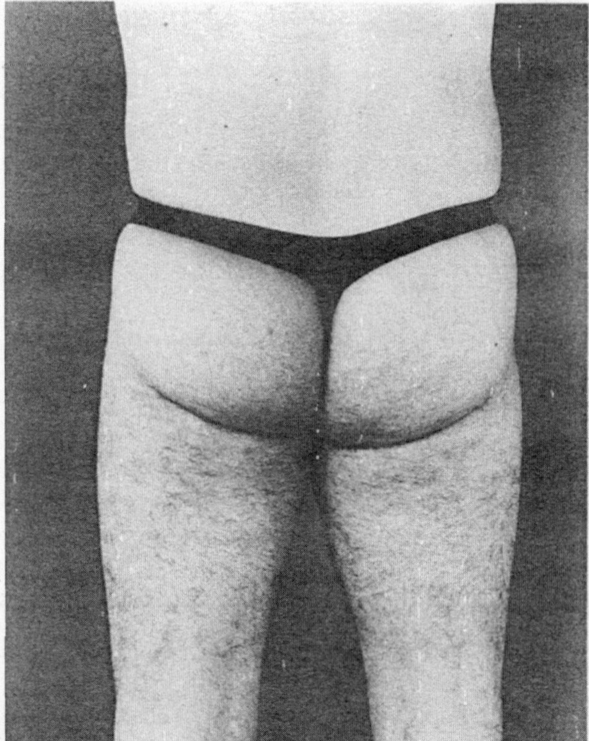

After 9th Class

JEANNE

Age: 32

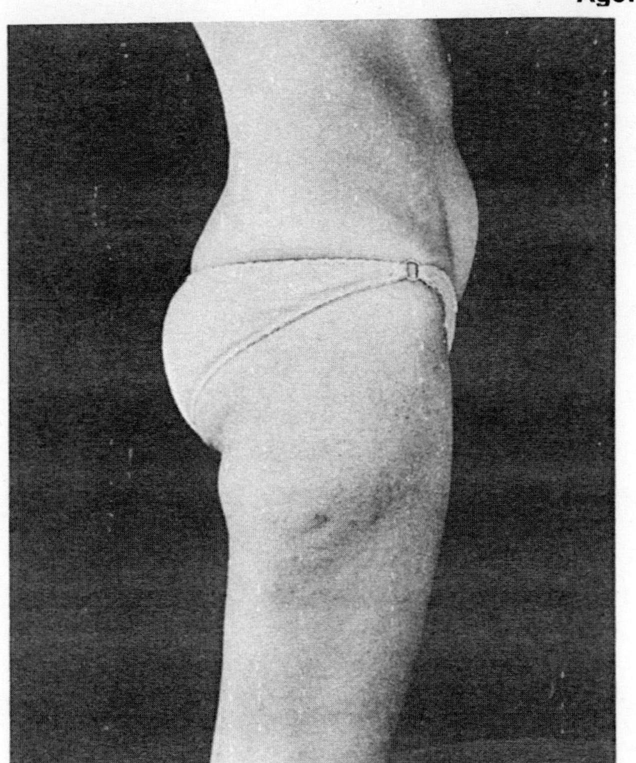

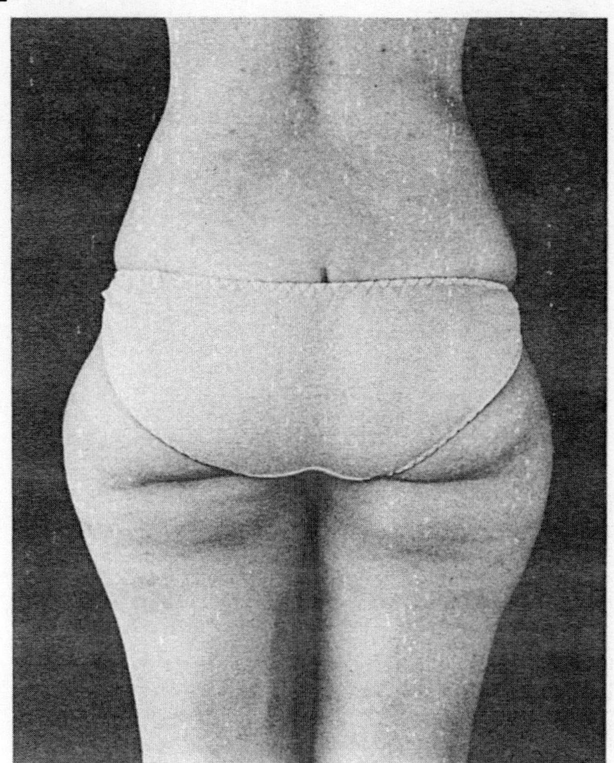

After 1st Class

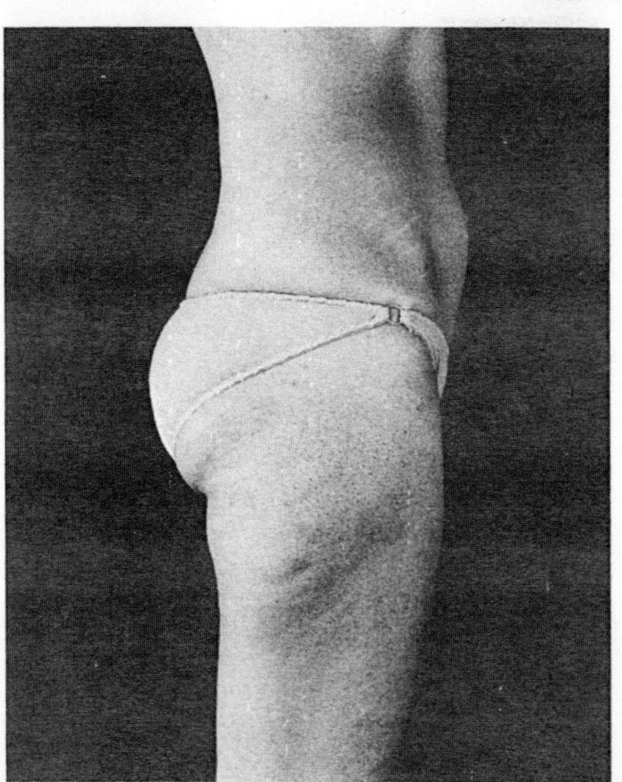

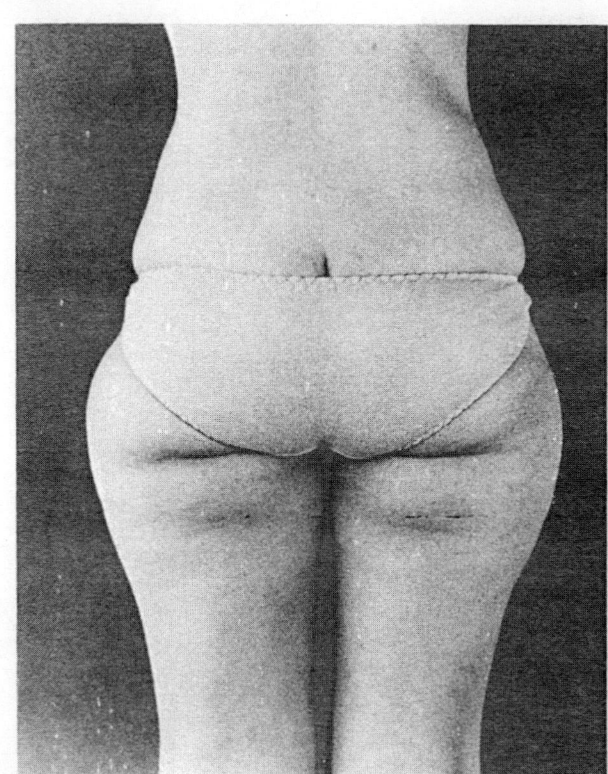

After 2nd Class

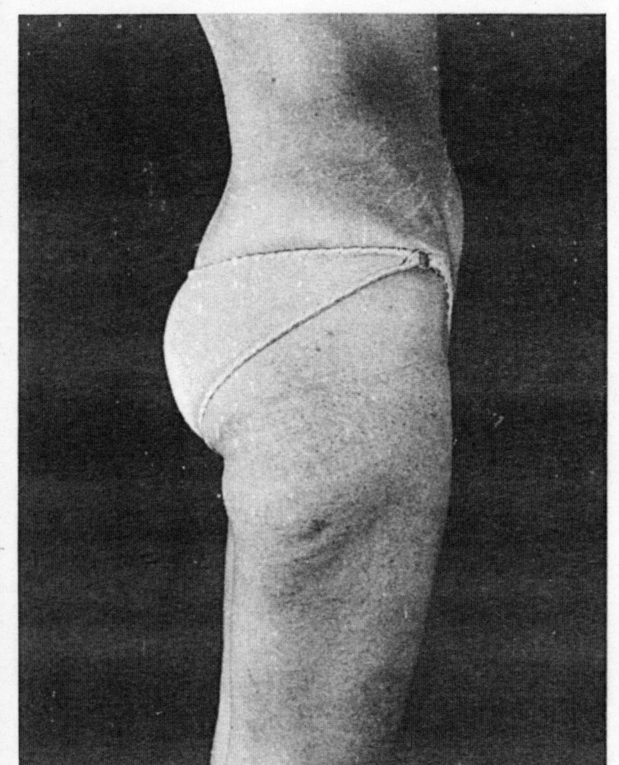

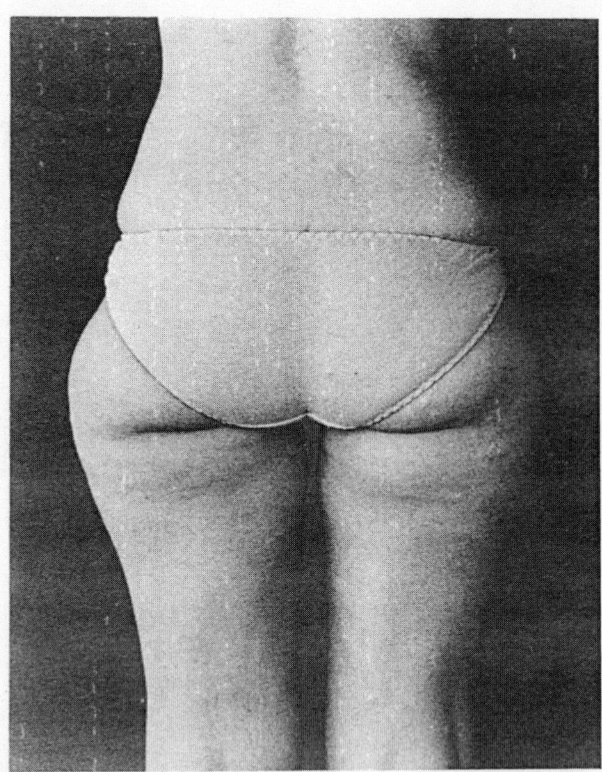

After 4th Class

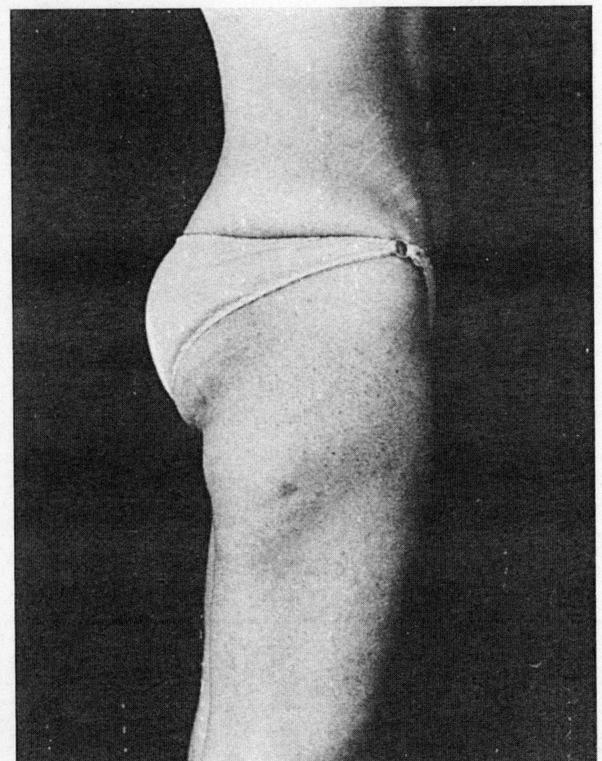

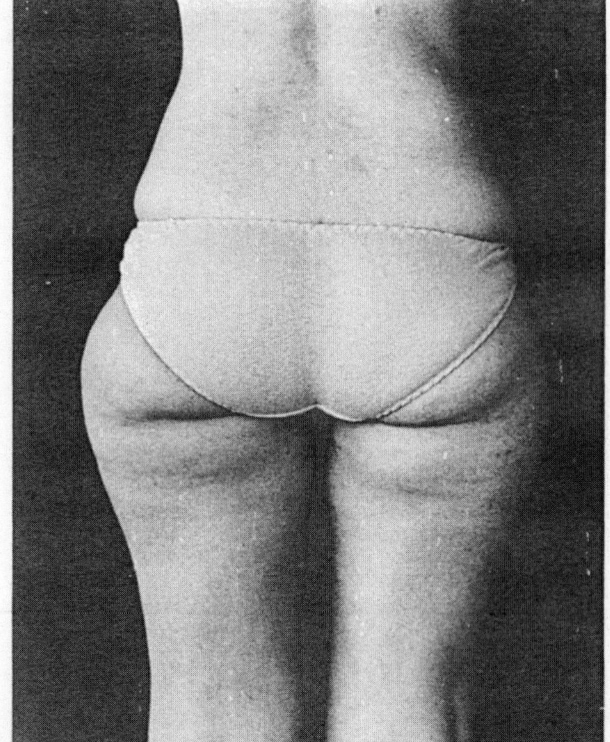

After 6th Class

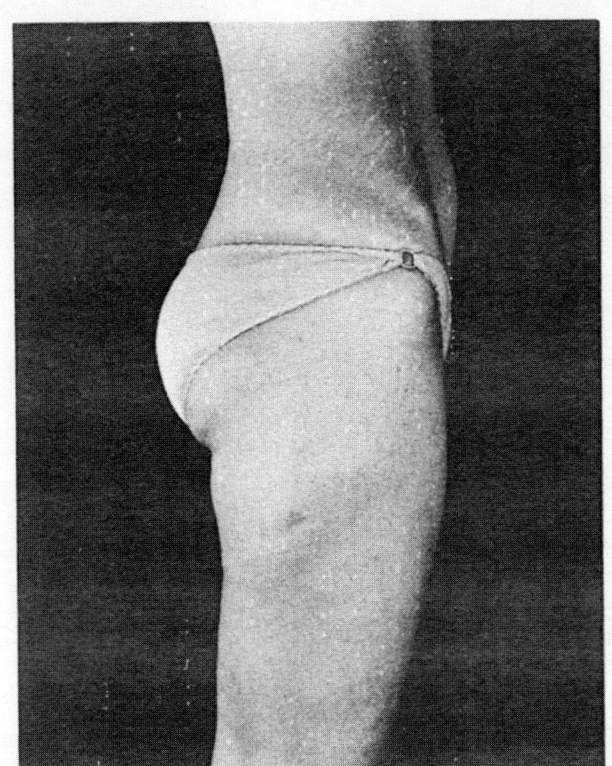
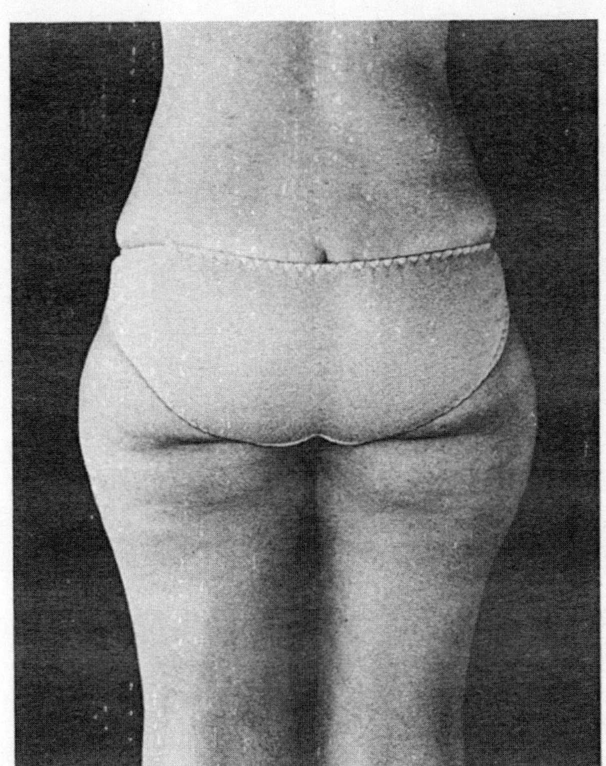

After 7th Class

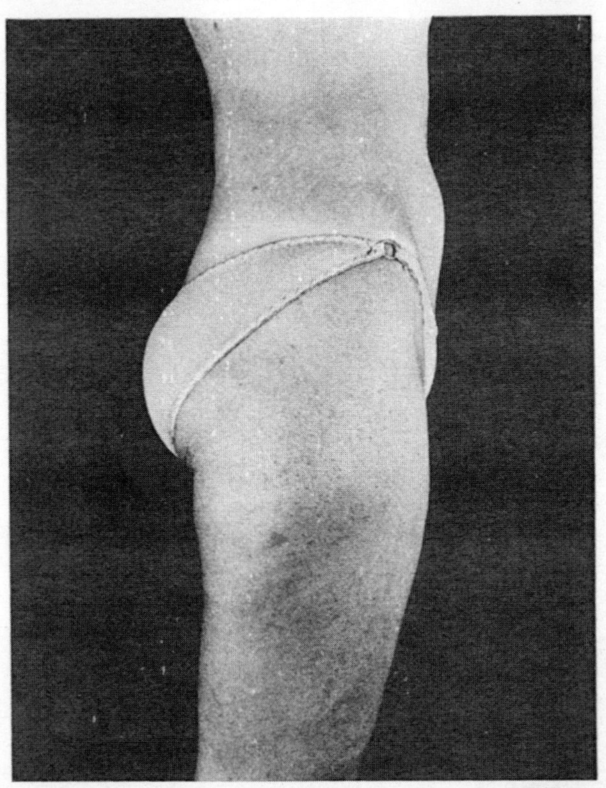
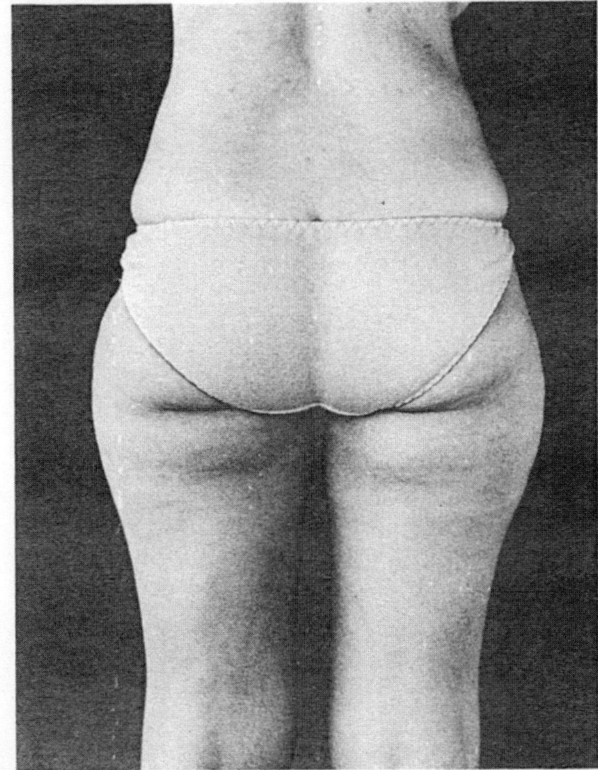

After 10th Class

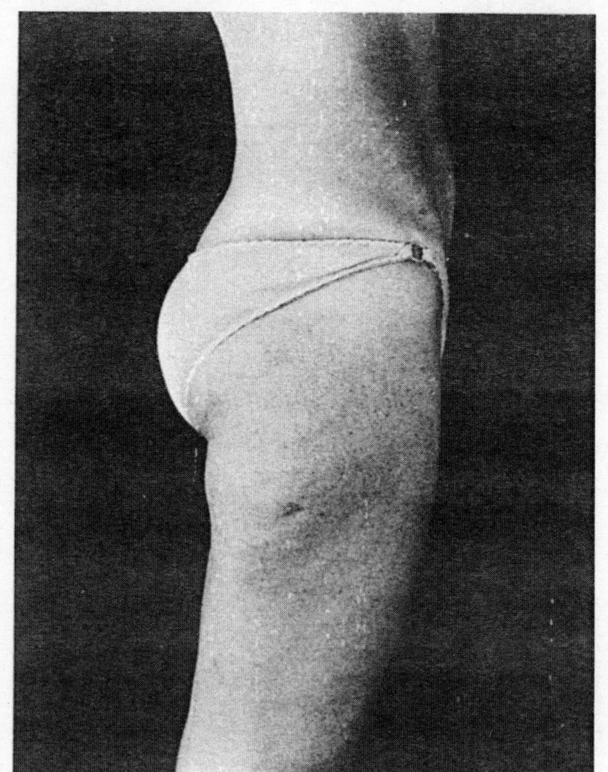

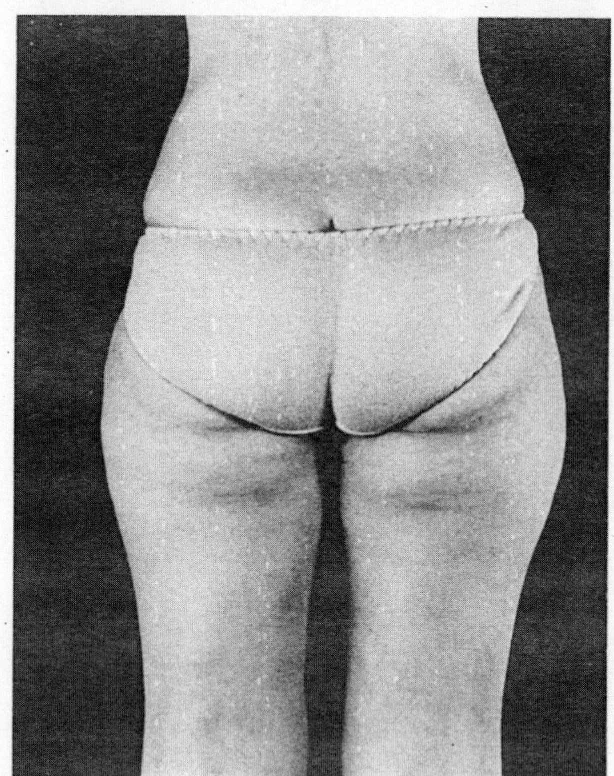

After 11th Class

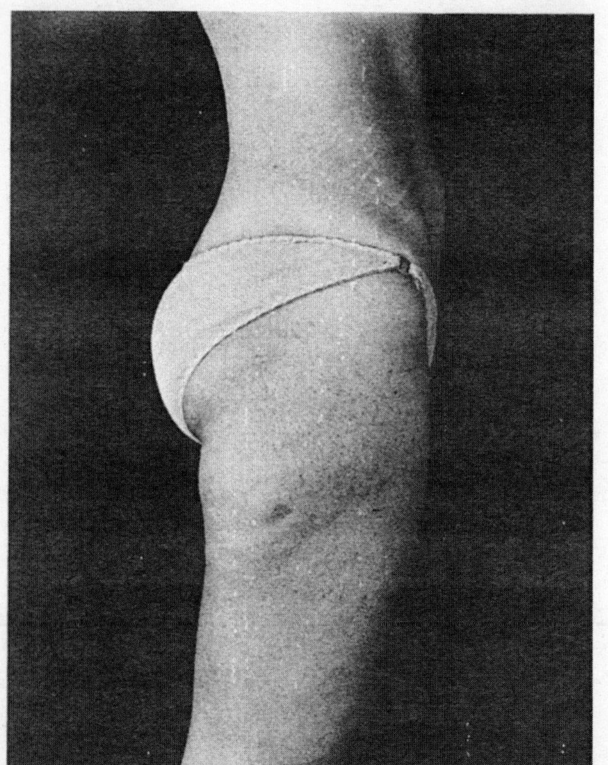

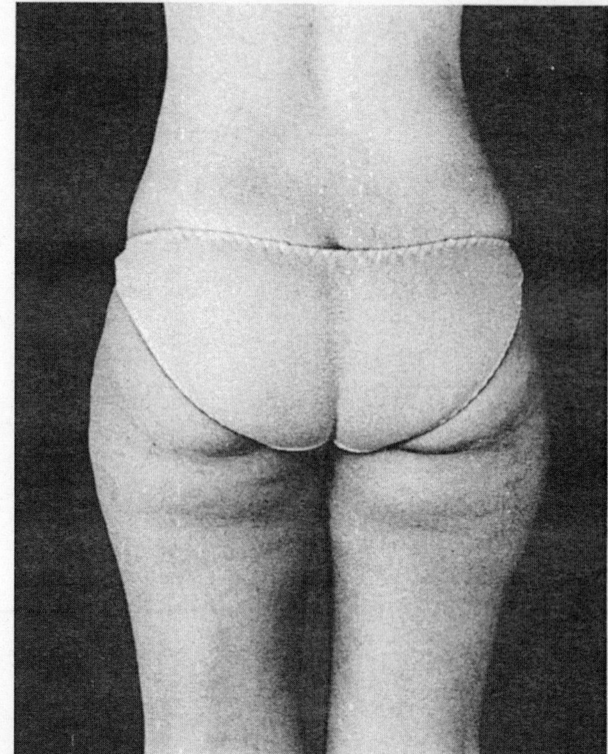

After 13th Class

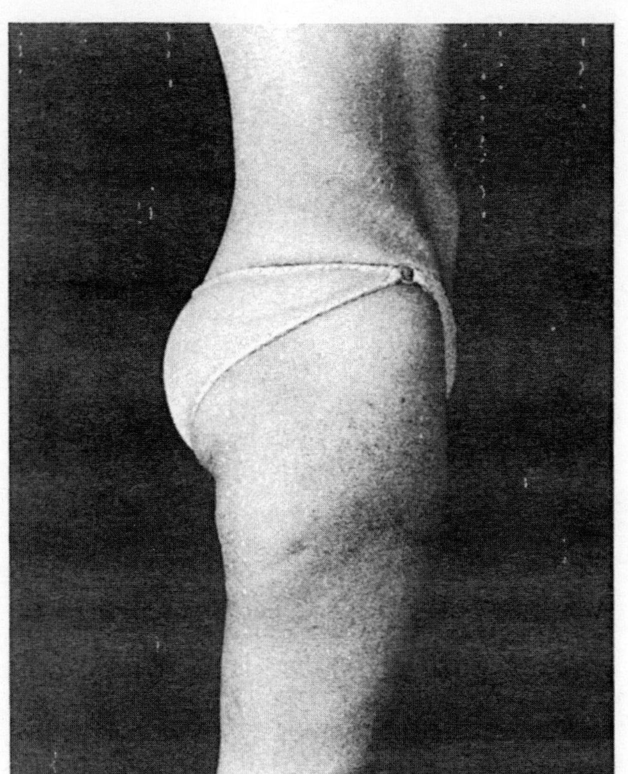

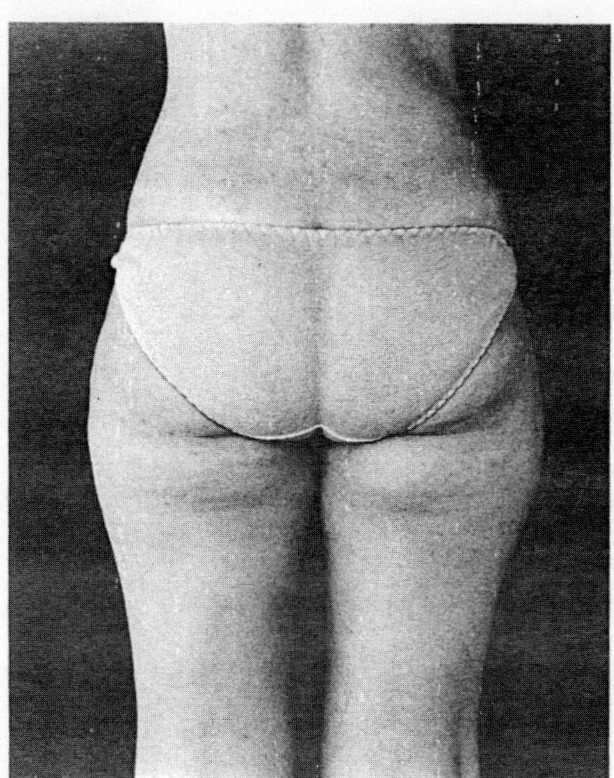

After 14th Class

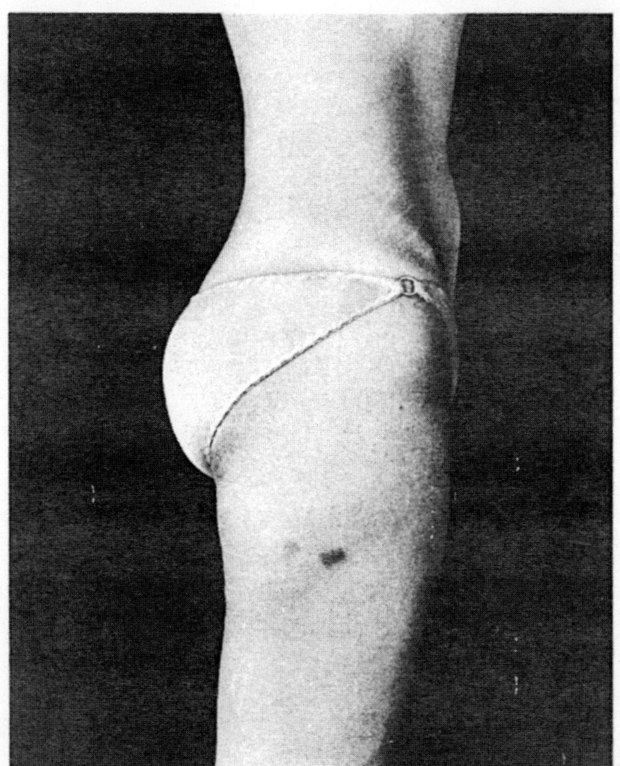

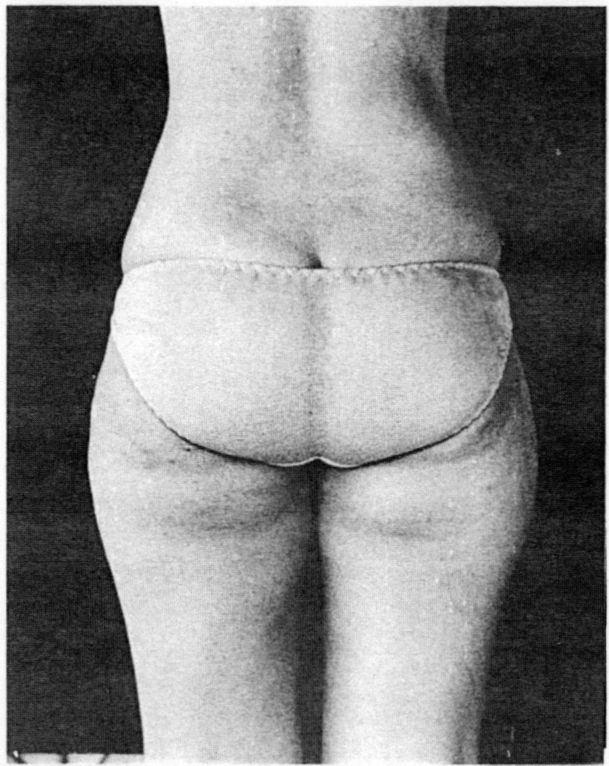

After 15th Class

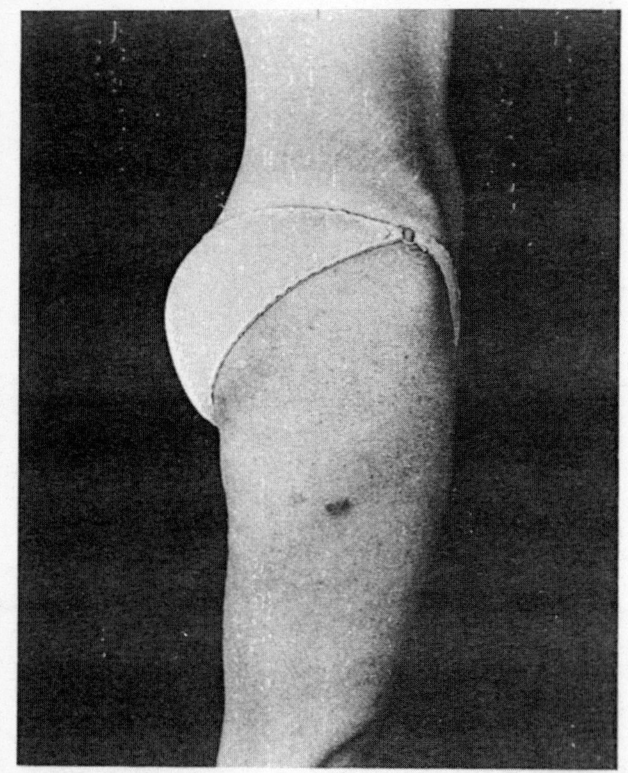
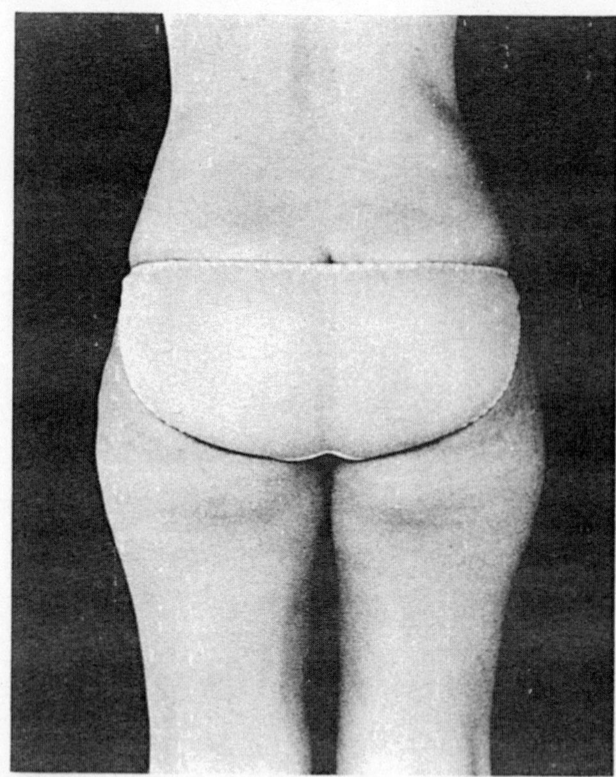

After 16th Class

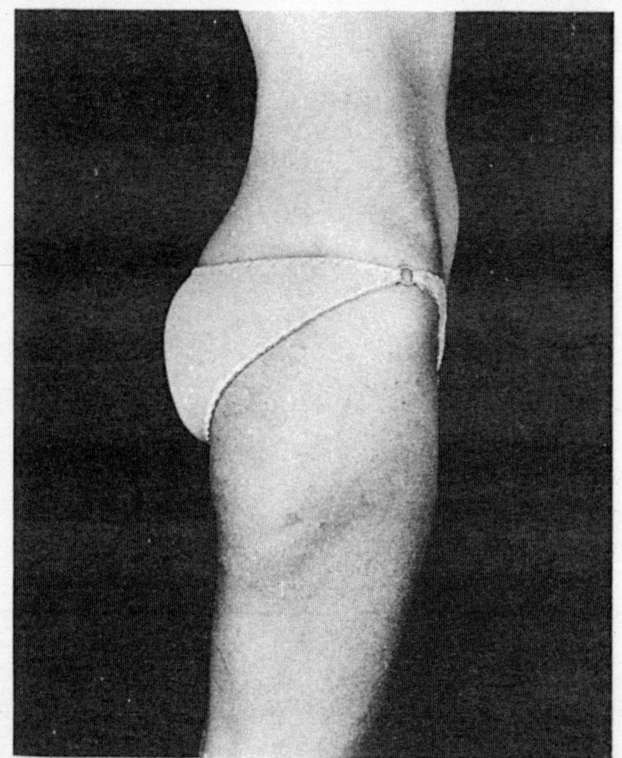
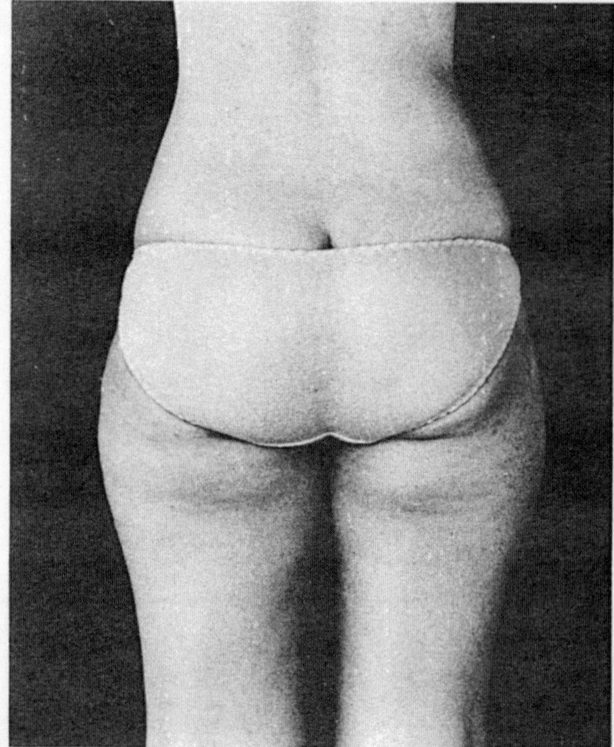

After 17th Class

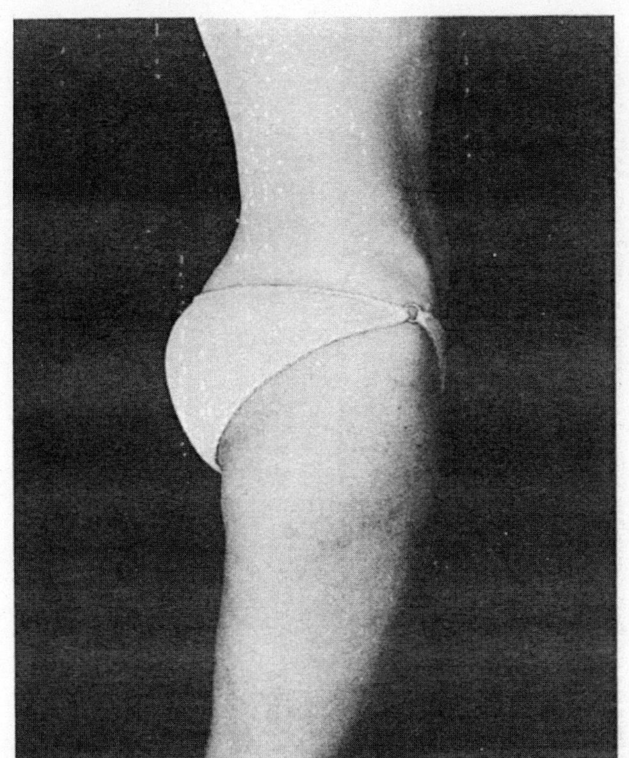

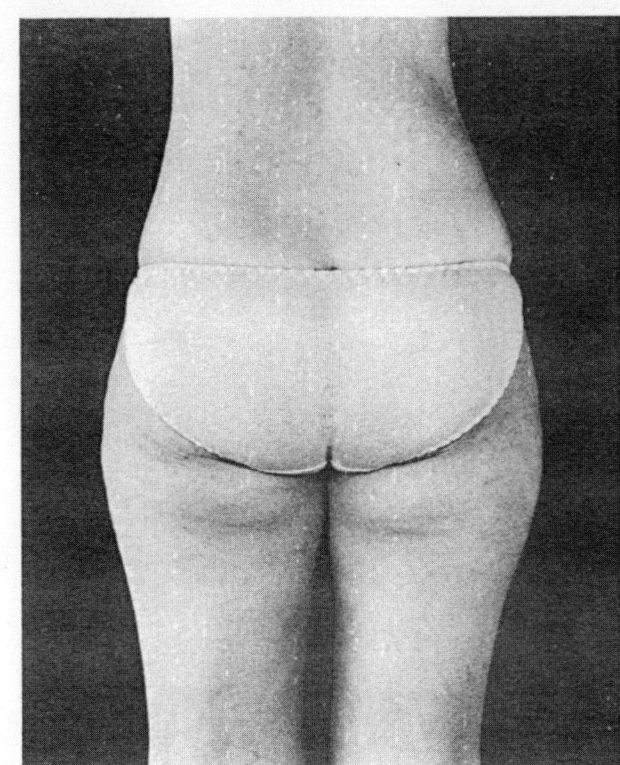

After 18th Class

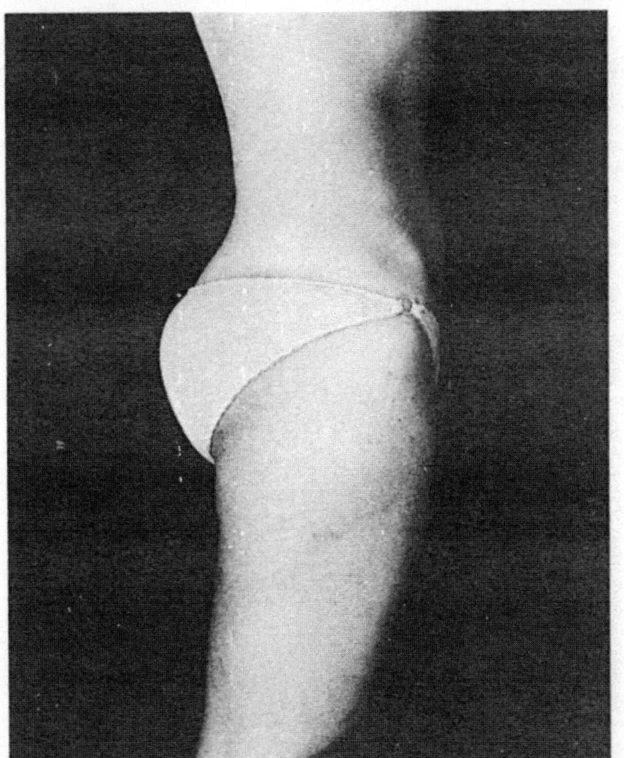

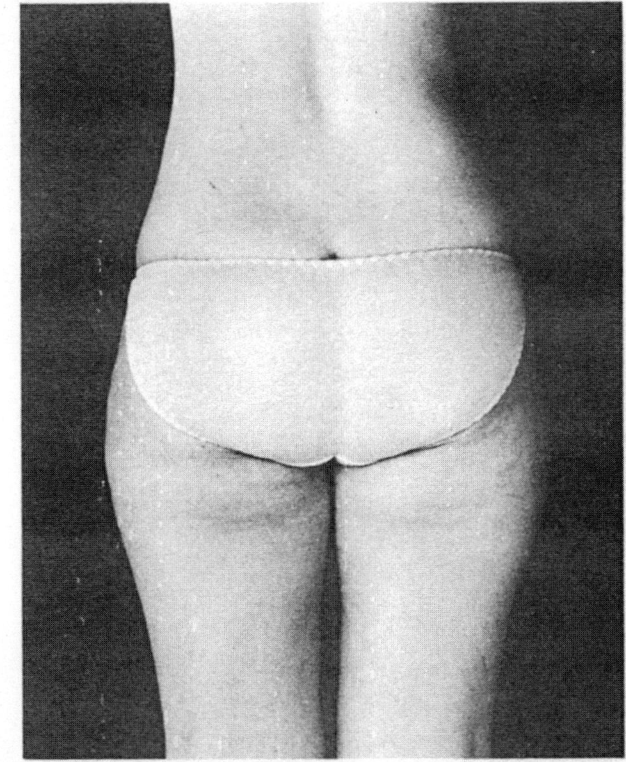

After 19th Class

JEANNE
Age: 32

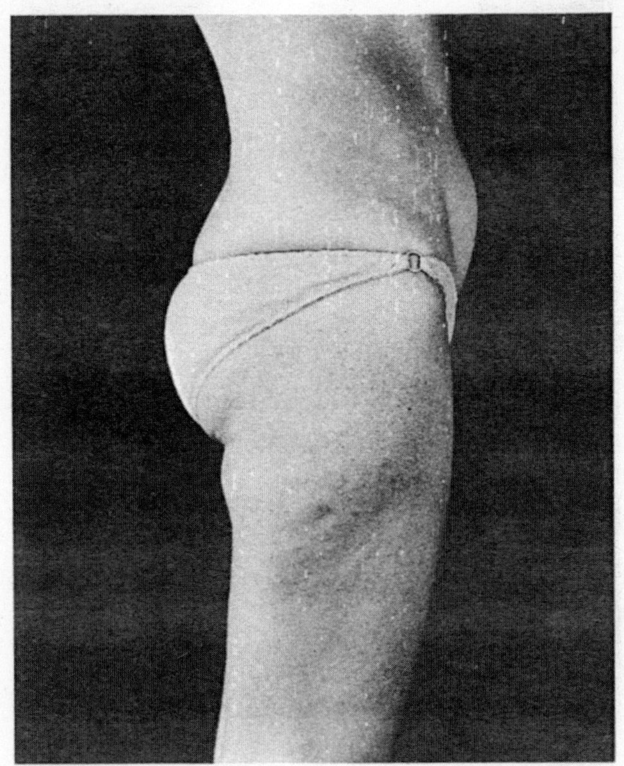
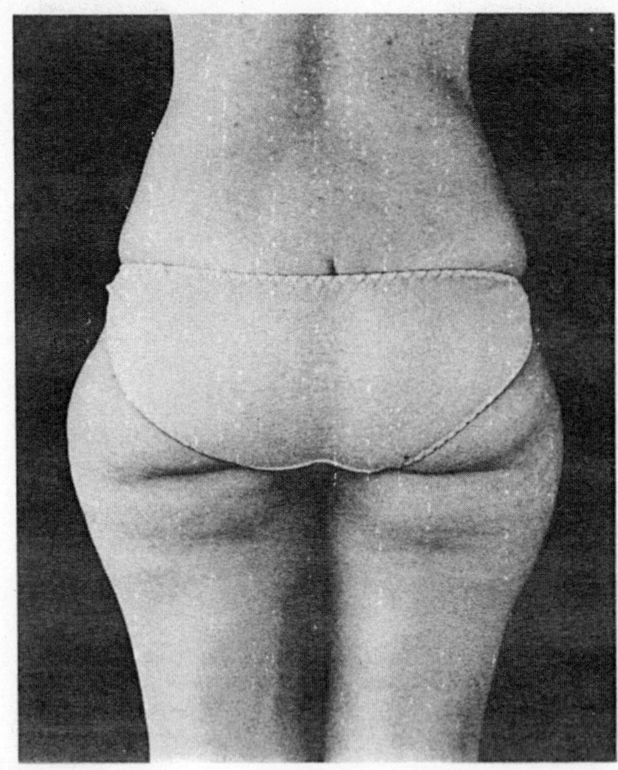

After 1st Class

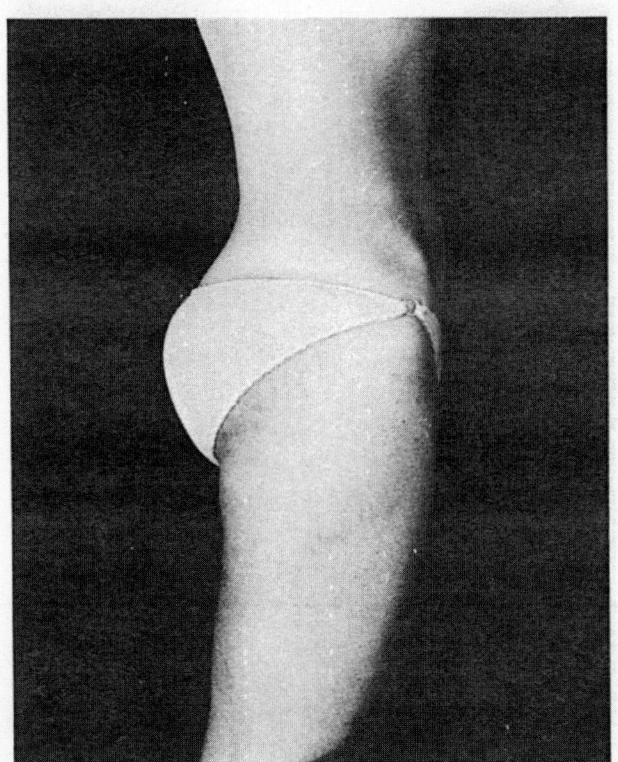
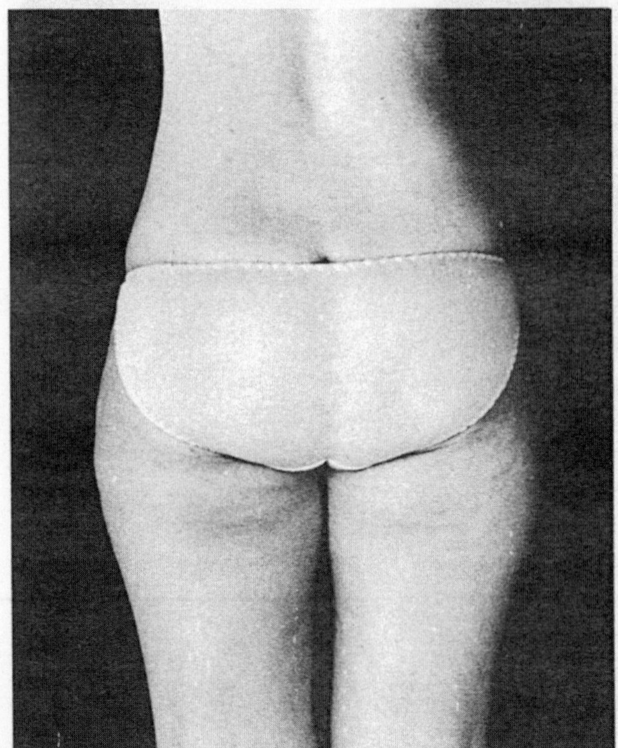

After 19th Class

CHAPTER FIVE

What Makes These Exercises Special?

Exercising should not be a second job with no salary, a chore with no reward. Time is money. Energy is precious. Why squander them on something futile?

I have taught exercise to thousands of people, ranging in age from eight to eighty-plus, during the past twelve years, with magnificent, rapid success. The movements I teach produce results in *hours,* not days, weeks, or months. The term "year" is unheard of when discussing getting in shape by this plan.

My impatience with the unnecessary effort and time demanded by conventional figure-trimming programs—aerobic dance, weights and exercise machines, calisthenics and ordinary isometrics included—prompted me to write this book. Life is too short to spend in a gym.

My students don't spend an hour a day working out. Who has that kind of time? Exercising is boring, boring, boring! Why be bored when you can get on with life? Spend your time on something that works. After the first hour of class, my students *feel* a difference in their bodies; after the second, most actually *see* it.

It's quite an adventure. In no time at all you will have restored your body to its lithe, firm, young form without injury—especially to your back—and without going to a gym or investing in expensive equipment.

If you're interested in rejuvenating your body and reclaiming your right to have a fantastic figure, it's not too late to start, no matter your age, sex, or physical condition. When I first began exercising, I felt like I had a toothache all over

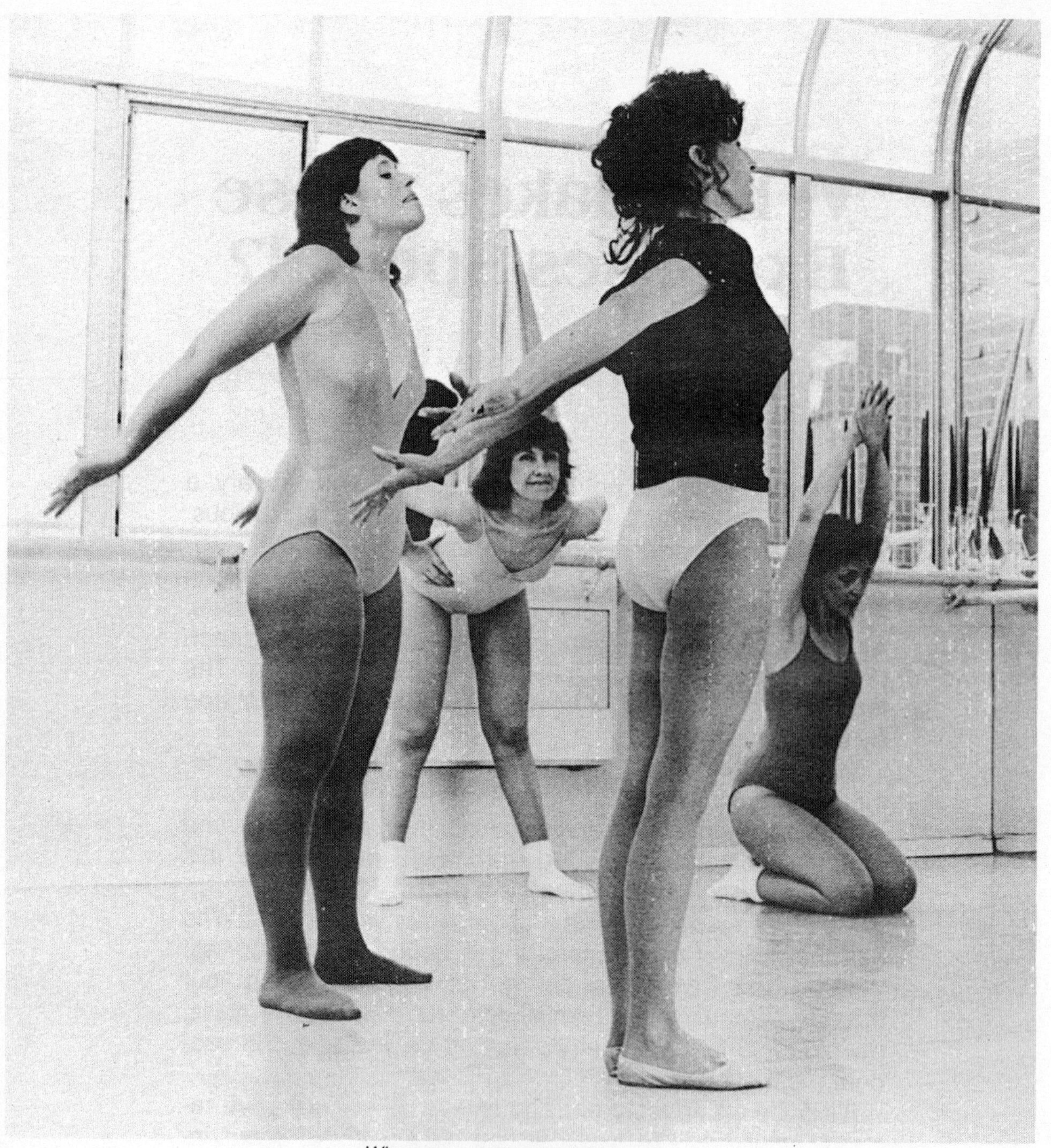

When you start exercising, do the complete program, from warm-up to inner thigh squeeze. In most classes, someone may be starting the warm-ups while another student may be working on her hips and behind, and another, her pelvis. Exercising is a very personal experience. Make the time you spend working on your body work for you. ▲

my body. Dancing, and most other activities I enjoyed, were out of the question because of my back pain and overall lack of muscle tone. Now look at me. You too can have the body you deserve if you're willing to work for it.

First, throw away your scales, or at least stash them in a closet where you won't be tempted to weigh every time you walk past them. Your body will quickly begin to go through some rather impressive changes. If you weigh yourself to check your daily progress, you may be in for quite a shock. The scale will not reflect your success as truthfully as your mirror and your clothes.

The important thing is how your body responds to the care it gets from your exercising. Exercise, in general, promises strength, endurance, and flexibility. This program has nine additional benefits:

- Coordination
- Balance
- Comprehensive body awareness
- Body control
- Discipline
- Speed
- Physical and mental relaxation
- Builds stamina
- Decreases appetite

When you start doing these exercises, you will no doubt discover more important pluses of your own. As you start to pull in, you will experience some surprising changes. For one, you may even show a weight *gain* of up to six or seven pounds. The trauma of putting on poundage could be so startling that it might throw you off your program. It is not uncommon for students to gain pounds, according to the scale, while dropping two or even three dress sizes. Every pound you lose looks like two.

There is a very rational explanation to this rather irrational occurrence. There is less muscle than flab to a pound. (Remember your high school science: A pound of feathers and a pound of steel weigh the same, but the pound of feathers takes up more room than the pound of steel because of the *volume* of feathers needed to make up that pound.)

Don't be frightened by the wonderful changes taking place within your body. These initial fluctuations are immaterial when you consider how beautiful your body is becoming.

WHAT MY STUDENTS AND I WEAR TO EXERCISE

An exercise session is *not* a fashion show. I personally don't care what anyone wears, as long as they are comfortable. You can wear a burlap bag, as long as your body is not restricted by what you have on.

When the pictures were being taken for this book, some of my students had to buy leotards or borrow from friends, because most of them do not wear them in class. Their usual garb is decidedly less photogenic: gym shorts and torn T-shirts, jogging suits, loose sweatshirts over dance shorts. Instead of leg warmers, most wear crew socks. We're a motley crew!

No one would have minded being photographed in their ordinary class clothes, but aesthetic wisdom prevailed. It was important to show the precise movements of the exercises as clearly as possible. That would have been impossible if everyone wore baggy warm-up suits.

Students of all sizes and shapes demonstrate the exercises and are in the group pictures. Most are new students.

Another reason I advise my students not to bother with dancewear for exercise is that people tend to spend too much time comparing what they have on with the latest status leotard-and-tights look.

Work on your body, not on your wardrobe of exercise clothes. Save your money for a few weeks and splurge on a gorgeous dress or a beautifully fitted pair of pants! Save your fashion energy for when you get your body looking beautiful, are going out with the man of your dreams, and you want to look and feel like a queen!

Tights are not essential to proper exercise either. In fact they can be a detriment to the full benefits of your program. Tights are appropriately named, indeed, especially those of Lycra and spandex, which are like leg girdles. They press your leg muscles and lessen the contractions of the exercises. They also inhibit circulation while hiding what you should be seeing.

Belted exercise uniforms are more fashionable than functional. I have seen women cinch their belts so tightly that their waists look gorgeous, but they can hardly breathe properly, much less bend over. The purpose of exercise is to make your waist smaller. The purpose of wearing a belted exercise costume is to make it *look* smaller.

WHAT, NO SOUNDS OF MUSIC?

Music may be exciting or soothing, but I prefer to teach without this distraction. The music gets between you and your mastery of your body.

When learning these movements, pay attention to your movements. If you are playing music with a driving beat, you instinctively move your body in time. Therefore, you forfeit control of the exercises.

Until you have perfected the techniques of these exercises, silence is golden indeed.

A WORD ABOUT TEMPERATURES

Leave your sweaty gym mentality with your scales when you begin this program! You won't need it to shape up.

Unless the temperature and the humidity are hideously high, I do not turn on the air-conditioners in my studio. I have the windows open and I use a ceiling fan that cools the air without stirring up a draft.

Exercising in an air-conditioned room can cause you to get a chill and, as a result, experience painful muscle cramps. Stay out of drafts, regardless of how hot you get. Dry off and get out of your exercise clothes before you become chilled and your muscles cramp.

The perspiration generated by exercise is one way the body regulates its temperature. It has very little to do with long-term weight loss. The weight loss by heavy perspiration is only temporary because it is, in truth, water loss.

Often my students sip water in between sets of exercises because they feel thirsty. Fruit juices and soft drinks, however, defeat the purpose of exercise. Juices and sodas are usually too sweet to quench your thirst. (Juices are also higher in calories than fruits.)

WHERE SHOULD YOU EXERCISE?

These exercises can be done anywhere, anytime. As long as you are comfortable.

Ideally, you should have a mirror—a big one—so that you can see how your body is positioned. Don't be intimidated. I lived in my mirrored apartment for a year before I really looked at myself. I was very conscious of avoiding my reflection. I was afraid that my body wouldn't look as youthful and tight as I wanted. One day I was exercising alone. It was summer. The sun was streaming through the greenhouse walls, bathing my body in a brutal light. I could see every lump and bump . . . only there weren't any. At last I felt wonderful about my body.

While you don't need any special equipment to do these exercises properly, you will need a secure *barre* for some of the exercises you do to trim and firm your legs and, especially, for working on your behind and hips. Rather than install rigging as I have done in my studio, use your imagination—a kitchen counter, a strong table, the back of your couch, or even your bureau top.

Find something other than a towel rack for support. Even the ones that are cemented in tile to the walls of your bathroom are too insecure to bear more weight than a couple of wet towels. The type that is screwed into the wall is even more dangerous, especially since you may be tempted to hold on for dear life until you build up your strength enough to use the *barre*—or whatever substitute you adopt—for balance.

Anyone can do these exercises. Even people who consider themselves Super Klutzes—they can't walk and talk at the same time—gain control of their bodies. Every person I have taught, regardless of his or her age or condition, who had the determination to have a strong, fit, and beautiful body, now has it.

The complete program, as it is constructed, can be done in less than an hour, once you have gained enough strength to do the exercises. This can be divided to fit your day's schedule. Break it up so that it suits you.

You will want to do the One-Hour Program twice a week at first. Once you have your figure the way you want it, you may adopt the 15-Minute Maintenance Plan as your primary exercise routine, doing the complete workout once a week . . . or when it's time to whip your body back into shape—after the holidays, for example.

Once you experience the deep contractions of these innovative exercises and see how quickly your body pulls in, you will *make* time for yourself. These exercises will become the highlight of your day.

CHAPTER SIX

The One-Hour Program

You are now ready to give yourself one of the most wonderful gifts in the world: a fabulous, tight, *fit* figure. It is only hours away if you follow the plan detailed in the pages ahead.

The One-Hour Program I teach is explained in detail in the following chapters in such a way that you will be able to follow the instructions and photographs movement by movement. These are not your ordinary exercises, therefore I have been very explicit, almost repetitious, in explaining how every exercise should be done. Since I won't be there to demonstrate and to position your body before you start, I have taken every care that you will know what to do.

Each set of exercises is designed to work on a specific part of the body. In each chapter you will see precisely how to execute the delicate movements and deep contractions that give the exercises their power, and you will see the exact parts of your body that will benefit from each section.

The people demonstrating the program had been to fewer than four classes at the time we took their photos. They are doing the exercises as best as their bodies will allow—or, I should say, *allowed*—when the pictures were taken.

That is all I ask of anyone who does this program. Do what you can. As you become stronger, you will be able to do more and more with ease. You will feel your muscles contract more deeply and you will stretch more fully when your body is ready.

Do not force your body to do anything it is not prepared to

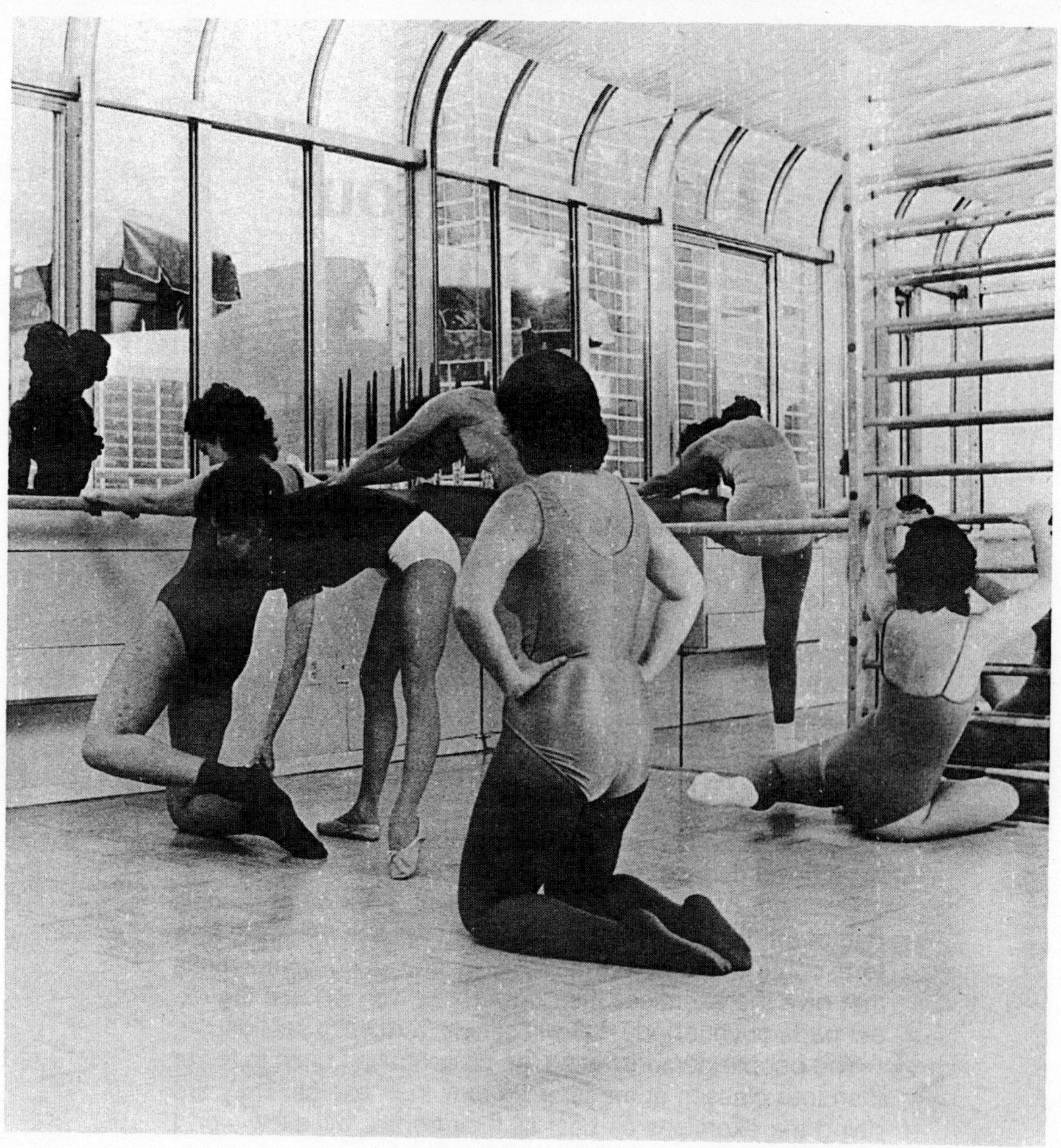

Classes are a free-for-all at my studio. Everyone works at their own pace and sees and feels results in hours, not weeks or months or more. There is no music, no dance routine and no machine and weight program—just a program of very personal, very practical body movements. ▲

do. If instructions say "Put your foot on the *barre*" and you cannot lift your leg all the way up to the kitchen counter that you are using as your exercise *barre,* don't even attempt it. Rest your foot on a sturdy, low chair. Once your hamstrings and spine are stretched and your entire body is ready for you to raise your leg as high as that counter, you will be able to accomplish it with graceful ease.

Take frequent breathers at first. If you feel a burning sensation in muscles after you have done twenty-five or thirty repetitions when instructions say you are to do one hundred, stop what you are doing and shift your position. This may mean your muscles aren't strong enough yet. Try working on the opposite side, so that your muscles can rest. Or, it may mean that you need to lie down flat and rest for a few minutes.

When you stop an exercise, rest and then start over again *from the original starting position.* Repeat it step by step. In this way, you will be certain that your body is properly positioned for safety and the success of the exercise.

I do not teach any special breathing technique because I have found that people pay so much attention to their breathing that they forget to exercise. Just remember to breathe naturally. If you hold your breath you are only denying your body the oxygen it must have to cleanse the blood and nourish your muscles. Without it you won't have the stamina you deserve.

I have two very specific words of warning. Please take them to heart.

To Pregnant Women: Under no circumstances should any woman in the first trimester of pregnancy do the stomach exercises unless her doctor has actually gotten down on the floor and done them to feel how deep the contractions are. Don't just show your Ob-Gyn the book. The exercises appear to be very easy, but looks, in this case, are terribly deceiving.

This is not to say that expectant mothers cannot do the program. I will take a woman after her fourth month if she will agree to make an appointment for the two of us to show the exercises to her gynecologist or obstetrician. I have the doctor get down and do them.

Mothers who have been in the program before *they* became pregnant or began it after their fourth month tell me that they had incredibly easy deliveries and amazing recovery rates.

To Everyone: I ask you to have your doctor check you over before you begin this, or any other, physical fitness regimen. We have all heard this warning before and all of us have gone ahead and exercised without benefit of a checkup. A lot of people have been severely injured. Because of the nature of these exercises, I ask that this time you pay attention; get your doctor's go-ahead. I have had no known injuries as a result of these exercises in the twelve years I have been teaching, but I won't be there to supervise you.

Now, we are ready to begin.

You will probably notice that your body is shifting after your second hour if you follow the program exactly, from warm-up to inner thigh squeeze, with everything in between, each time you exercise.

To say it another way: If you want with all your heart to get rid of your thunder thighs and think you can do *only* the exercises for the behind and hips and have your dream come true, you are only fooling yourself.

Follow the program as it is written. That works.

If you have weak stomach muscles, your stomach may appear larger at first, even though your waist is already smaller. You are working on your upper stomach muscles first. Also your hips are pulling in and your behind is rising. Keep working. All of a sudden your abdominal muscles will catch up with the rest of your newly-firm body and be beautifully flat.

As your hips and behind pull in and up, you may notice a lump of flesh just below your waist in the back, where you feel when you put your hands on your hips. Don't get hysterical like I did. As everything tightens, all that gooshy mass on your hips is being lifted and tightened to be a high, round, firm behind! Keep at it.

Here are more surprises that you may have ahead:

- One morning you will notice in the mirror that your neck is longer and narrower.
- As if by magic, your inner thighs will look smooth and part of your legs, not something mushy and separate.
- Your legs will look longer and leaner and you will feel as though you have the spring of a gazelle.
- One night you will roll over in bed and feel as if your cat had left a toy under the covers and it is poking into your

hip. It's your hipbone. Your stomach has become so tight and flat that your hipbones show.

You are truly able to resculpt your body into an image of beauty. It won't be a breeze, but it will be fast.

Laugh at yourself if your body won't cooperate. Talk to your muscles, caress them, cajole them, tease them, and soon you will be able to get them to do anything you ask. Each hour of exercise you do, your body becomes stronger and firmer . . . and lovelier.

It's so exciting.

One Final Word: Please read the instructions for each exercise thoroughly before beginning the movements.

CHAPTER SEVEN

Warming Up

Don't think you can let yourself off easy if you skip over these warm-ups and right into the real body work. If you do, you are asking for trouble.

Contrary to the casual-sounding name, warm-ups are not "nonexercises" that are done before you do an exercise program. Quite literally, warming up means that you warm up your muscles. You elevate your body temperature and increase cardiovascular activity to send blood and oxygen throughout your body.

Many years ago, I asked doctors and therapists what should be done in a warm-up and could not get a straight answer. So I tried my own experiment. For two weeks I had one particular class do only stretches to "warm up," while the rest of my classes did my regular program of warm-up exercises and stretches. The test class did not perform well at all. I concluded that their muscles were stretched but they certainly weren't warmed up.

Dancers are known to spend forty-five minutes or more *limbering* up before a performance. One high kick could tear an unprepared hamstring to shreds. A muscle spasm might cause a fall that could end a career.

This heightened activity prepares the muscles for the more strenuous, demanding activity ahead. Muscles are gently stretched and flexed, joints are put through their range of motion, all to protect the body from injury. Because you have given your body a taste of the delicious results of exercise, you will be able to work safely and completely on your entire body.

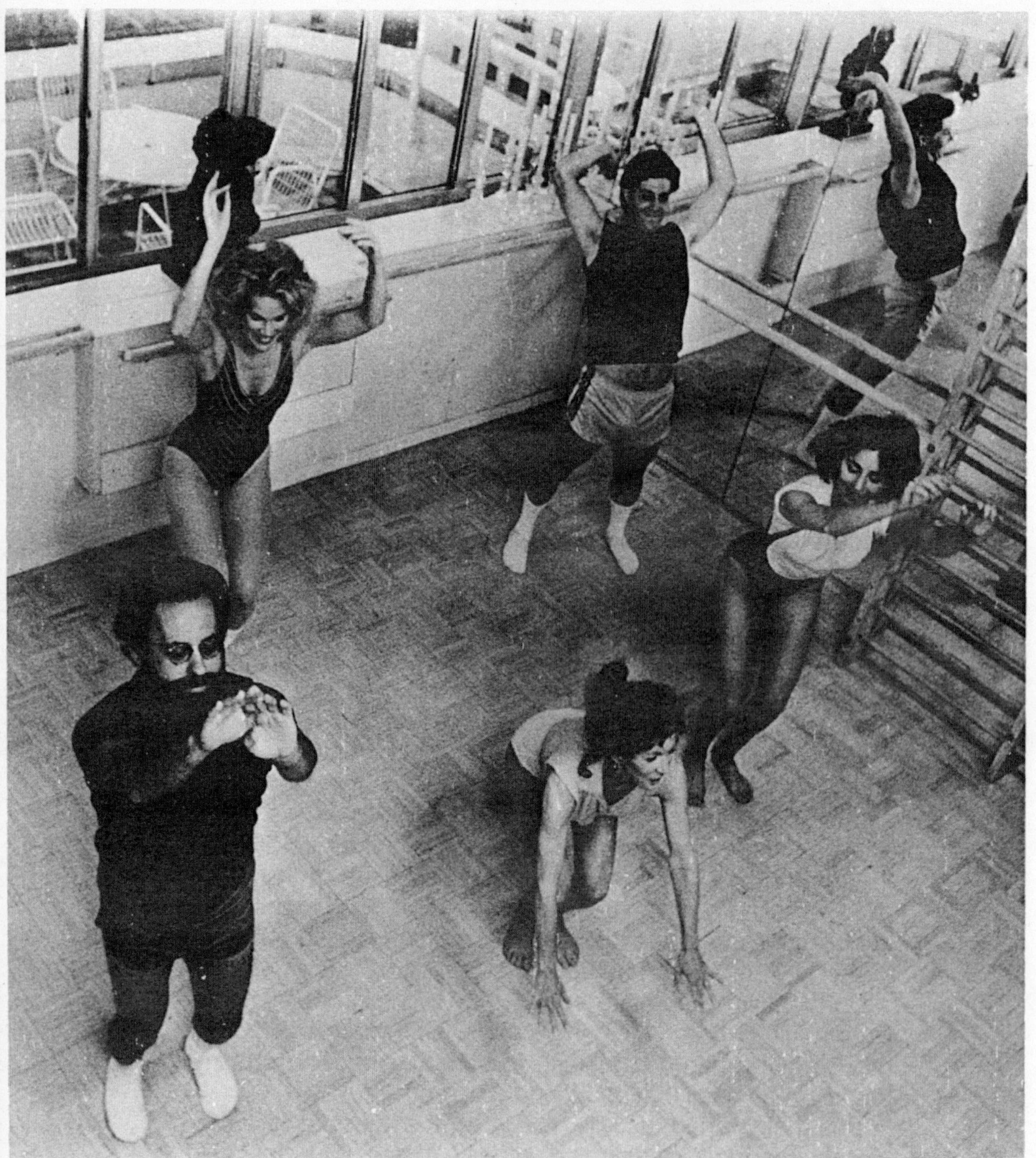

My classes are informal, intimate. It is a safe, comfortable environment for my students to work on their bodies. Classes small—seven students, tops—and there's nothing regimented to force anyone to do something they aren't ready for. You could easily create the same secure intimacy in your home, or at the home of a friend, and start your own exercise group. There is something about having a specific time and place, where you regularly join the same group of friends, that makes starting an exercise program fun. ▲

Each of these gentle, seemingly simple warm-ups is perfect preparation for the deep contractions and the precise, accurate movements inherent in the remainder of this one-hour program.

Pat, who is demonstrating this part of the program, had completed three classes at the time of the photography session. She is in her mid-fifties, a highly-motivated professional woman who is also the mother of teenagers.

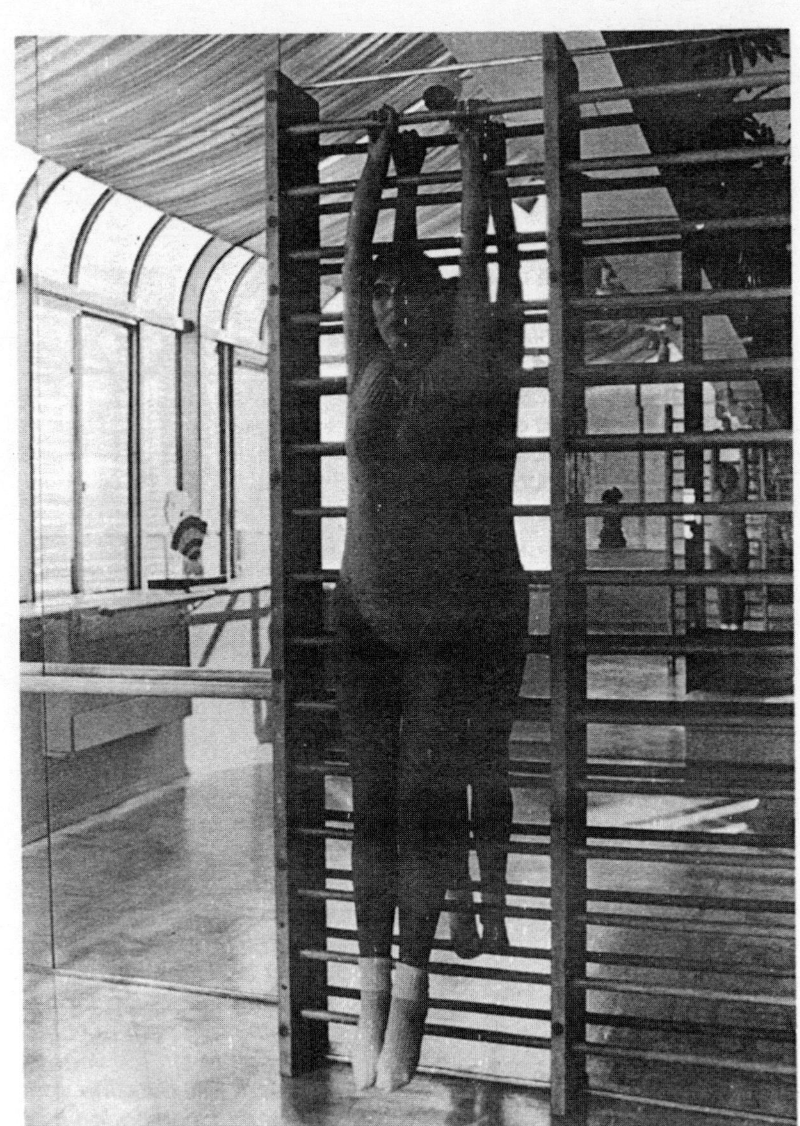

WARM-UP #1 *Stretch your spine by hanging. Let your body drip to the floor like melting wax. If you don't have access to a ladder, as I have in my studio, or a chinning bar, grasp the top of a sturdy door braced open against a wall and covered with a towel to protect your hands. If you use a door, you will have to face it in order to hold on. Otherwise, reach around the bar and hold as Pat is doing. Don't be afraid that you will fall, or you will make the mistake of tensing your entire body. That defeats the purpose of the stretch. Hold as long as you can—even if only for a second—with your feet off the floor. If you're too tall, bend your knees. Point your toes if you can. Feel your body stretch and lengthen. When I started hanging, I could only hold for a fast count of 5. Now, my wrists and arms are so strong, I can hang for a slow count of 75 or more. If you are lucky enough to live near a playground or schoolyard, you can hang from the swings or jungle gym.* ▶

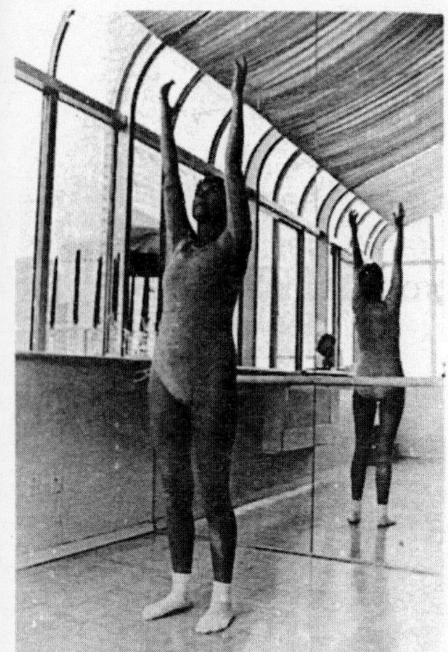

WARM-UP #2 *Stand erect with your feet about a foot apart—but never more than 15 inches—and raise your chest upward. Lift both arms over your head, reaching high. Keep reaching. You want to stretch your stomach, making you feel as if your torso is 2 inches longer than it really is.*

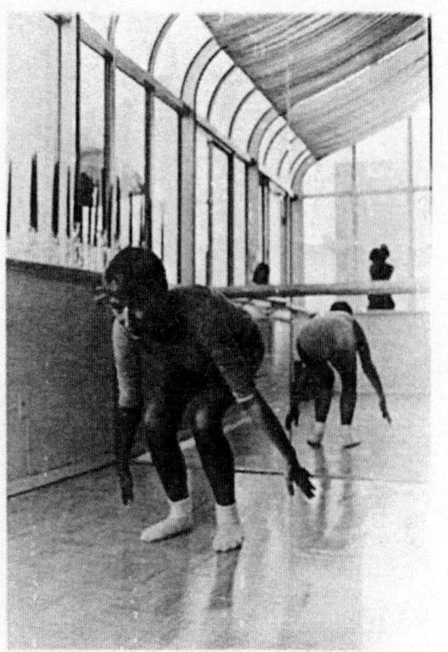

Bend your knees, keeping your feet flat on the floor. Continue stretching upward. Bend your upper body forward, arms out, as though reaching for something in front of you. Continue to stretch your torso outward. Still bending your knees and leaning forward, bring your arms to your sides, even with your calves. ▲

Continue to raise your arms up behind your body, stretching your neck out as you do this. Keep knees relaxed and body bent over. Do not arch your back. Keep shoulders relaxed and rounded. Complete this exercise by reversing the movements to the starting position. Do 5, returning the arms to the initial stretching position between each combination. ▼

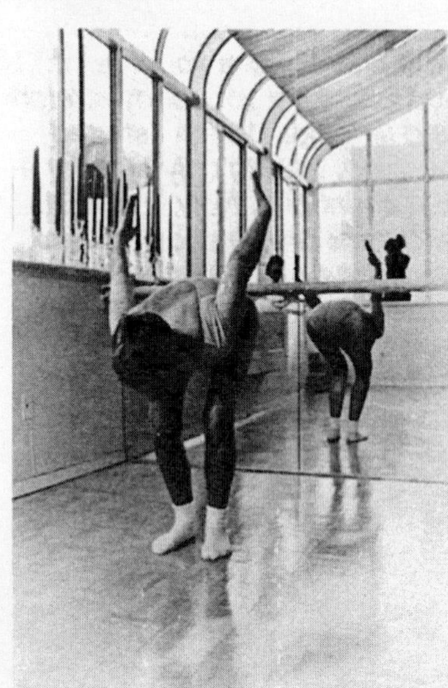

FOR TIGHTENING THE UNDERARMS *This is the* only *underarm exercise you need to do. Standing erect, as for the initial warm-up, reach arms outward to the sides at shoulder level and roll them forward so that the palms face upward. The more you turn your arms so that your palms are pointing to the sky, the more you will feel. Gently take your arms behind you, as if you were trying to make your shoulder blades meet. Move only a half inch at a time back and forth behind you. Do not jerk. Hold your head and shoulders back. Tighten your behind and hold your stomach in as you tip your pelvis upward. Relax your legs. Do 100, trying to touch thumbs. Keep your arms turned over behind your back and keep your thumbs up. The higher you can hold your arms straight the more you will feel the muscle working. Do not bend your elbows. Done properly, this exercise tightens your underarms and pectoral muscles, which raises the bustline and loosens tension in the muscles between your shoulder blades and neck.* ▼

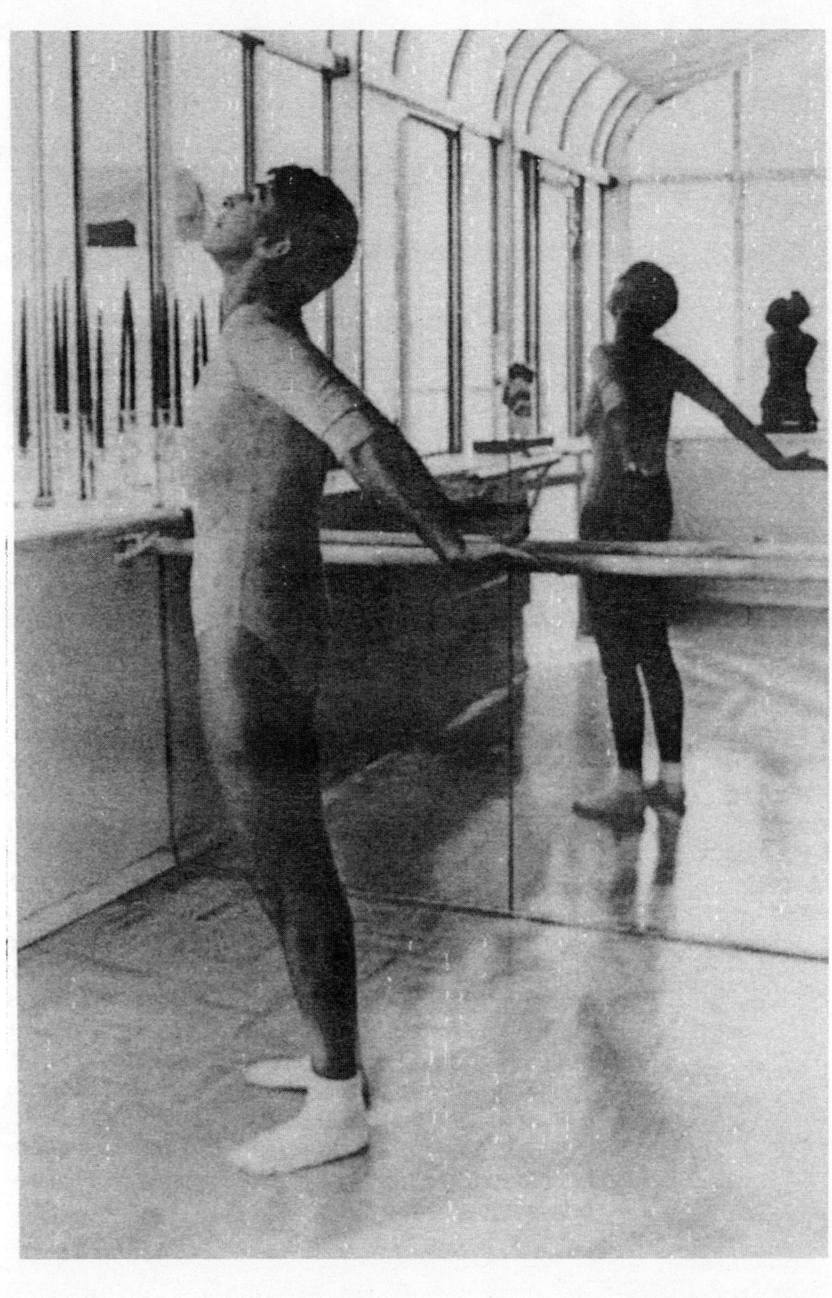

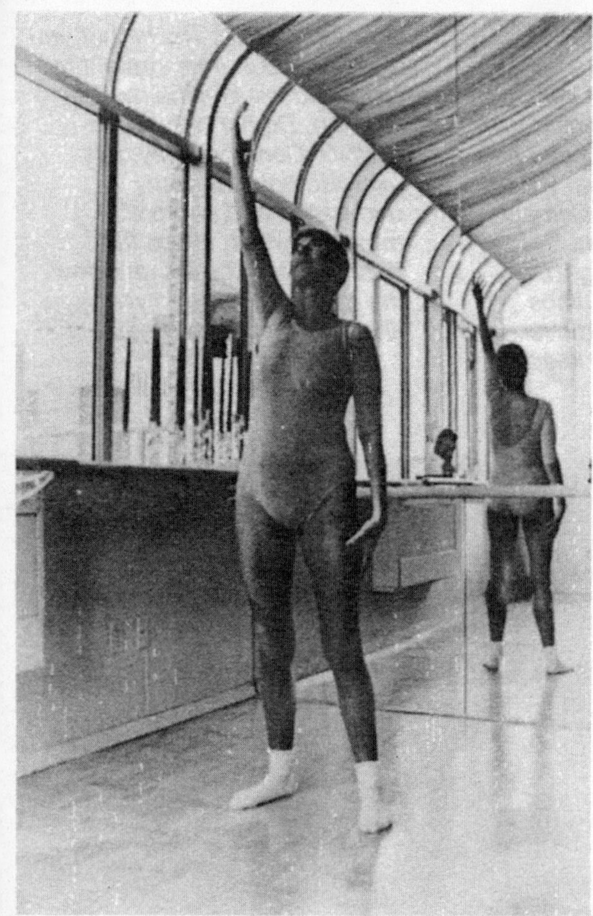

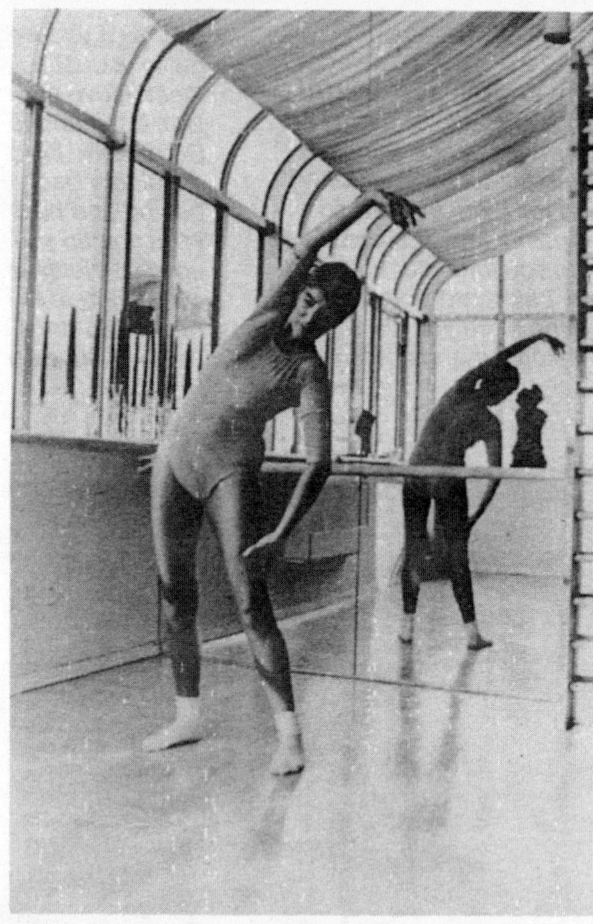

WAIST STRETCH *Stand with feet about a foot apart and arms at your sides. Raise your right arm high over your head and place your left hand on the outside of your left leg. Stretch your right arm and the right side of your body upward, straightening your right elbow. Reach your right arm about 2 inches higher than you think you can. Do not arch your back. Tighten your behind and tip your pelvis upward. Hold position.* ▲

Stretch your right arm up and over to the left side, bending your left elbow as you lean. Keep reaching over your head with your right arm, keeping it straight to stretch your underarm and the back of your shoulders. Reach over your head as though you are trying to touch something on a table at your left side with your right hand. Soon you will be stretching so far that you will be reaching for something on the floor. Keep your pelvis tilted forward and your behind tucked and tight at all times to stretch the spine. From that point, reach over a half inch more, gently moving up and down, a half inch each way, 100 times. Do not bounce or throw your hip out to the side. Hips and pelvis never leave their starting positions. Do not allow your left elbow to slip to the back or to the front. To change sides, gently reach forward with your right arm, bending your body from the waist to the front. Keep your left hand on your left leg and turn your entire upper body to the right, gently returning to a standing position. Put your right hand on your right leg and raise your left arm high over your head. Proceed from there, repeating 100 times in each direction. Done properly, this waist stretch will stretch your underarms, the backs of your shoulders, and your waist and spine. It's essential to learn to do this properly because as your hips become smaller, you have to work harder to keep your waist looking small. ▲

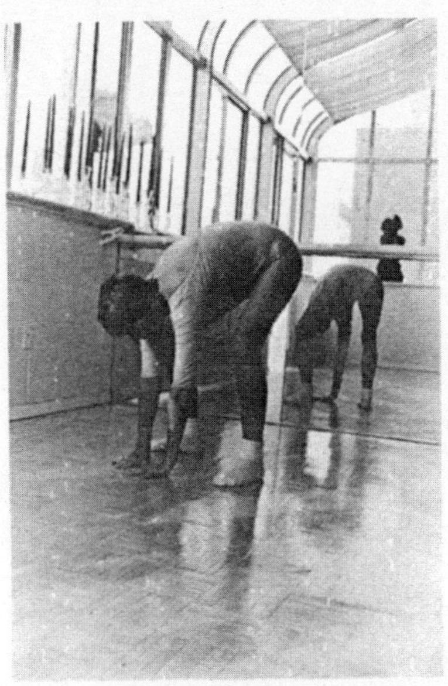

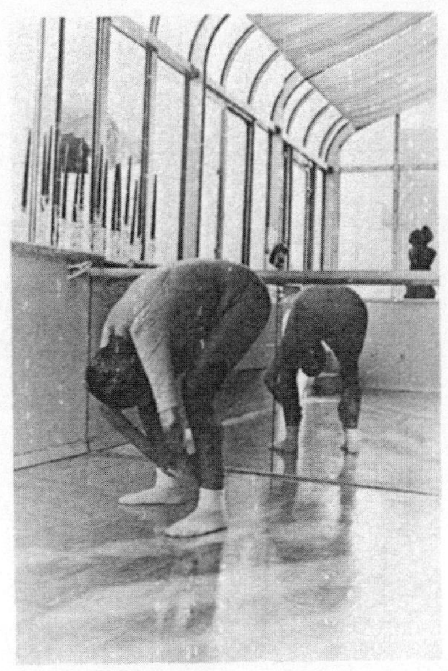

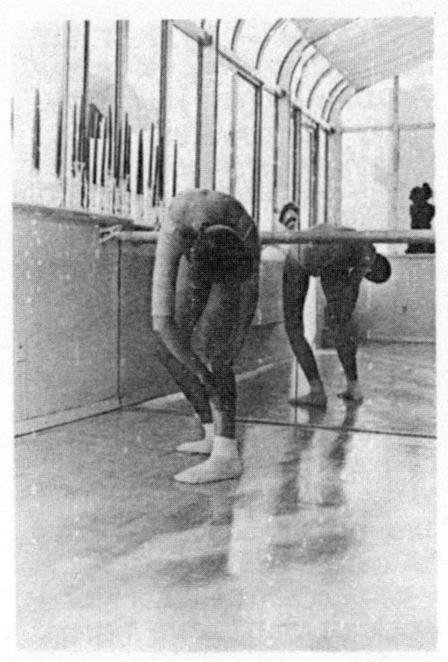

HAMSTRING STRETCH *This is a classic, though controversial, stretching exercise. Some experts advise people with back trouble to avoid it, and others recommend it. I, with my history of back problems, do it with no difficulty. Similarly, my students who have back problems report that their backs feel wonderful once they learn it correctly. From a standing position—the basic starting position—bend forward from the waist with your arms out in front of you. Keep knees bent. Gently touch your palms to the floor, if you can. Pat could not do this at first. However, after only three classes, she was able to. Never lock your knees. If you are not* stretched *enough to touch the floor with ease, bend your knees, as Pat is doing in the pictures. Although she was already able to straighten her legs while touching the floor, I felt it essential to show you how beginners start. All I ask is that you do what you can.* ▲

Gently grasp the insides of your legs, as low as you can, with your hands. Keep your body relaxed, shoulders rounded, and head tucked under. Bend your elbows outward to stretch between your shoulder blades. Gently move your torso a half inch, or as close to that as you can, between your legs. Do not bounce. *Relax your neck. Do 20.* ▲

Do not *come back up. Move your left hand behind the left calf and bring your right arm over, clasping your left leg just below your left hand, above your left ankle. Bend your elbows out like a duck's wings. Tuck your head between your left leg and right arm, as though you were trying to look behind you. Stretch as far as you can without straining, then relax. Count to 20.* Without standing up, *change to your right side, gently and slowly moving to that side, and repeat for 20 counts. Return both hands to the floor in front of you without forcing and arch your back upward like a cat, slowly straightening one vertebra at a time, until you are standing erect. This hamstring stretch also gives your calves, waist, lower back, and the muscles between your shoulder blades a good workout.* Remember: *Practice keeping your knees relaxed, not locked, throughout the exercise or you are inviting damage to your knee-joint complexes. The more stretched your hamstrings become, the more you will be able to straighten your legs.* ▲

NECK EXERCISE #1 *From the initial stance, slowly lower your head, chin to chest. Relax your shoulders. Tighten your behind and tip your pelvis upward. Tighten your stomach as you stretch your neck upward.* ▶

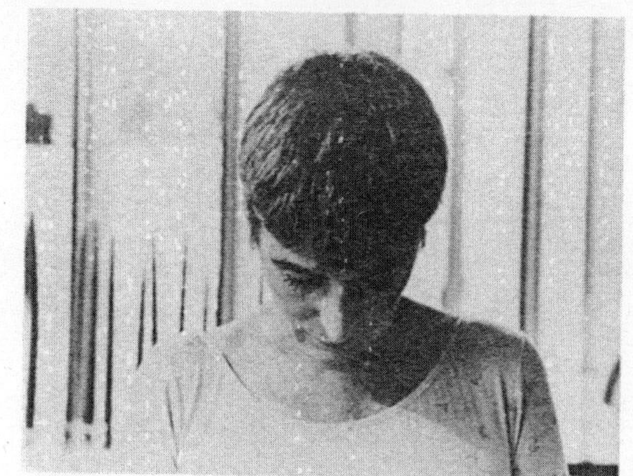

Slowly and smoothly roll your head to one side, lifting your chin as far as you can toward the ceiling. Keep your shoulders relaxed and your behind tight. Remember to make all movements extremely gently. Your neck is a delicate construction of bone and tissue that can be damaged by hard or jerky movements. Let your shoulders drop toward the floor. This is a common mistake—tensing the shoulders and holding them up. Still moving slowly and gently, roll your head to the opposite side, lifting your chin as far as you can to that side. Do 5 in each direction. ▶

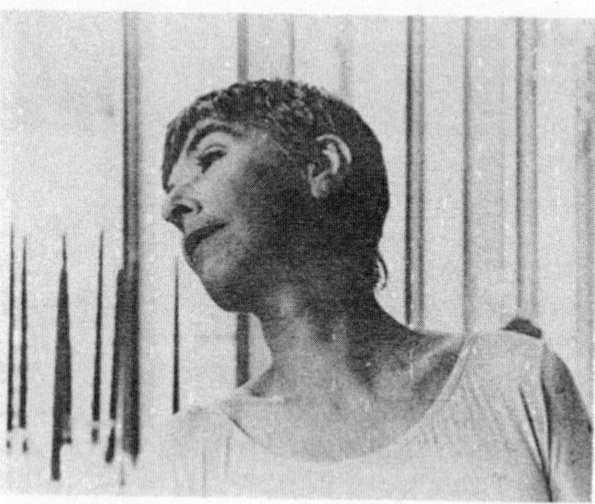

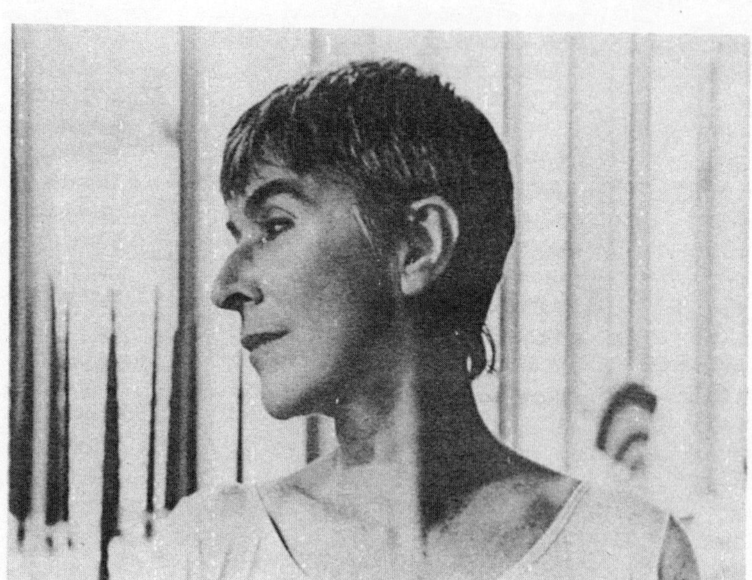

NECK EXERCISE #2 *As in the preceding exercise, this is for pure relaxation while loosening the neck and shoulders. Stand straight, tummy tight and behind and pelvis tipped forward and up. Relax your shoulders and arms and stretch your body upward. Hold your head and neck as high as you can. Then, as slowly as you can, move your head to one side without moving your body or shoulders. Pretend you are trying to look behind you without moving anything but your head. Hold for a slow count of 5 and gently move your head to the other direction. Do 5 in each direction.* ▲

CHAPTER EIGHT

For the Stomach

At first glance, these look like many other stomach exercises you have seen in magazines and books. However, you will find that they are very different indeed.

They are not sit-ups, nor are they backward rolls. They are precise, concentrated movements that contract and release the entire network of muscles that lace across the stomach from breast to pubis. The effect is so powerful that it benefits the body all the way to the chin in sixteen very specific ways. The following exercises:

- Tighten all four sections of the abdominal muscles, from breastbone to crotch.
- Release tension in the back of the neck.
- Lengthen the neck.
- Release tension across the shoulder blades.
- Expand breathing capacity by expanding the chest.
- Lift the breasts by working the pectoral muscles.
- Eliminate double chins.
- Release tension and stretch the *entire* back, including the sacrum.
- Usually relieve menstrual cramping for most women who experience this.
- Benefit the cardiovascular system.
- Usually regulate bowel movements for most people with irregularity and diarrhea.
- Increase body awareness.
- Teach coordination.
- Enable you to relax.
- Decrease appetite.
- Increase your sexual drive—like it or not!

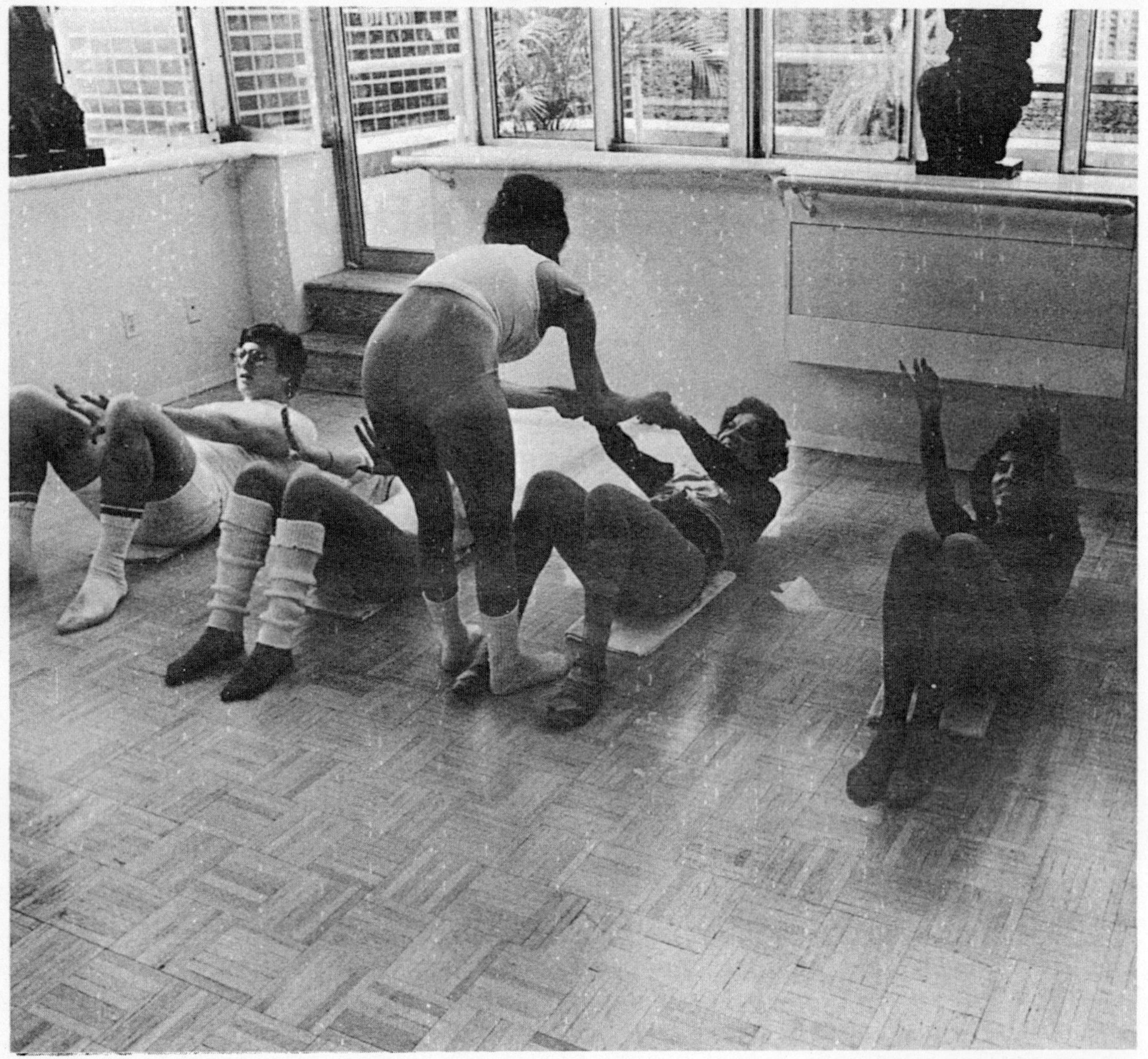

These powerful exercises are not simple to do. Often, I pass among my students and lend a hand where I am needed, or correct students who are not executing the movements properly or safely. It is important that you move your head, shoulders, and arms as one unit, without rocking your body back and forth. ▲

Each one of these exercises does all this. As with all the exercises you will see here, they build stamina, endurance, and strength.

What makes them so special is that *you* have complete control over each movement. Regardless of the basic starting position, you determine when and how much you move. You control the movement, rather than letting the movement control you.

For most of us, once we reach a certain point in a backward roll, we no longer have control over how fast we roll our bodies back. Gravity takes over. When we do a series of sit-ups, we begin by pulling upright and easing down to the floor, never realizing that a sit-up involves, conservatively, 80 to 85 percent of the back muscles. Once we gather momentum, we yank our torsos to a sitting position and collapse back to the floor.

With this series, you won't find your body or even gravity taking over the activity. Once you have learned to position your body and move properly, you will be able to feel every contraction and every release of every muscle involved, regardless of how deep. This is because you learn to isolate your muscles and move only certain groups to achieve specific results.

The more you control your muscles, the more you will be able to tighten and trim your stomach. The abdominal muscles will form a taut resilient girdle that holds you flat and young-looking regardless of your age or sex. Even women who have had children experience a tightening that they won't get from aerobic dancing or yoga.

I know of no other exercise program that gives contractions as deep and powerful as these. That is why they work so well. I have had students who were extremely overweight when they started classes. Every one of them who stuck with me found positive, dramatic results from following these essential stomach exercises. Others who, once they were past their first trimesters, exercised through their pregnancies, felt fabulous for it. Every one of them reported easy deliveries and each was able to get her firm figure back much faster than her friends who did other exercises.

These exercises may feel a bit unusual at first. You may not feel the contractions in your stomach muscles at all because you are concentrating on the tension—the ache—in the back of your neck. Unless you are *really* tense, this disappears after your first hour; whatever tightness you may feel in the sides of your neck, gone after the second. By your third hour, you should feel no pain in any part of your neck. Then you will really get a sense of how strong the contractions in your stomach are.

Tension in the neck and upper body may also be felt between or across the shoulder blades after the first few hours. As you exercise, this tension is released and you acquire full movement in your shoulders and upper torso. (If this continues past the fourth hour, your body might be telling you to see your doctor about possible disc problems.)

The deeper the muscles work, the less you will be able to do. When your muscles become stronger at a deeper level, the more repetitions you will be able to do. When one layer of muscles have been completely worked, the layer below will take over.

If you have weak stomach muscles, the contractions will begin under your bustline. The stronger, more relaxed these muscles are, the higher you will be able to pull your shoulders and upper body, which will result in deeper, lower contractions of the stomach and abdomen.

I cannot remind you enough: Each movement you make is gentle, small. Move no more than half an inch in either direction where movement is called for. Your head, shoulders, and upper torso are a unit. Do not rock your body back and forth or tighten your behind. These are not exercises to be done with your head. Relax. You may find this difficult at first, but practice keeping your legs loosened and relaxed.

As your hips and thighs tighten and your upper stomach muscles become firm and flat, your lower abdomen may appear to be puffier than when you started. This is an illusion. After very few sessions, you will find that the muscles flatten right across your tummy and your hipbones will show.

Don't worry about your breathing. Exhale as you pull yourself up; otherwise, breathe naturally.

I start students out with one hundred of each exercise. As each section of muscle is strengthened, you may feel that you are starting all over again and can only do a fourth of what you did the class before, because your muscles are working more deeply. You have progressed to another level. Keep going. Soon you will be able to do the full number again.

Twenty-two-year-old Lisa is a transplanted Texan who came to New York to expand her career as an actress. She had had only three classes when these pictures were taken.

Note: Common mistakes at first are bouncing your head, only moving your arms, rocking your body back and forth, holding your breath, not relaxing your body, and tightening your behind.

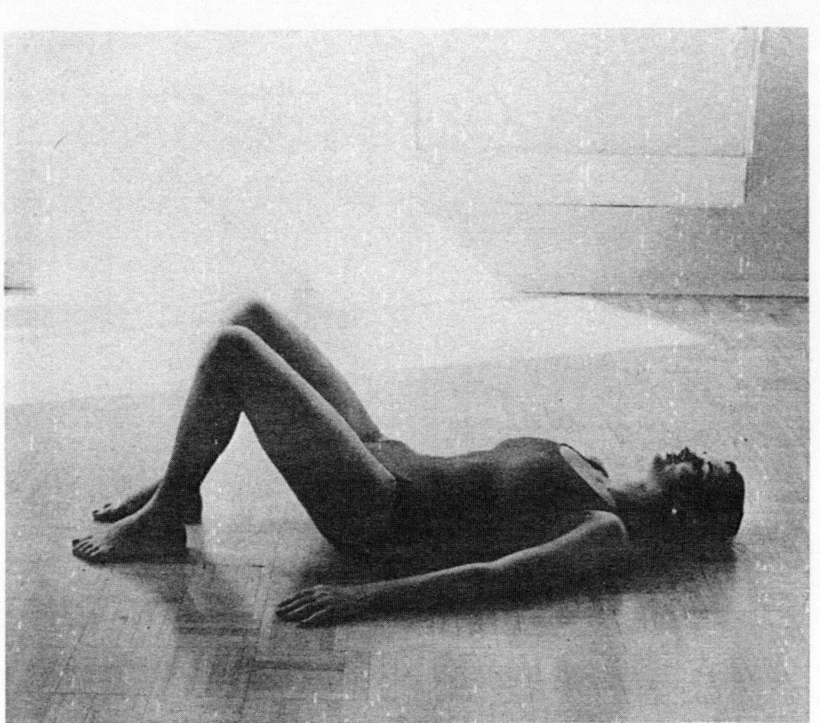

FOR THE STOMACH #1 *Lie on the floor, relaxing your entire body, with your arms at your sides and your knees up. Feet should be 3 to 5 inches apart. Push the small of your back into the floor.* ◄

With your head and shoulders still on the floor, firmly grab hold of your inner thighs and raise your elbows up and out to each side to stretch between shoulder blades. Don't be gentle—grab. ►

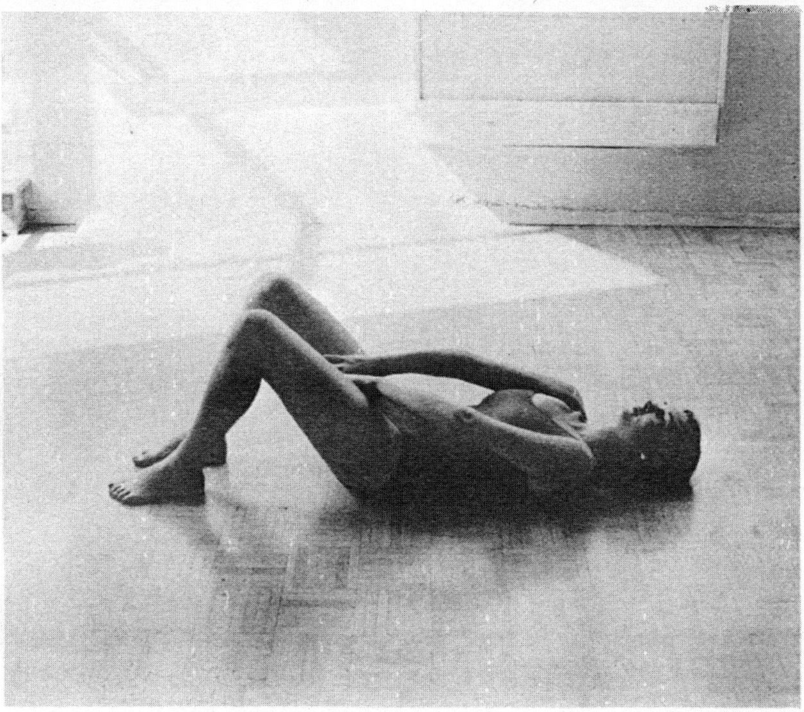

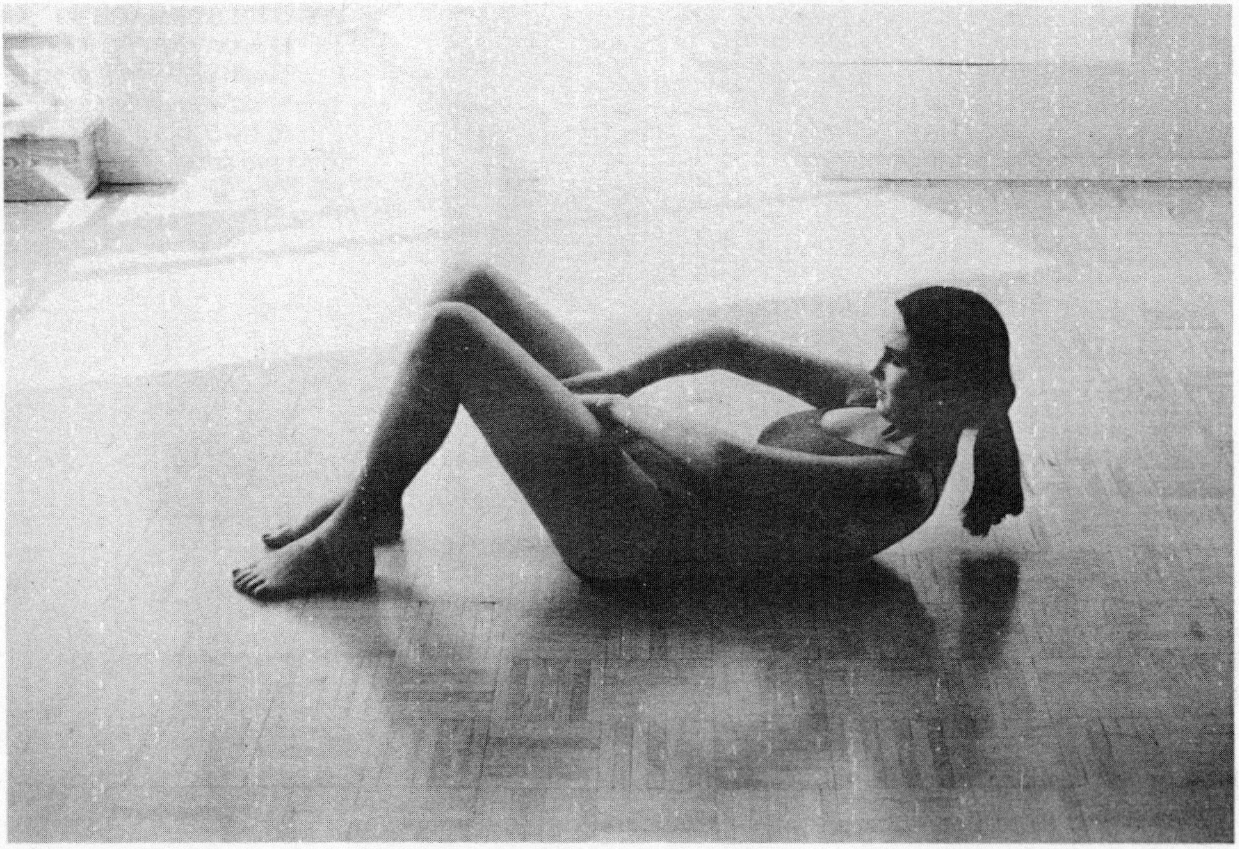

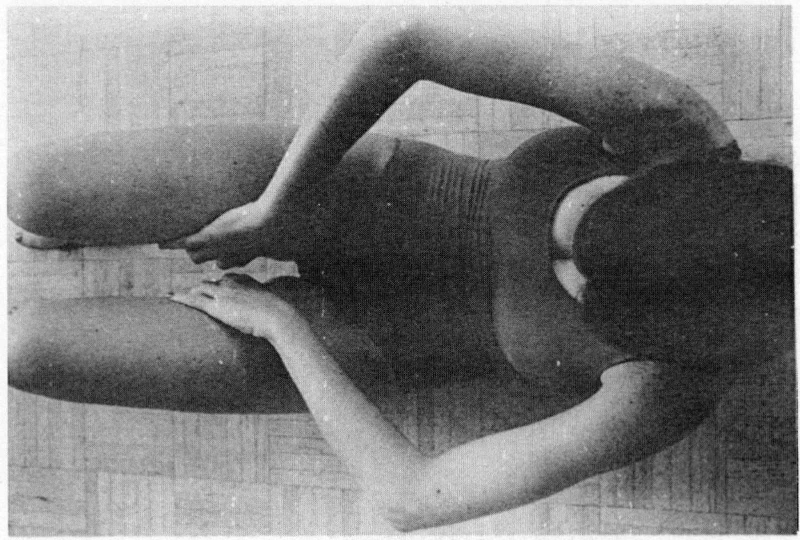

Pulling on your inner thighs, pull your head and shoulders off the floor, rounding upward from under the bust. The small of your back should still be pushed into the floor. ▲

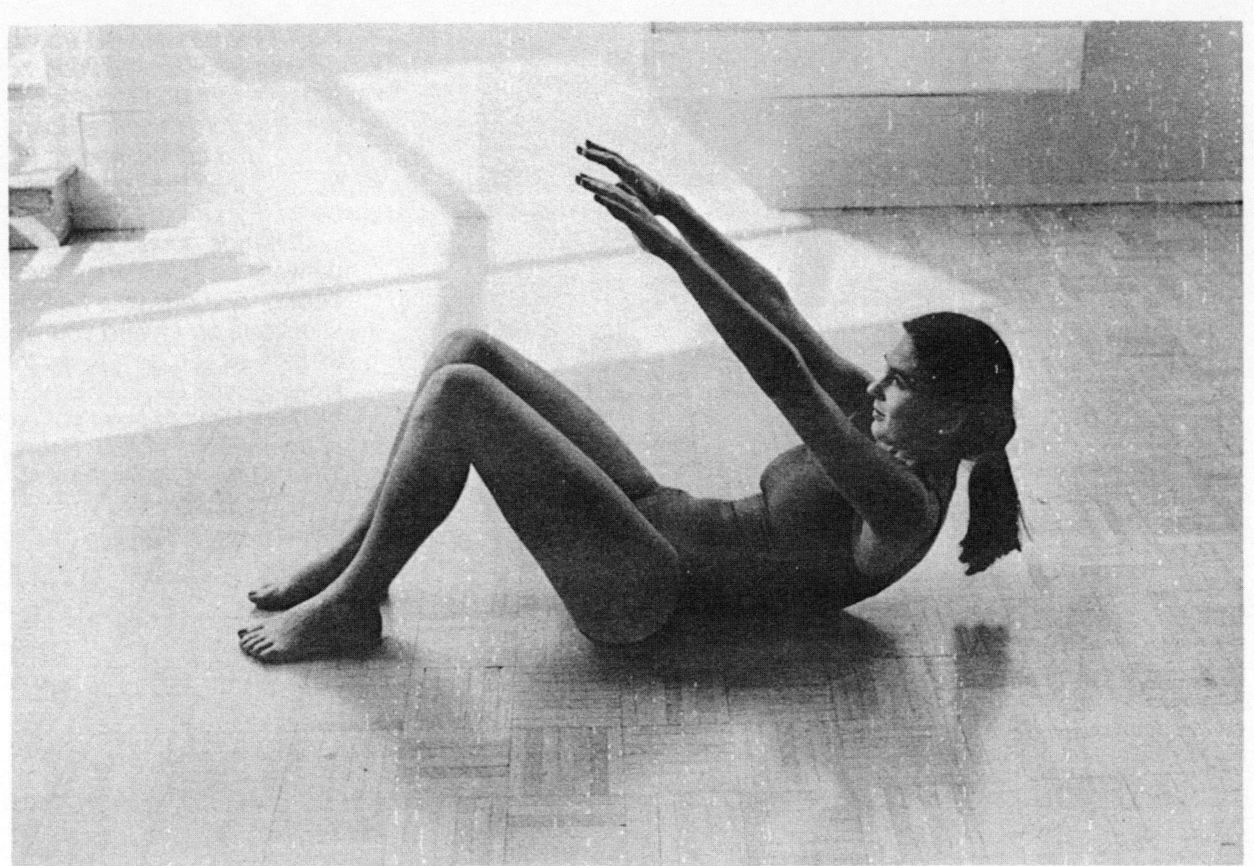

Release hands from inner thighs and raise arms parallel with your thighs and knees. Do not let your head and shoulders fall back to the floor. From that position, lift your arms, shoulders, and head as one unit a half inch further from the floor. Only the top *of your body moves. Move slowly back a half inch, again using only the top part of your body. Move upper torso back and forth, in* triple *slow motion, a half inch in each direction; do this 2 more times than you think you can. Then rest. Aim for 75 at your first class, but stop when you feel you must. When you feel that you can do no more, gently let your body roll down to the floor, vertebra by vertebra, and take a breather. Then, repeating each step from the beginning, come back up and continue.* Do not rock back and forth. *Keep behind still. If you feel this in the back of your neck at first, this is natural. You are beginning to loosen up stored tension. If it* really *hurts, clasp your hands behind your head, just above your neck, and let your head rest in the palms of your hands. Take your elbows out to the sides as far as you can.* ▲

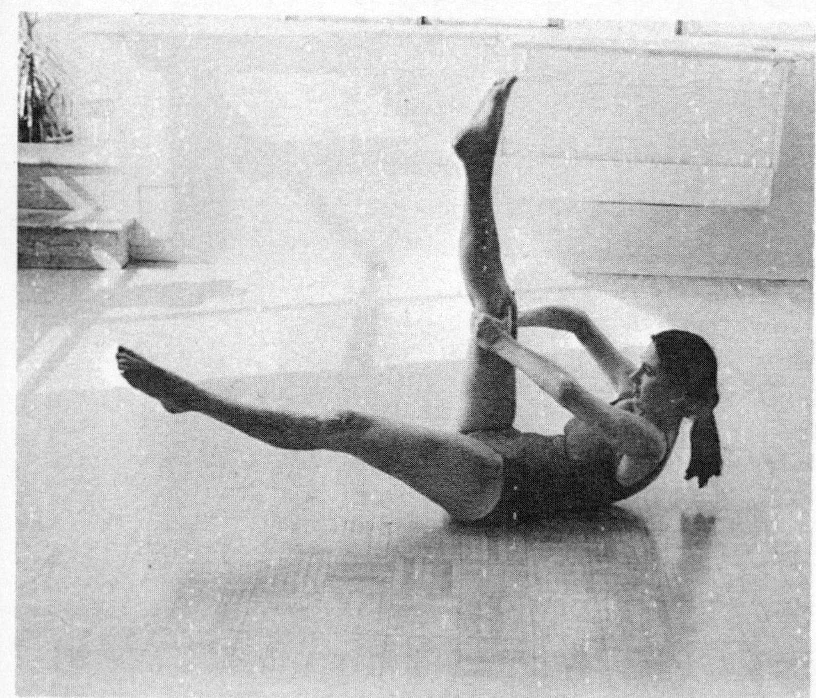

FOR THE STOMACH #2 *Lie on your back on the floor, both legs straight and together. From that position, raise the right leg toward the ceiling and lift left leg a foot off the floor. Grab the back of your right knee with both hands, round your elbows outward and up toward the ceiling, and pull your head and shoulders up toward your knee as high as you can. Keep the small of your back pressed into the floor. Do not point your toes or tighten legs at first. Relax. Think of them as feathers.* ◄

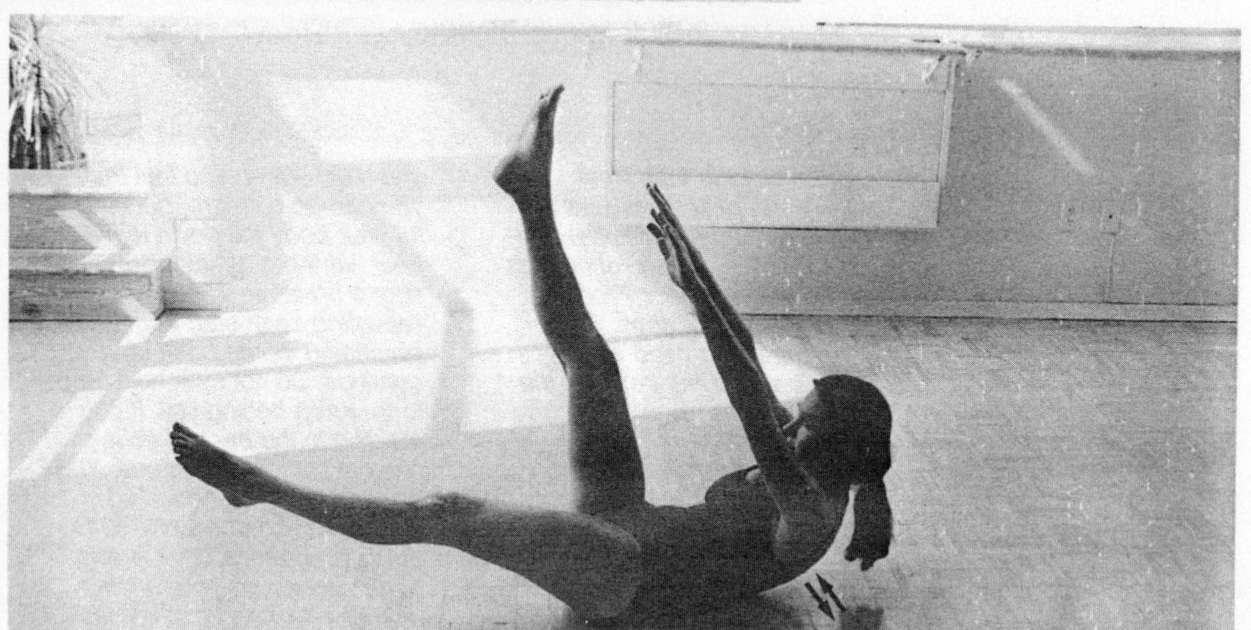

When you feel you can't bring your head and shoulders any higher, let go of your raised knee and stretch arms toward your right foot. Move your upper torso back and forth a half inch in triple slow motion. Do 100 times with each leg raised, taking breathers when necessary. If you have average stomach muscles, you will only be able to move up and down a half inch. Keep your back pressed into the floor. The important thing about this exercise is not to see how high you can move your chest but how rounded you can curl your upper body. If you feel your lower back working for this exercise, either rest your left leg on the floor or put your left foot on the floor and bend your knee upward. Keep your raised leg high to discourage your lower back muscles from assisting your abdominals. When your stomach muscles are strong enough, you can lower your legs as low as you wish. If you feel a burning sensation between your shoulder blades, nine times out of ten it simply means that your muscles are tight and are beginning to loosen up. ▲

Note: When you are lying on your back, always bend your knees and then straighten your legs upward; otherwise, you will exert pressure on your lower back.

FOR THE STOMACH #3 *Lie on the floor with both legs in the air. Grab the outer thighs with your hands and, rounding your shoulders and elbows out, pull your head and shoulders up toward your knees. Pull as high as you can, with your lower back pushed into the floor.* ▸

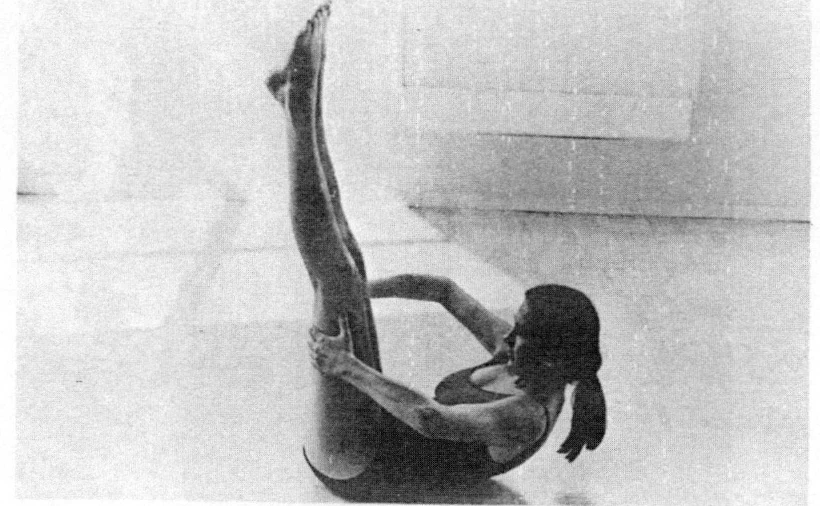

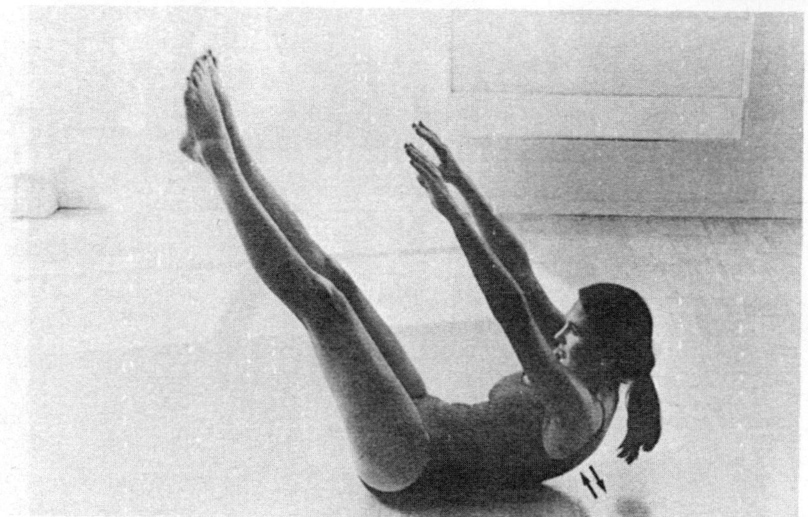

Let go of your legs and stretch hands and arms toward your toes. Do not let your head and shoulders fall back to the floor. Gently lift the top of your body up and down a half inch to an inch for a count of 100. Again, keep your legs relaxed. If you have weak legs, you can bend your knees. At first, you will probably not be able to let your legs go down as far as Lisa can. Your legs will be up higher. ◂

For People Who Find It Difficult to Keep Their Legs Up *Rest your feet on a wall, as shown, again pulling yourself up on your outer thighs. Let go and stretch your hands toward your feet. Gently move up and down. Keep your knees bent to avoid pressure on your legs. When you are strong enough to take your legs off the wall, they should feel like feathers.* ▸

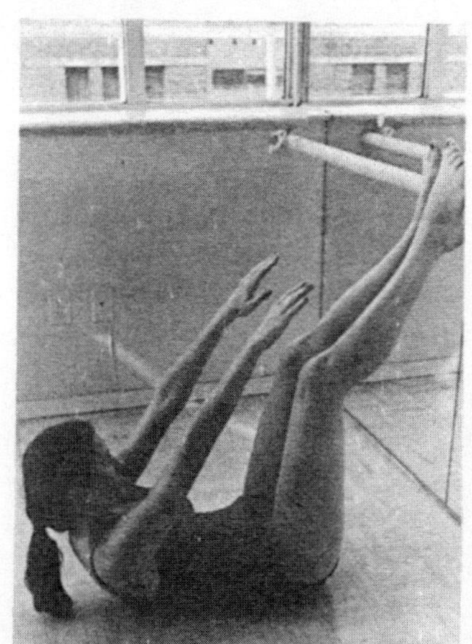

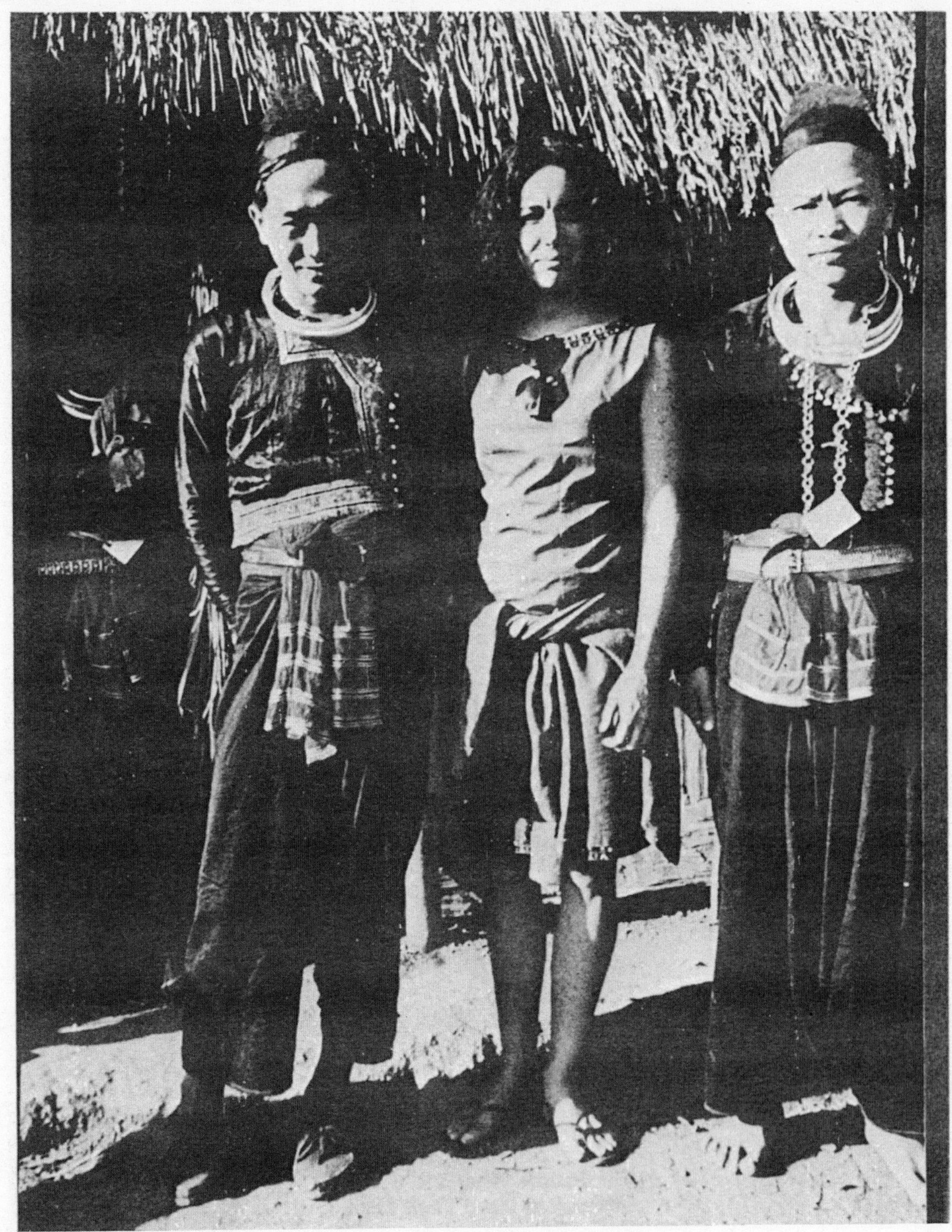

My stomach was distended from malnutrition and, though I weighed only about 80 pounds, I was so bloated that I looked larger than I am now. (I wore a Size 6 dress then. Today, I fluctuate between 100 and 105 pounds, but my body is so tight I wear a Size 2.) My mother showed this photo, taken among a Laotian mountain tribe, for several months before she recognized me by the crease in my brow. My body had deteriorated so much that I had no muscle tone and no strength. Still in my twenties, I looked and felt 120! ▲

CHAPTER NINE

For the Legs

I tell my students that we all can have long, thin, tight-looking legs like Cyd Charisse. It's all in the exercises we do.

The legs are the one part of a woman's body that can be overdeveloped in a very short time. All it takes is certain body movements—too much contraction, the use of weights, even the wrong exercises. In a matter of days, thighs and calves can become hard and mannishly muscular. Or, they can become long looking and thin.

I know this firsthand. A nurse asked if she might use two-and-a-half-pound ankle weights so that the exercises for the hips and behind might work faster. Against my better judgment, I decided to give them a try. We both questioned how this might affect the knees and hip joints, but I went ahead with the experiment. In a total of thirty minutes of exercise over a three-day period, my knees became terribly swollen and painful. My right hip hurt so much that I had to use a hot, moist heating pad to relieve the ache. If that wasn't bad enough, varicose veins appeared behind my knees and on the sides. I had aggravated my knee problems, which I had not experienced in years. My knees were so distorted, and legs larger, from this small amount of weight work, that twice I had to cancel photography sessions for this book. I feared that my knees might never return to their better shape.

Needless to say, my students who witnessed this are nervous about weights now—especially when they saw how bad my knees looked! It took at least a month for all the swelling to go down.

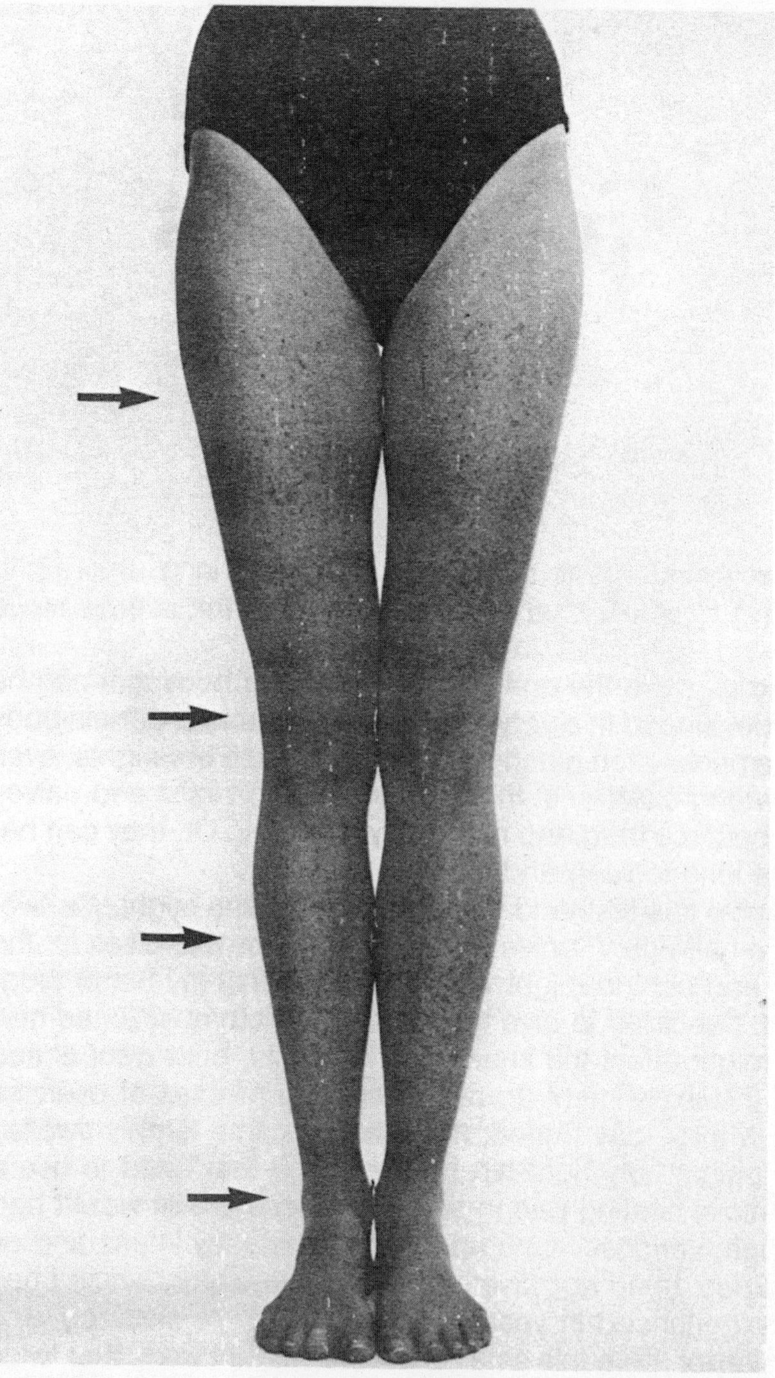

When I was a child, I saw a large photograph in Life *magazine of what was supposed to be "The Perfect Legs." Four 50-cent pieces were placed between the model's legs at the four places where a woman's legs should touch: thighs, knees, calves, and ankles. I never forgot that image and have strived to achieve that look through the years. Now, at age forty-five, I can honestly say that I have not merely acquired the look in the magazine, I have surpassed it. Through the proper stretching and contractions, I have rid myself of the knotty calf muscles that so many ballet dancers get.* ▲

A man, on the other hand, could double the work that I did with weights, and his legs would generally look better for doing it.

The exercises I teach do not build bulk or increase your thighs and cause hamstring bulge. They do just enough to create a light, firm, long look without hulking, protruding muscles. We short women must be especially careful about becoming too muscular because, on us, bulky muscles make our legs look wide and shorter than they already are. As a result, our *bodies* look stubby and ugly.

To some extent, these leg exercises come from my ballet training—*pliés* and *barre* work, in particular—yet they are designed to care for the delicate mechanisms of the knees, hips, and ankles.

I must caution anyone who has had knee problems to see their doctor before attempting these, or any other, exercises that use the legs. Out of hundreds of students who have come to me with bad knees, all but one experienced relief. The one who did not get noticeably better did admit that although she had not experienced any *improvement* while doing the exercises, she had not gotten any worse. She then admitted that when she stopped doing the exercises altogether, her pain increased.

I can't remind you enough: Do what you can. Don't force your leg higher than it can easily reach. *Never* jerk your body. Abrupt movement is a primary cause of injury, no matter what kind of exercise you do. Don't expect to move and look like a prima ballerina—or even like Katie, my student who is demonstrating these exercises for you—the first time you try them. At first, you will find it impossible to keep your shoulders erect and your behind tight at the same time. You may also feel like you are clinging to the *barre* for dear life. Don't worry. As you become stronger, all this will become much easier.

Katie, a thirty-year-old mother with a small child, had completed three classes at the time of our pictures. She did the exercises as well as her body allowed at that time.

Note: I teach the first two exercises for the legs with the heels together, balancing on the balls of the feet. Katie, however, found it more comfortable to do them with her heels slightly apart. I have found that with the heels together you get more relief from pressure on the knees, since the body's weight is centered over the heels instead of through the knees. Also, with heels together, the inner thighs work more, taking pressure off the knees. At first, if you are uncomfortable, like Katie, in that position, you may feel free to take them apart to achieve a balanced stance. The exercises will still work.

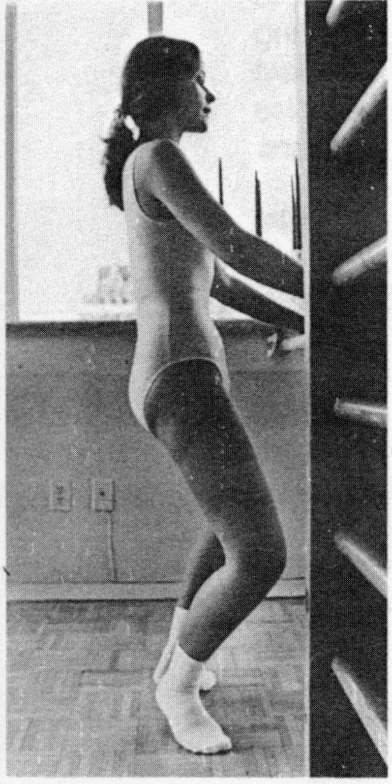

FOR THE LEGS #1 *Gently clasp the back of a sturdy chair or sofa, or even the kitchen counter, with both hands at shoulder width. Stand on the balls of your feet, feet and knees facing out to the sides, heels together. Keep your back erect if you can, and shoulders relaxed and even. Lift your head high, as if you were a prima ballerina.* ▲

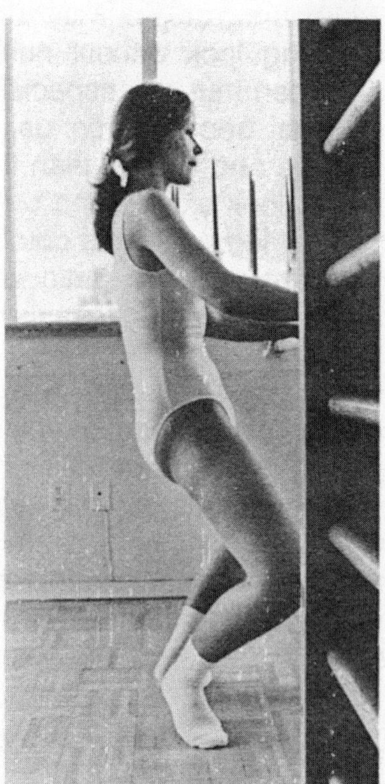

Tighten your behind and tip your pelvis up as high as you can. Return your pelvis to the straight starting position. Lower your body an inch, still keeping heels together and balancing on toes. Remember: *Do not stick out your behind. That puts pressure on the lower back.* ▲

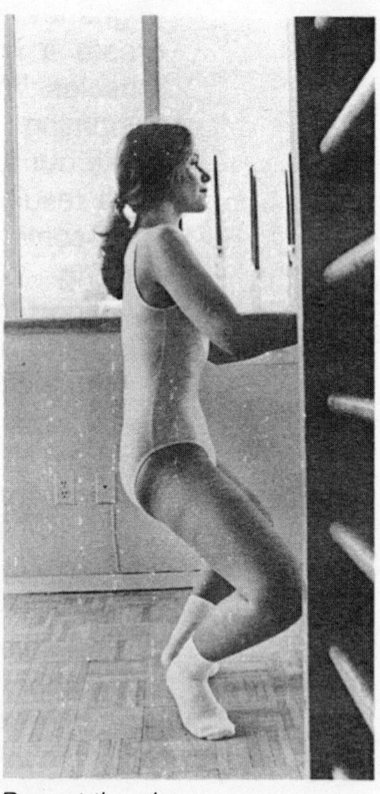

Repeat the above process, tipping your pelvis forward and moving it back, then lowering your body another inch. Do combination again lowering 1 inch more. Shoulders should be as even as you can keep them and, if you have to hold onto the barre tightly, that's all right. Reverse the process until you have returned to your middle position. Do this combination 2 more times. When your legs are strong enough, you will be able to stand up straight. ▲

Note: *Each combination of moving the pelvis up and back and lowering your body counts as 1 movement.*

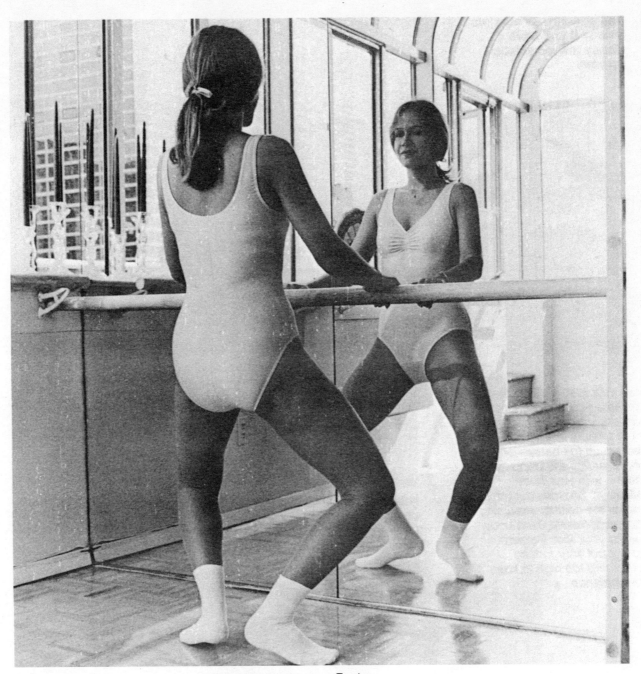

FOR THE LEGS #2 *Facing the* barre, *hold on with both hands at shoulder width. Go up on the balls of your feet, knees and feet facing outward, heels together. Keep your back straight, if possible. Hold your head high. Lower your body 3 inches* and no more. *Do not drop your heels. Keep your body straight. Go back to your original position and repeat for a total of 10 times.* ▲

Do not attempt the next two exercises if you have a tendency toward sciatica syndrome.

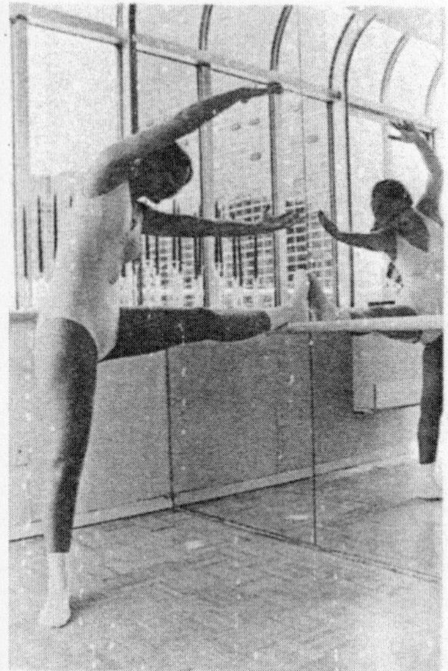

FOR THE LEGS #3 Note: *Do not force your leg higher than it can easily reach.* See stretch #1 in Chapter 12. *Put your left heel up on the* barre*—or whatever you are using as a* barre*—with your body sideways. Stretch your arms up toward the ceiling, stretching your abdominals. Turn body toward your foot.* Remember: *Do not put your foot on something too high to keep your balance.* ▲

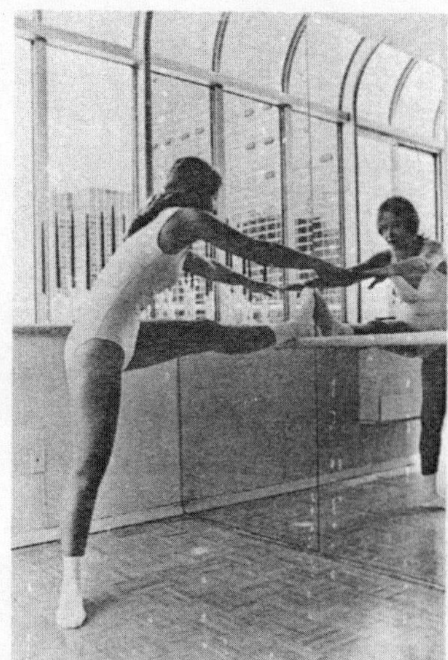

With arms outstretched, continue to lean your torso over your leg. Keep back stretched toward your raised foot. Beware that you do not lock your knees. ▲

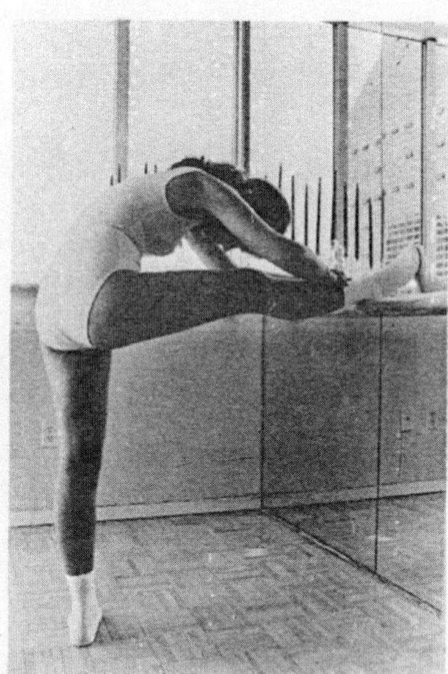

Rest your hands across the shin of your raised leg, as close to your foot as you can comfortably reach. Gently move your torso a quarter of an inch toward your knee and back. Do 50. If you already feel a strong stretch, do not move. Simply hold that stretched position for a count of 50. Keep your entire body relaxed. Repeat with other leg. Do not force knee down with your hands. *Don't worry if you can't straighten your raised leg. Bending like this is fine. Your leg will straighten when it is ready. It does not need your assistance.* ▲

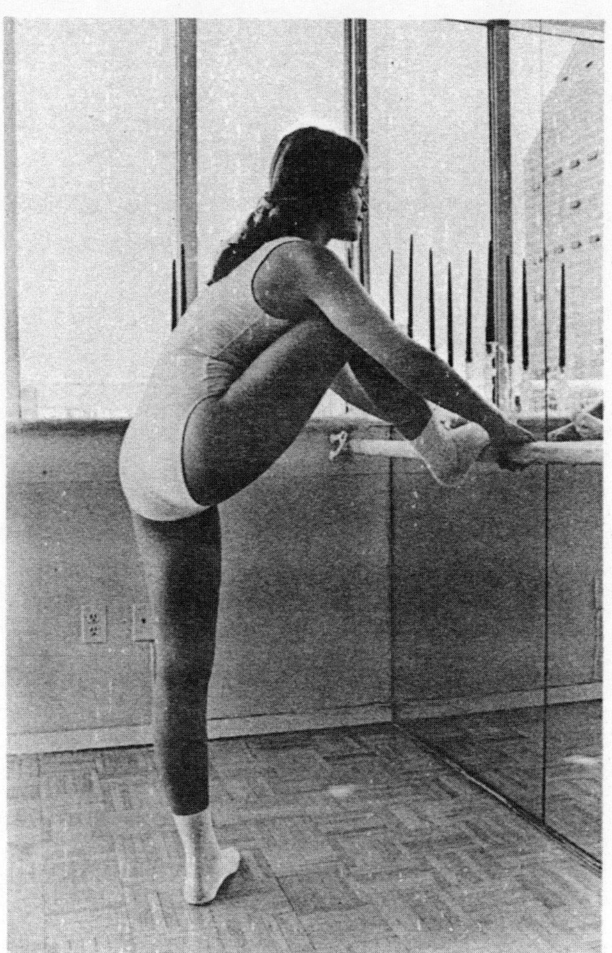

FOR THE LEGS #4 *Raise your right leg to the* barre, *placing the arch on the* barre. *Hold the* barre *with your hands on both sides of the foot, bending the right knee. Scoot forward with your left foot from 1 to 5 inches.* ▲

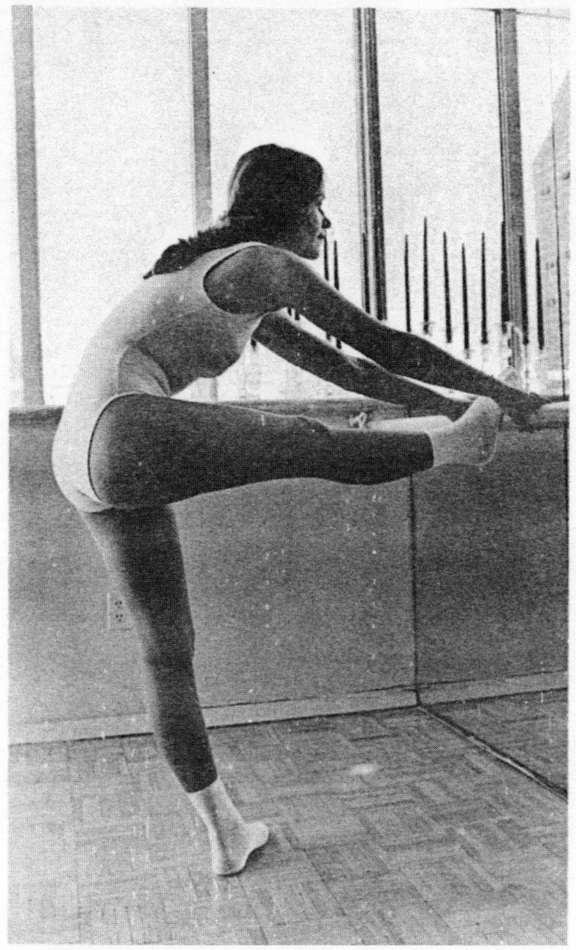

Straighten your raised leg as far as possible without pulling on the barre *with your hands. You should only use the* barre *for balance. Do not lock your knees on either leg, and do not force your raised leg to straighten. When your hamstrings are ready, you will be able to do this with ease. Hold for a count of 50. Repeat on the other side.* ▲

CHAPTER TEN

For the Behind and Hips

I had to fight the temptation to call this chapter "Gone with the Goosh" because that is exactly what happens when you do these exercises.

I've never kept a written record of the complaints my new students have about their bodies, but if I did, nine out of ten would be about their hips and behinds. You will be surprised at how conscious of your own behind and hips you become once you begin these exercises. I know of one student who missed a bus because she had become so preoccupied with studying the reflection of her pretty new shape in a nearby window.

I continually warn students not to invest money in expensive clothes for the time being. When their hips start pulling in and their behinds move in and up, their inner thighs also become smaller. In short, their whole proportion changes. Turn back to the Portfolio of Proof (Chapter 4) if you have any doubts. When your body changes shape like this, the cut of your slacks must change as well.

Most of the popular pants designed for American women are cut to cover the wide hips and pear-shaped spread that is so prevalent today. Once you have gotten your slim, tight hips and high, young-looking behind, you will find that your favorite pants' label is now your *former* favorite. You will have a grand time trying on different styles of clothes and noticing your body's wonderful new curves.

Even my male students (some in their early twenties) are excited by the changes in their derrières. They will *get fast* results from these exercises, but it won't look as dramatic as

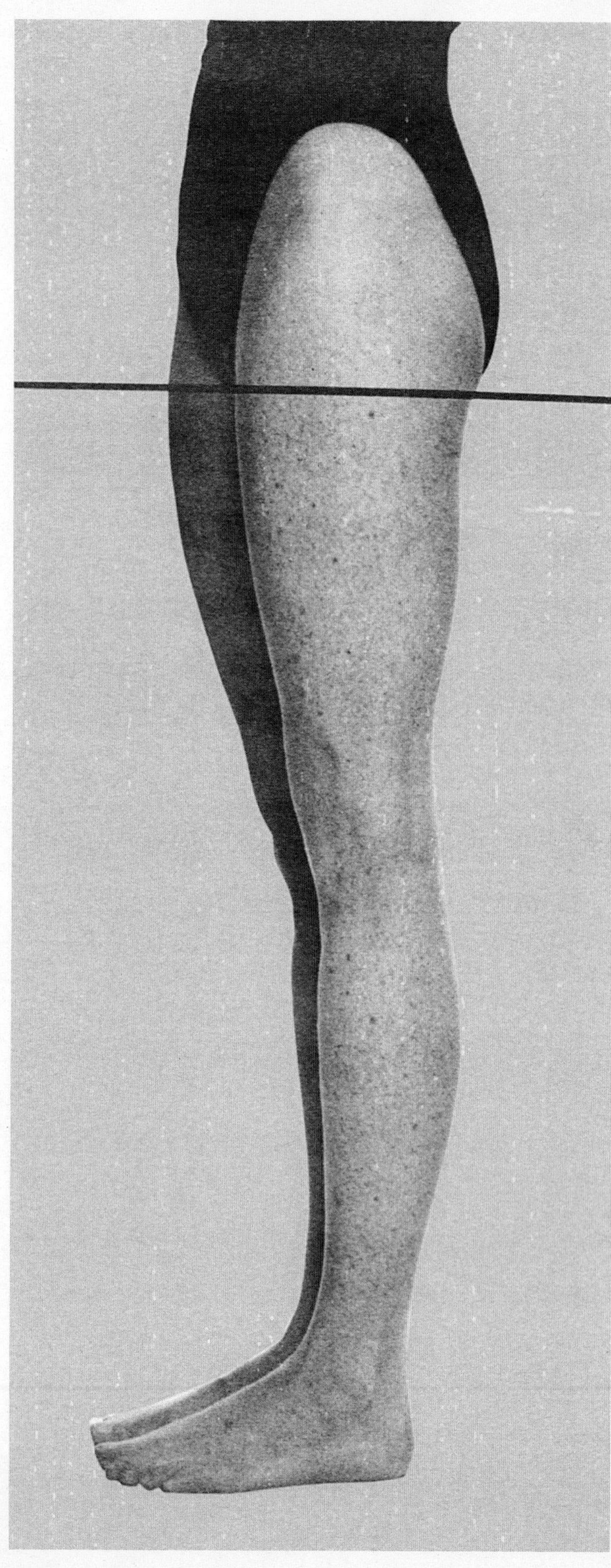

This is the perfect bottom line—drawn front to back, level from the pubic bone to the rear. It runs just below the hip joints, highlighting both hips and behind. See how my behind is firm and round? It's even higher *than the line. This is what you see people comparing in the mirrors when they think no one is looking. If your behind drops below this imaginary line in back, you know you have to get to work on tightening the muscles and lifting everything, as I have done.* ◄

it does for women, yet they feel it just the same.

These exercises work because they concentrate on the very muscles you must tighten to have thin thighs and a well-shaped behind. I see no reason to spend time doing one set of exercises for the behind and another for the hips when this one group of movements will:

- Resculpt the behind.
- Round and lift the buttocks.
- Restore firmness.
- Erase saddlebags.
- Tighten inner thighs.
- Develop the behind without harming the lower back.
- Stretch the spine.

In addition, these exercises allow you to use your arms and upper back just enough to make them beautiful. You will find that none of the movements I teach will add bulk to your arms and shoulders. Instead, they tighten to give you that youthful, firm look. It only seems like magic.

New students actually laugh at their legs in disbelief when they find that they are unable to lift them off the floor. They tell me there's no way they can move them back and forth. I remind them to talk sweetly to their muscles and to keep trying. Keep concentrating. You'll be able to do it sooner or later.

If you have positioned your body correctly, with your hip rolled forward and your pelvis tipped up to the front, you may have some difficulty in coordinating these tiny little movements. Once you have taught your body to accept this as a natural position, your movements will become easy and your muscles will respond automatically for you.

I have seen long lists of exercises that are supposed to decrease the size of the buttocks—jogging, aerobic dancing, swimming, weights—the works. They may do some good if you are sixteen, but once your body has begun to slip, there is no way that running around a track or jerking your body about to disco music can halt the ravages of time. You need drastic measures: *deep* contractions. Just tightening and releasing your behind muscles is not enough. It is merely preparation for exercise and nothing more.

Soon you will see a true sign of fitness—a slight hollow along the sides of your hips as your thighs and behind are made tighter. Look at a picture of a dancer or gymnast. This little dent is at the juncture of the hip and thigh muscles. When both sets are taut and firm there is a lovely definition that sets them off.

These exercises are so special I have used two models, with two very different body types, to demonstrate how to do them. Lane, the little blonde, is my twenty-one-year-old niece. Like me, she has scoliosis and swayback and, as a child, had the same problems with her legs and feet as I did. I had shown her the exercises several years ago. She only did them when her back hurt, but she never did the program seriously until she visited me in New York. She took only two classes and was photographed for the book!

Shelly is in her forties. This mother of a teenage daughter is one of those rare people who was *born* with a nice, tight body. However, one morning in her late thirties, Shelly woke up and saw nothing but goosh . . . almost overnight. Since then, she has exercised with me on and off for a year.

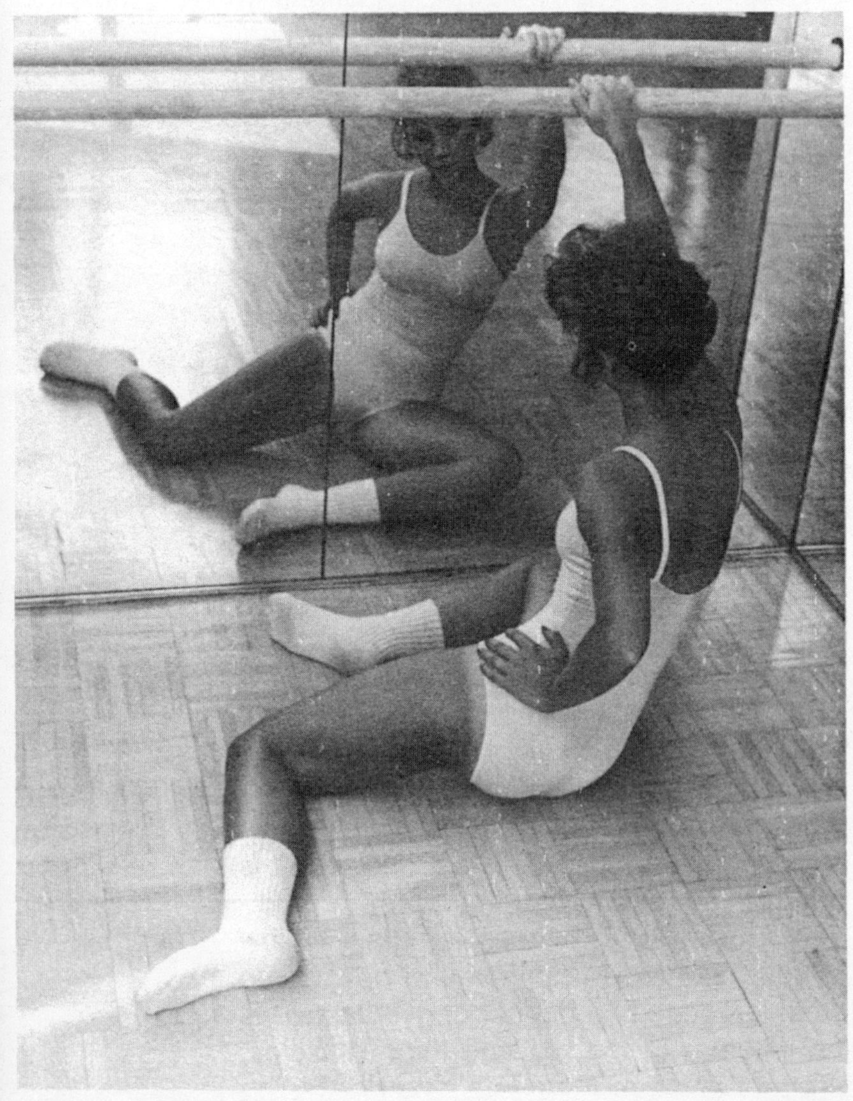

Note: *The mistake everyone makes at first is the failure to tighten behind muscles and curl pelvis up, keep arms straight, hips even, back erect, and stomach in. Do not arch back or stick behind out.* ◄

FOR THE BEHIND AND HIPS

#1 *Facing the* barre, *sit on the right side of your derrière. Right leg is positioned in front of you, bent at the knee, so that the right heel is even with your crotch, 8 or 10 inches from your body. The left leg is extended to the left, bent backward at the knee. The knee is even with the left hip and the left foot is behind you and relaxed. Hold* barre *with your right hand and rest left hand on left hip to ease it forward. Roll the left hip forward, pointing your left knee into the floor. Your foot will start to come off the floor.* ◄

Without letting your hip roll back, put your left hand on the barre. *Try to tighten your behind and tip your pelvis up. Try to keep your back straight. At first you may lean over and hold on to the* barre *for dear life, but once your behind muscles learn to work and become stronger, you will merely use the* barre *for balance, if at all.* ▸

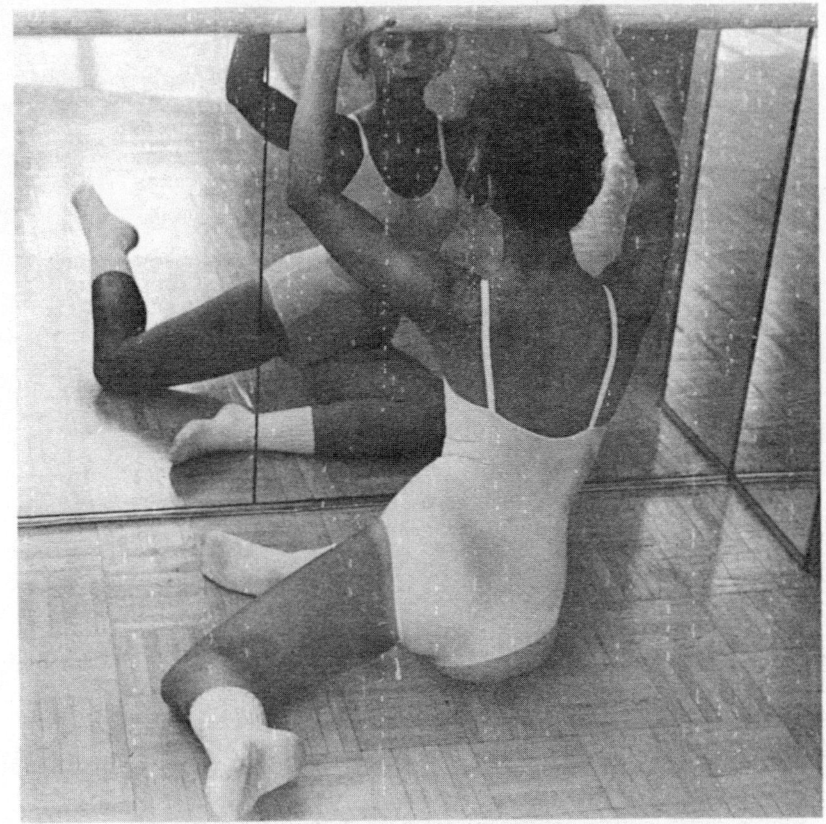

Lift left knee not more than 3 inches off the floor, keeping the knee turned to the floor and the foot up. Move raised leg back one-half inch, without letting your hip or pelvis change position. Slowly return your left knee one-half inch to its original position even with left hip. Gently move leg back and forth like this, 100 times on each side. I suggest that you do 20 on one side, switch, and do 20 on the other, back and forth. Work up to 100 on each side. If you feel too tired or are too uncomfortable to continue, take breathers. Do as many as you can. If you have raised your knee too high, you will throw your hip back and transfer the control to your front thigh muscles instead of letting your behind do the work. If you feel an ache going up your hip to your waist, either lean over to the opposite side, or switch sides to release it. There is nothing wrong. Your muscles are simply weak in the beginning. ▸

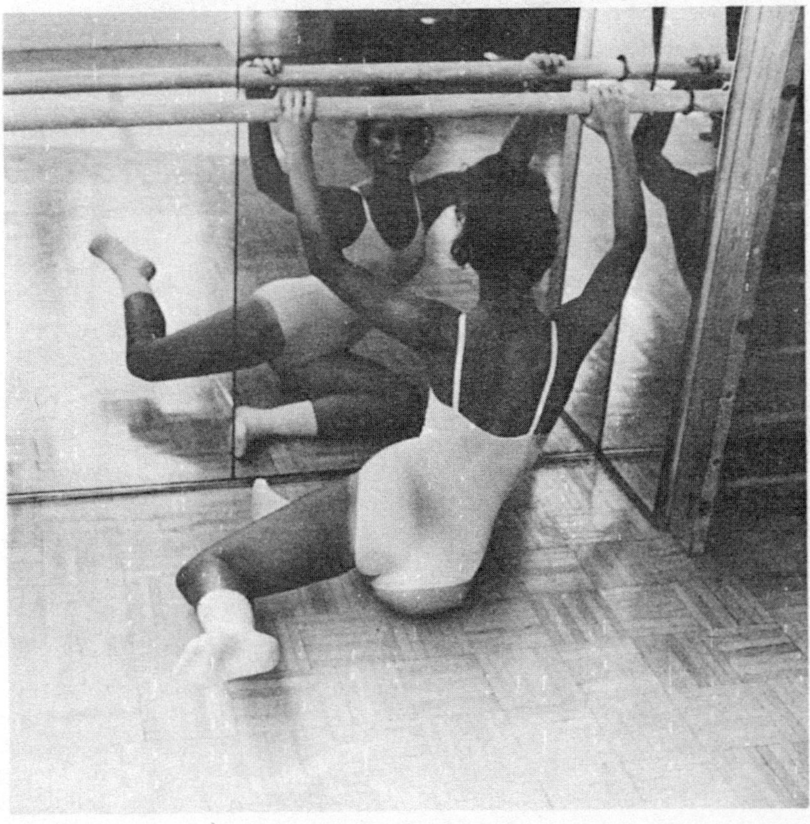

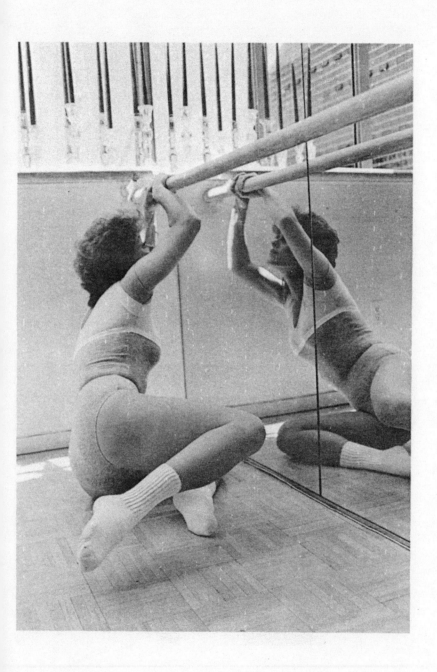

THE ALMOST WRONG WAY
Don't be upset if you start out in this position. Most people do. When your behind muscles get tighter, you will be able to sit up much straighter. People with especially weak behind muscles may need to hold the barre *with their hands close together on one side in order to maintain balance. The important thing is to* do *the exercise. Your style will improve as you get stronger.* ◄

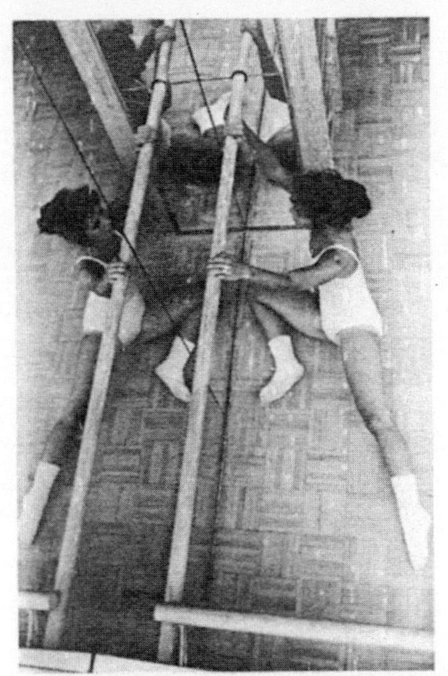

FOR THE BEHIND AND HIPS
#2 *After working on your right side, switch to the left to start the second exercise. In the same starting position, straighten the left leg to the left side, resting on the floor.* ◄

Roll your left hip forward, tightening the behind and curling the pelvis up. Try to turn your leg so that your toes are pointed to the floor. Do not lock the left knee. Relax your shoulders. ►

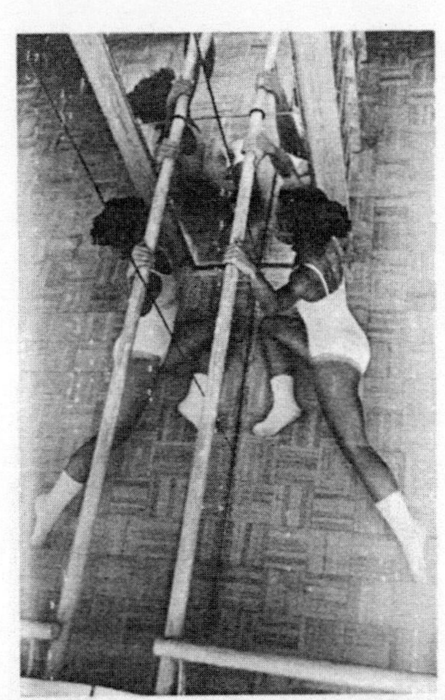

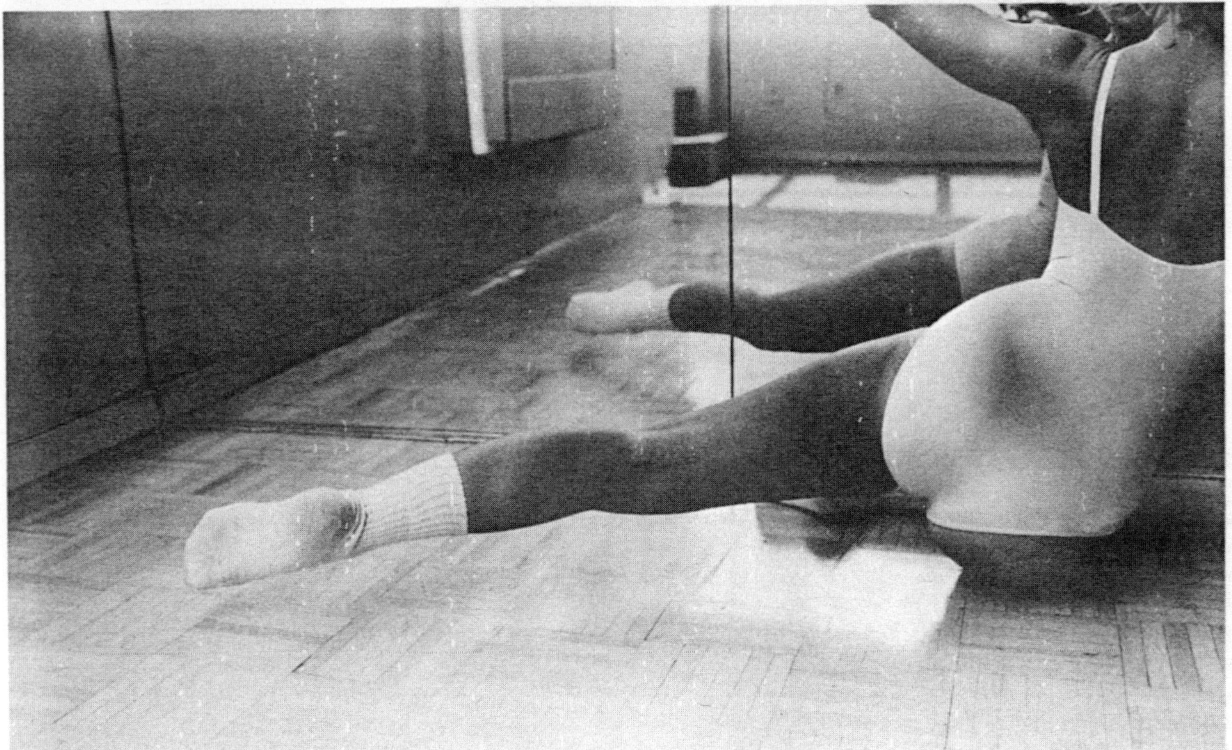

Keep your hip rolled forward and your behind tight. Your pelvis is curled upward. Raise your left leg not more than 3 inches off the floor and return. Just keep at it. Even if you can't lift it off the floor, keep trying. Eventually, it will lift. Do 20, alternate sides, working up to 100 on each side. Look at how rounded Lane's left cheek is compared to her right. You can actually see how you can look if you do this exercise in front of a mirror, with a second mirror behind you. If you don't have a mirror, feel your contracted behind with your hand to get some sense of how round, tight, and strong your bottom can be naturally. ▲

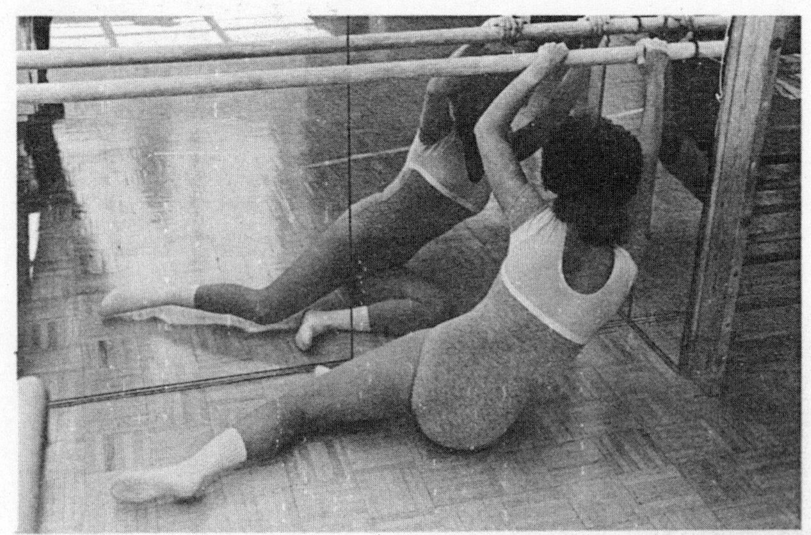

THE BEGINNER'S ALTERNATIVE *When you begin this exercise, you may find that you have to lean over like this, simply to be able to raise your leg. This is perfectly all right for now, if you remember not to continue that way once your muscles are strong enough . . . or you won't get the results you want.* ◀

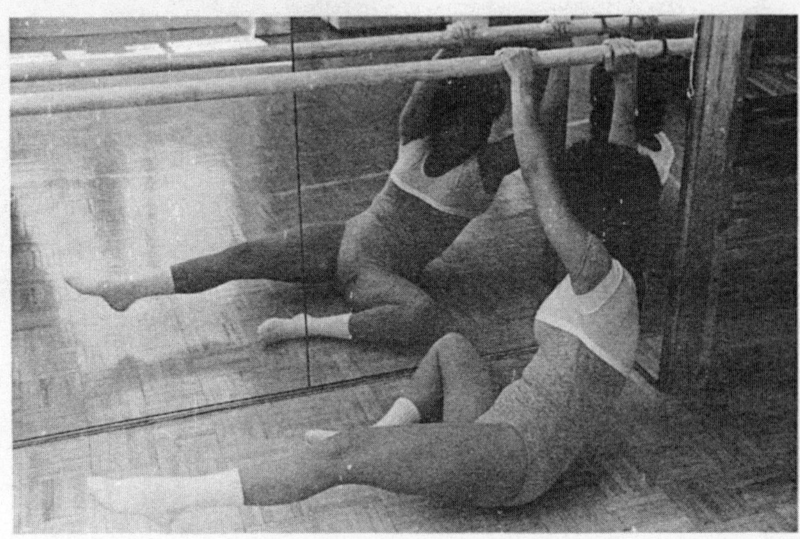

DRASTIC MEASURES *Shelly demonstrates another way that beginners attempt this exercise. If this is the only way you can get your leg off the floor, do it until you acquire enough coordination to do it properly. Know, however, that if you do the exercise this way, you use your thigh muscles more than your hips and behind.* ▶

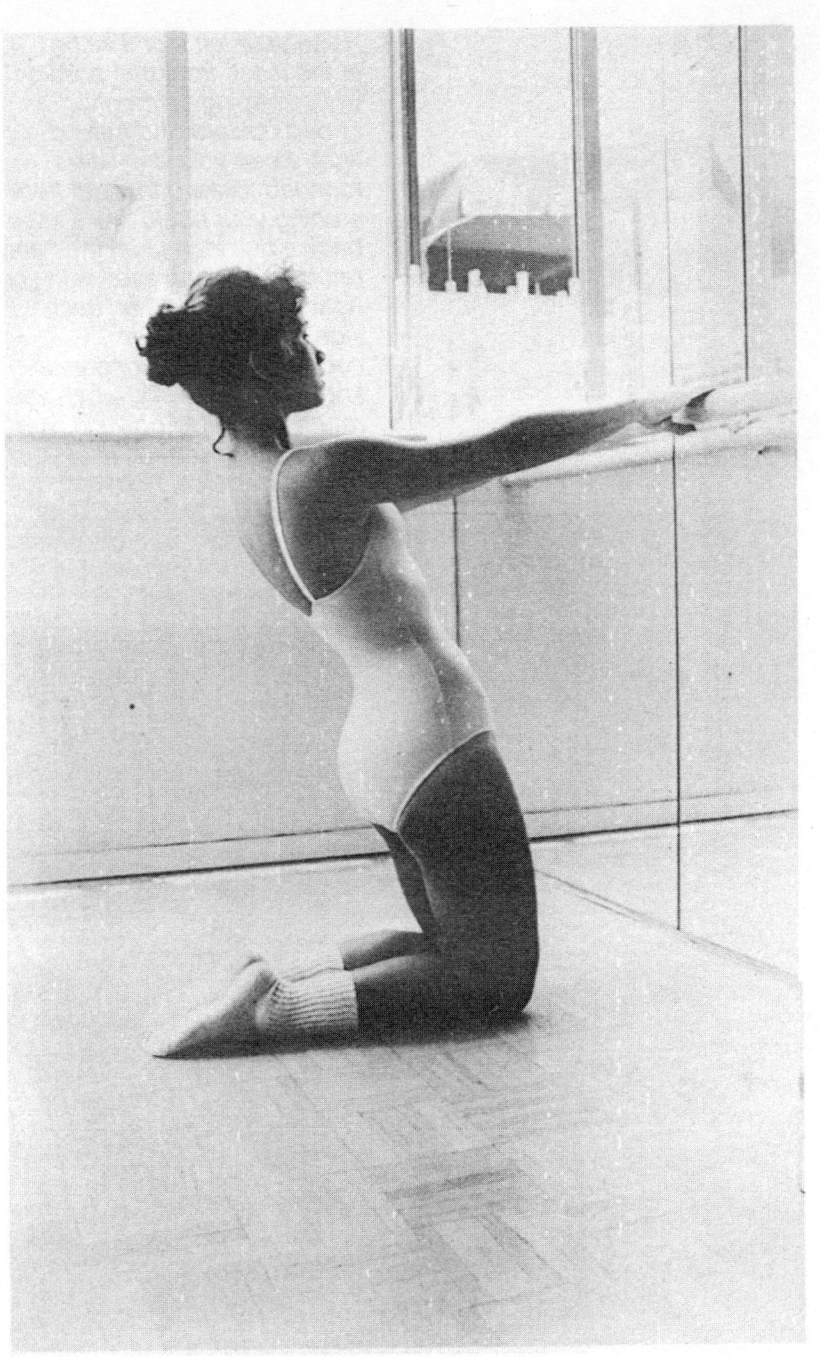

FOR THE BEHIND AND HIPS #3 *Kneel facing the* barre, *your knees away from the wall. (Always use padding under your knees for protection.) If you are unable to kneel, see detailed instructions in the Advanced Program, Chapter 22, Exercises #1 and #2. Lean back, so that your arms are straight. Tighten behind and curl pelvis up. This is the foundation for these exercises.* ◄

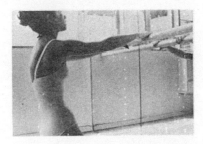

Round your shoulders forward in order to stretch your spine and keep your elbows straight. You will look and feel as if you are water skiing. It doesn't matter how high or low you hold your arms as long as you are able to lean back with straight arms and your pelvis tipped upward. If you bend your arms, you automatically arch your back and push out your behind. ▲

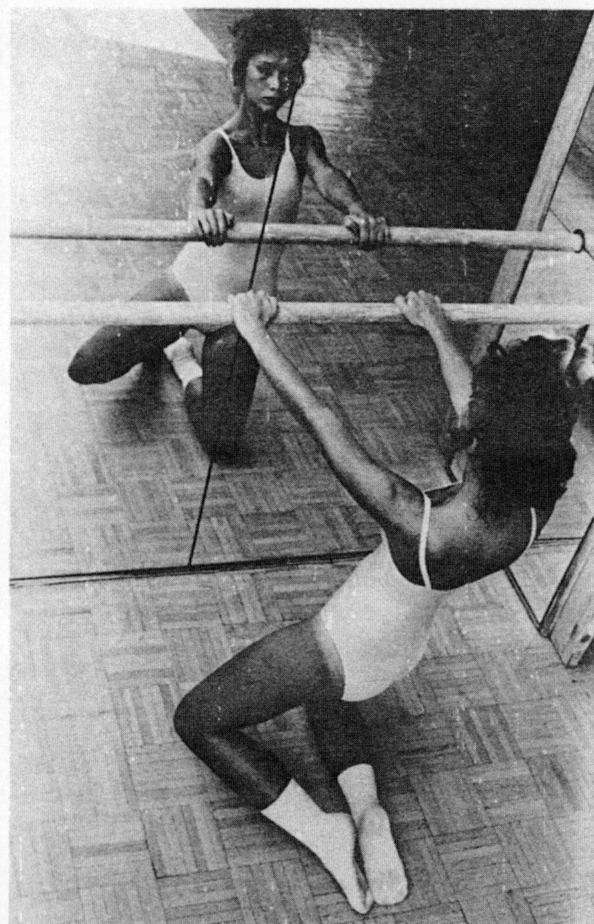

Slowly raise your left knee up to the left side, leaving your foot on the floor beside the right foot. (Because of her scoliosis, Lane has found that the only way she can keep her pelvis tipped is to turn her left hip slightly to one side.) Take the knee up as high as you can until your left foot starts to come off the floor. This is how most of you will do this exercise at first until you learn to keep your hips even. ▲

Raise your left foot 3 inches, 4 at the most, from that position while keeping your pelvis tipped upward and behind tight. Keep your shoulders rounded forward to keep from arching your back. Move knee back a half inch to an inch and return to position even with your right knee. Do 100 on each side, switching when necessary. If you bring your knee too far forward when you return to original position, you release the contraction of your behind muscles, lessening the benefit of the exercise. Until Lane's sacrum area becomes looser, she will not be able to keep both hips even. ▼

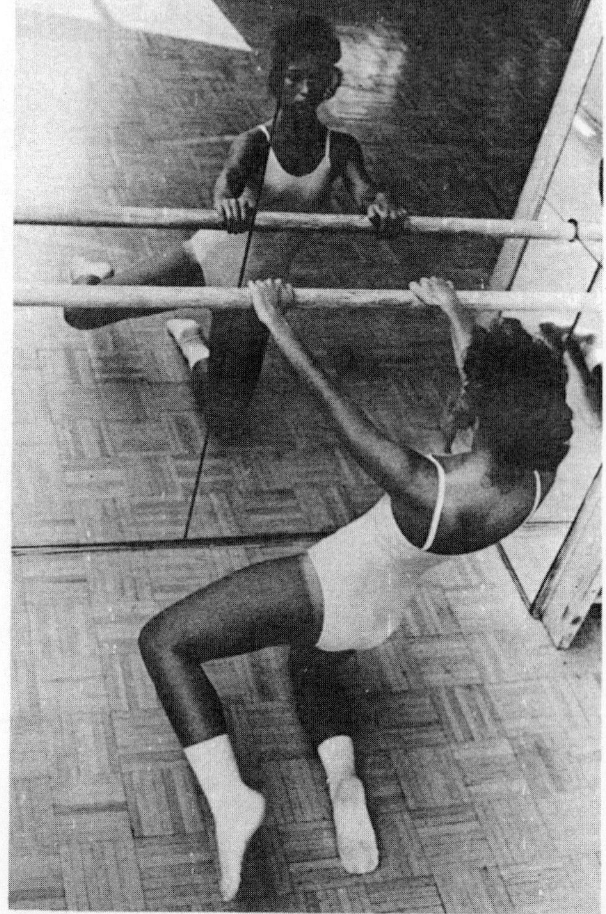

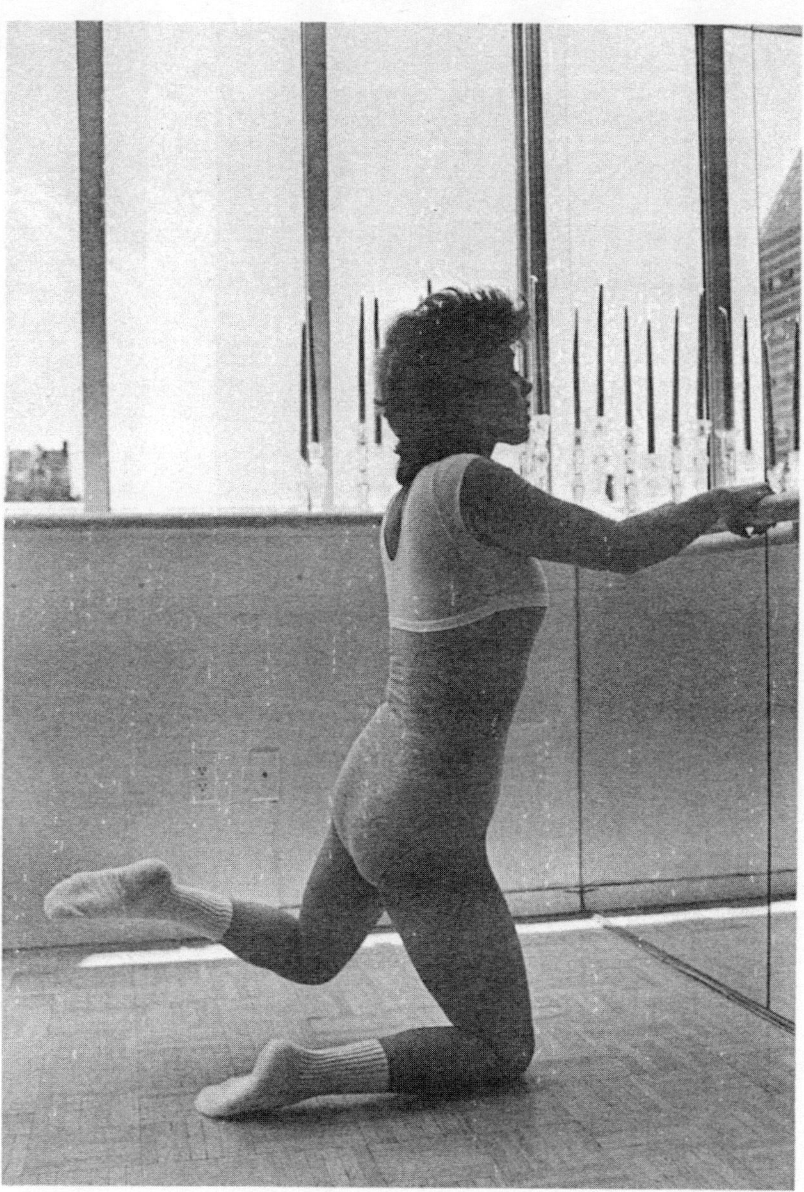

COMMON MISTAKES *Initially, you will be tempted to arch your back, stick out your behind, and bend your elbows. Once you overcome this, it is difficult to do it any other way but properly—your pelvis tipped up and forward, hips even, and shoulders rounded. Shelly had to concentrate to recall what it was like when she started out. She has become so strong and has such control over her movements that she found it difficult to revert to beginner's level for these pictures.* ▶

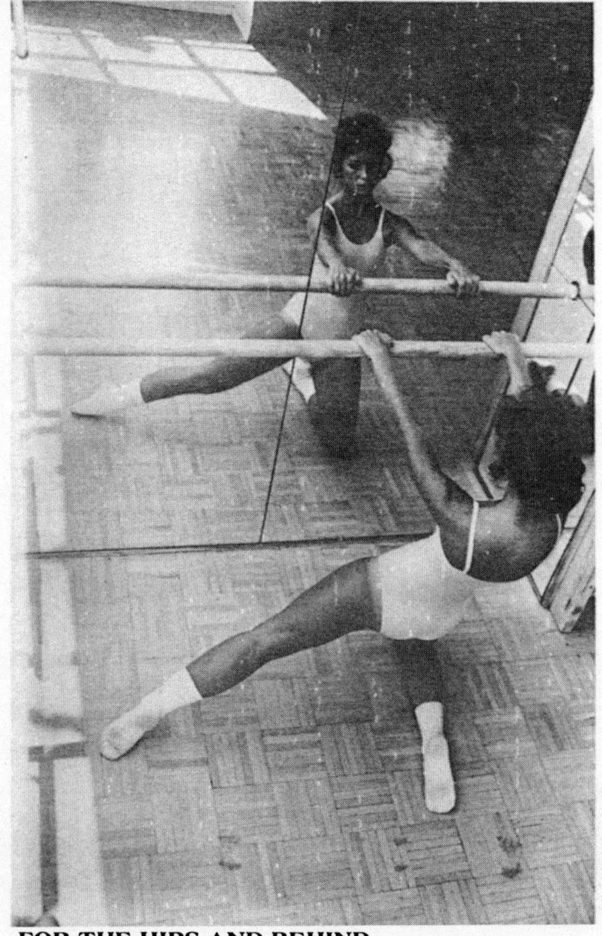

FOR THE HIPS AND BEHIND

#4 *As in the third exercise, kneel facing the* barre *with your hips even, left leg straight out to the side. Do not lock your knee. Lean back, holding the* barre *so that your arms are straight. Roll your left leg over so that your knee and the top of your foot face the floor, if possible. Relax and concentrate your energy on the part of the body involved.* ▲

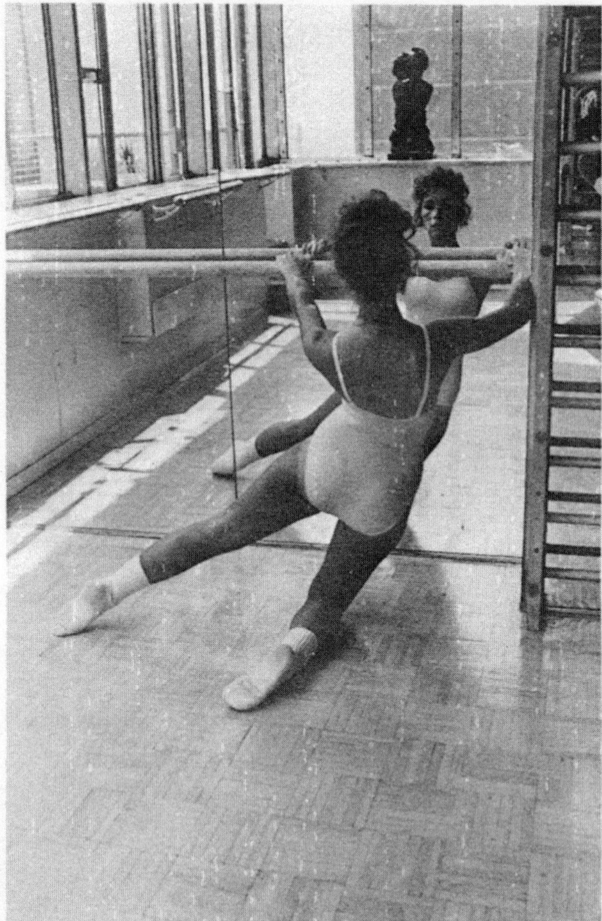

Without shifting the position of your hands on the barre, *pull your left leg to the right, toward your body, without bending your leg. Ease over onto the side of your right knee to lessen pressure there. Now tighten your behind and tip your pelvis up, more than you think you can. Round shoulders forward.* ▲

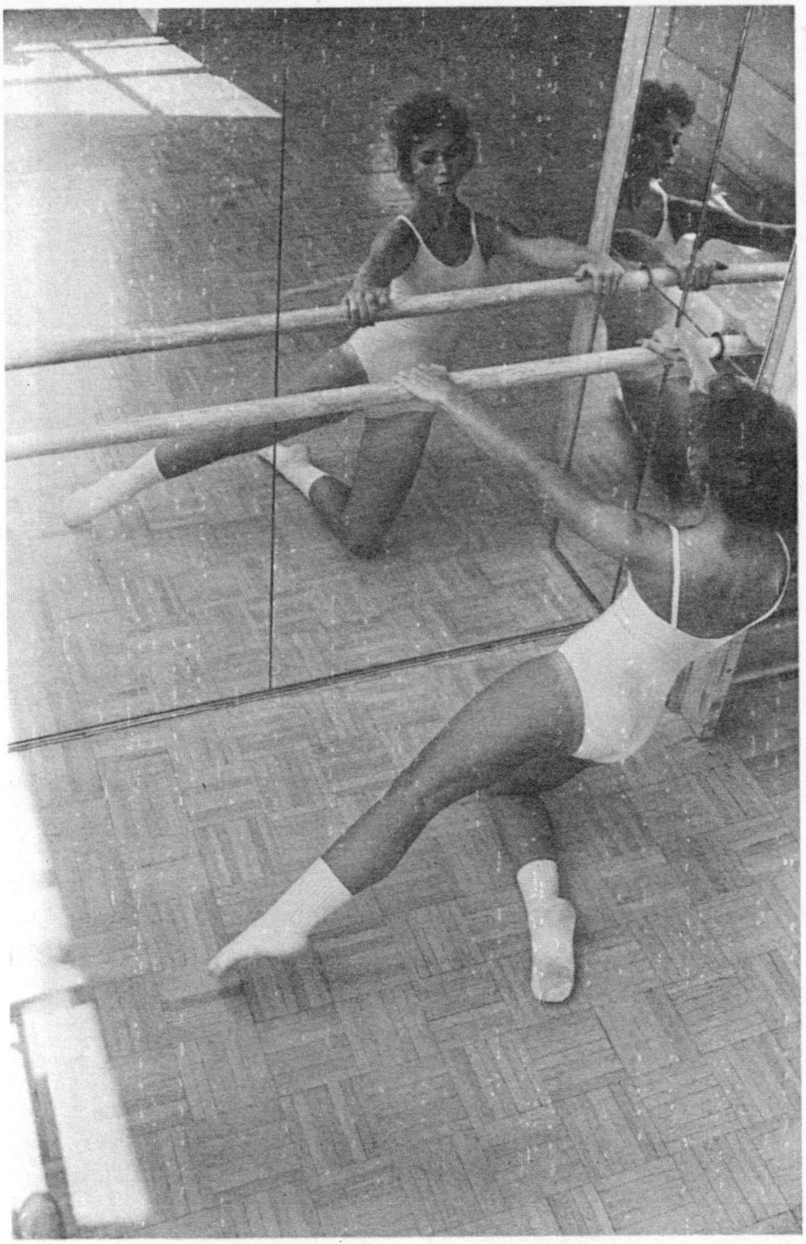

Without allowing your leg to turn upward, move foot and leg up and down, not more than 3 inches. Raise your leg and put it back to the floor 100 times with each leg—50 left, 50 right, 50 left, 50 right. Again, you will find it difficult in this position at first. However, if you talk to your muscles, coax them to cooperate, you will be able to master this move. Lane is not yet strong enough to do this without turning her leg over a bit. Warning: *You are not trying to see how high you can raise your leg. Do not bend elbows and lean into the* barre *or arch your back and stick out your behind.* ▲

We are in the "Decade of the Derrière." A Syracuse University sociologist reported that American women and men are more concerned with their hips and rear ends than with the bustline. However, with all this attention, many beautiful women have let their buttocks lose their peachlike roundness, settling for a pear-shaped bulge. I know that it is possible for anyone, regardless of age, to have a high, childlike behind and trim hips. ▼

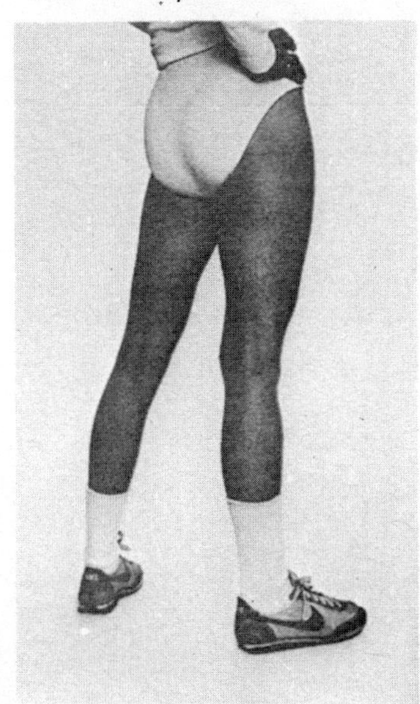

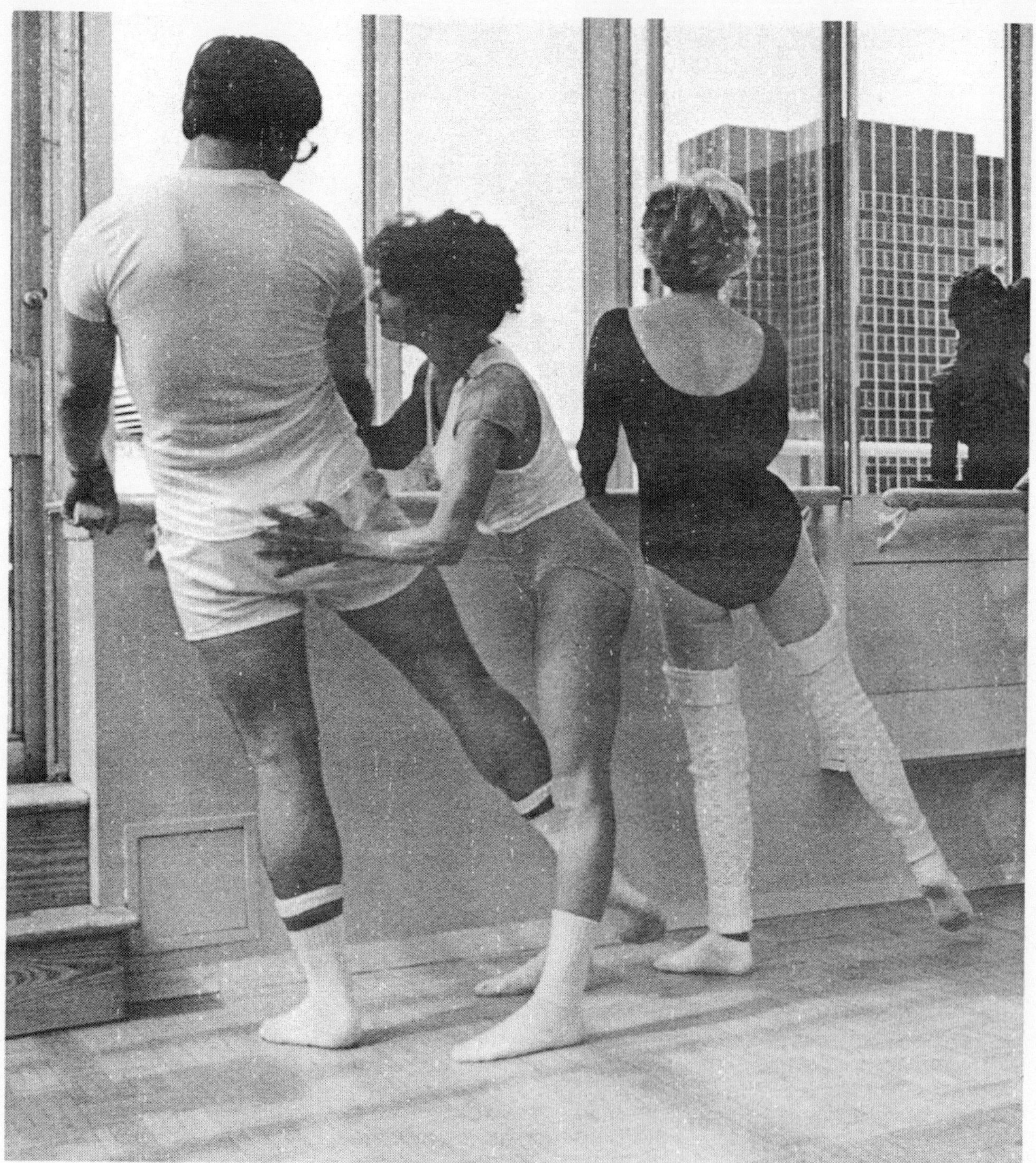

This exercise only appears *simple. It is for the advanced section. It is excellent for tightening and shaping the behind and hips and for stretching the lower back. It also contracts your stomach muscles.*

Students must learn to rotate their hips forward and tip their pelvises up for proper deep contraction of the muscles that make up the hip and behind. Hips should be kept even, parallel with the barre. ▲

CHAPTER ELEVEN

Open & Close

This is one of the most difficult exercises I teach, and it is also one of my favorites. Whenever I fall into a low-energy slump, I do fifty of these and it makes me feel as if I've had four hours of restful sleep. The results are incredibly fast because you are using several sets of muscles—from your chest, upper back, arms, stomach, abdomen, and even your thighs. At first you will only feel this in your thighs. However, the stronger your thighs become, the more you will notice how much your stomach has been working all along.

By sitting as you do with shoulders against the wall and behind five or six inches from the baseboard, you stretch the muscles up and down your spine. If you feel pressure in your lower back, lean your head forward, putting your chin to your chest, to release the tension in your spine. You may also lean against a sturdy chair or counter and grasp the top with your hands. Caution: people with back problems shouldn't do these exercises until the back is strengthened.

Jane, whom you see on these pages, was in a terrible automobile accident that left her unable to work, much less exercise. During the better part of her two-year convalescence, she was in pain and could not exercise. Only two months before these photos were taken, this forty-nine-year-old mother of four college-age children began to exercise again. Because of her medical history, I would not allow her to do this exercise without her doctor's approval. I was completely unaware that she was doing them on her own.

I wasn't surprised, however, when she told me how much better her back had begun to feel.

Anything is possible, as they say! I had been holding Jane back, solely because of my own fears of back pain.

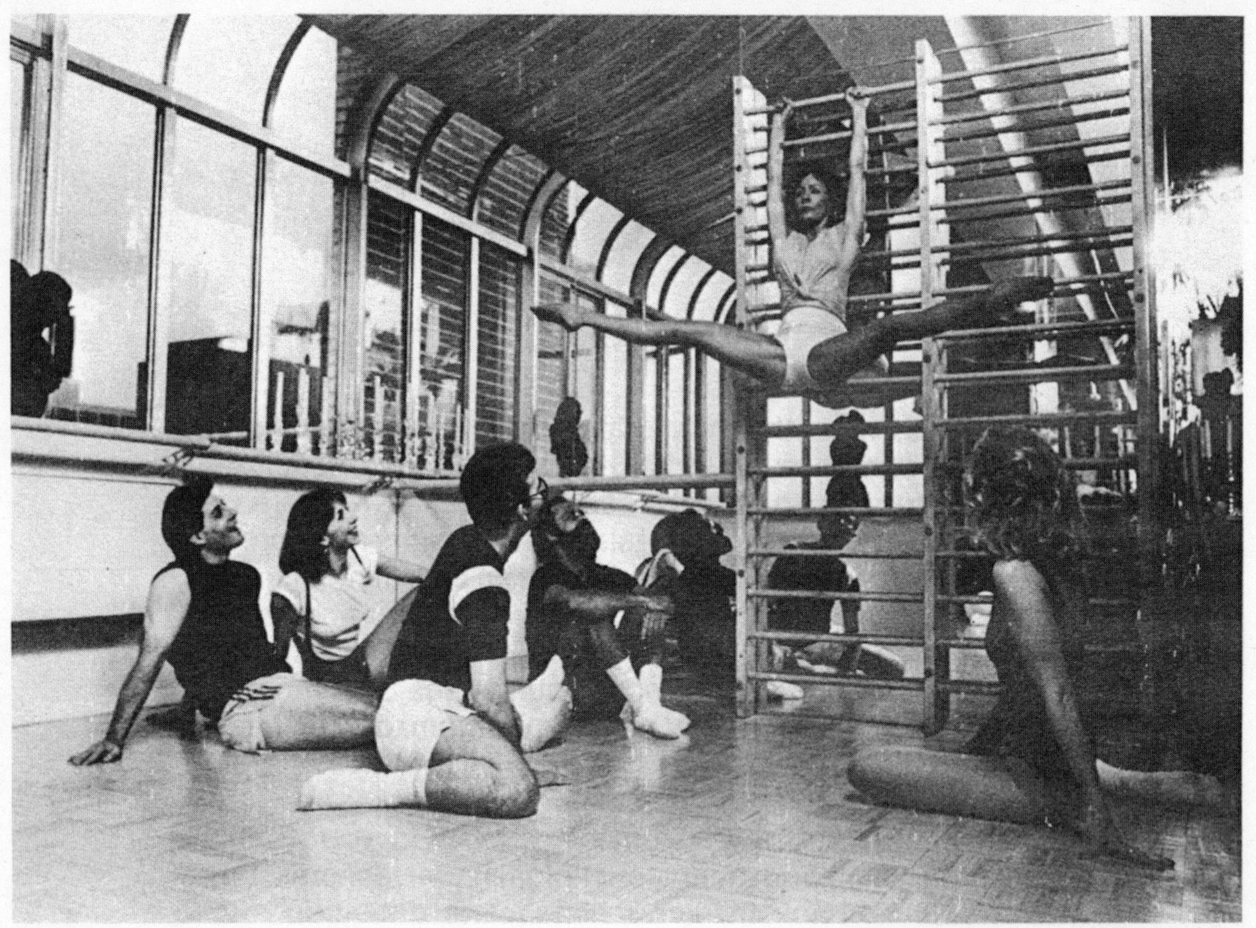

When I show new students after their first class how they will be able to do this Open & Close hanging from the barre *after 5 or 6 lessons (if their wrists are strong enough), they are very impressed by the physical strength required to support the body against gravity.* ▲

Sit with your shoulders against the wall—or the back of the couch, counter, or bureau front—so that your behind is about 5 or 6 inches from the surface. Reach your arms over your head and hold the edge, if there is one. The height of whatever you are using does not matter. With your legs together, bend them at the knees and pull up to your chest, leaving your toes on the floor. ▶

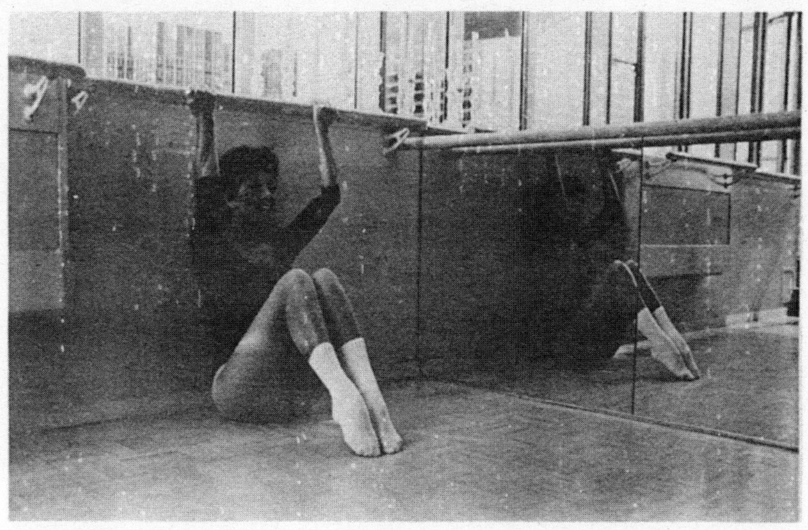

Clasping the barre firmly with both hands, relax your shoulders and neck. Lift your legs out straight in front of you, as far off the floor as you can hold them. The higher you can hold your legs, the more your stomach muscles will work, which means you'll see and feel results faster. If you feel pressure in your lower back, let your head gently roll forward and rest your chin on your chest, even closer than the model in the picture has her chin. ▶

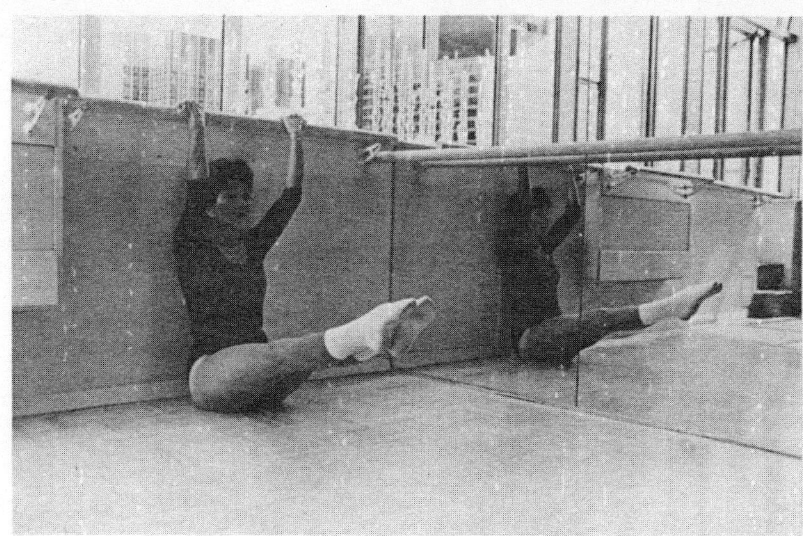

Open and close your legs, trying not to let them fall to the floor. Concentrate on keeping your neck and shoulders relaxed. Breathe normally. If at first you can't get your legs off the ground, much less make them move, don't worry. Drag them along the floor as you attempt to lift them. Bend your legs if you have to. As you get stronger, you'll be able to straighten them out. Do 4 sets of 5. Increase as you feel stronger. ▶

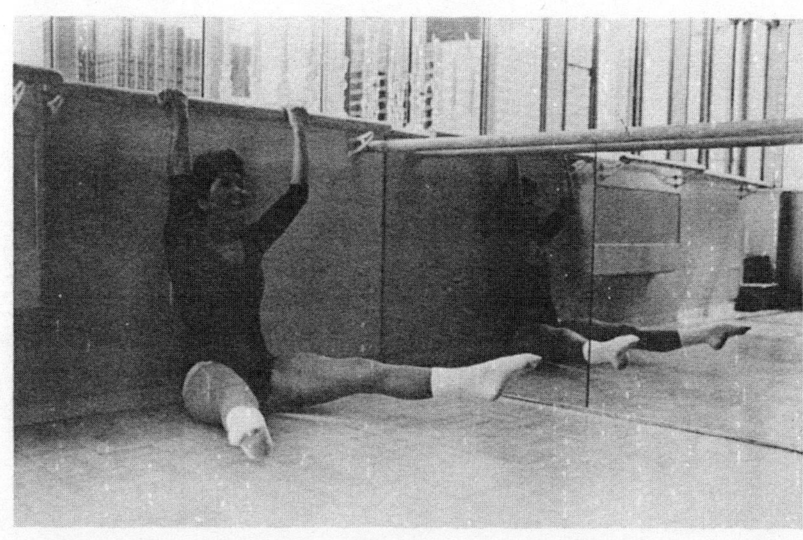

CHAPTER TWELVE

Stretching

Now you can stretch. Your muscles have been warmed up, even stretched, and put to work. They are ready to be stretched to keep them flexible. Stretching now lengthens muscles after they have been contracted. This is what prevents bulk.

I have positioned this stretching routine toward the end of the One-Hour Program rather than with the Warm-Ups because now is when you need them. You have been pushing your body. It needs the relaxation that stretching brings.

Stretching is essential to an exercise program. It not only helps to keep you flexible, but also to prevent common injuries, such as shin splints or Achilles tendinitis from jogging, or sore shoulders and elbows from tennis. It helps to improve your posture. Stretching is simple. It is not stressful. Done incorrectly, however, it can do more harm than good.

I tell my students to caress their muscles. Be gentle, kind, and respectful to them. I constantly remind them to let their bodies determine how far they stretch. Never *ever* compare your stretches to another person's. If you have to study any living creature, look at animals. Watch a cat or a dog. My students have my cats for inspiration. Pets instinctively know how much to stretch. They are spontaneous, never overstretching, never jerking or forcing their bodies into position.

Use the time you spend stretching to be alone with your body. Think positive, peaceful thoughts. Relax your spirit *and* your body. Do not *ever* stretch with a partner. Unless you and your partner are professional dancers or athletes,

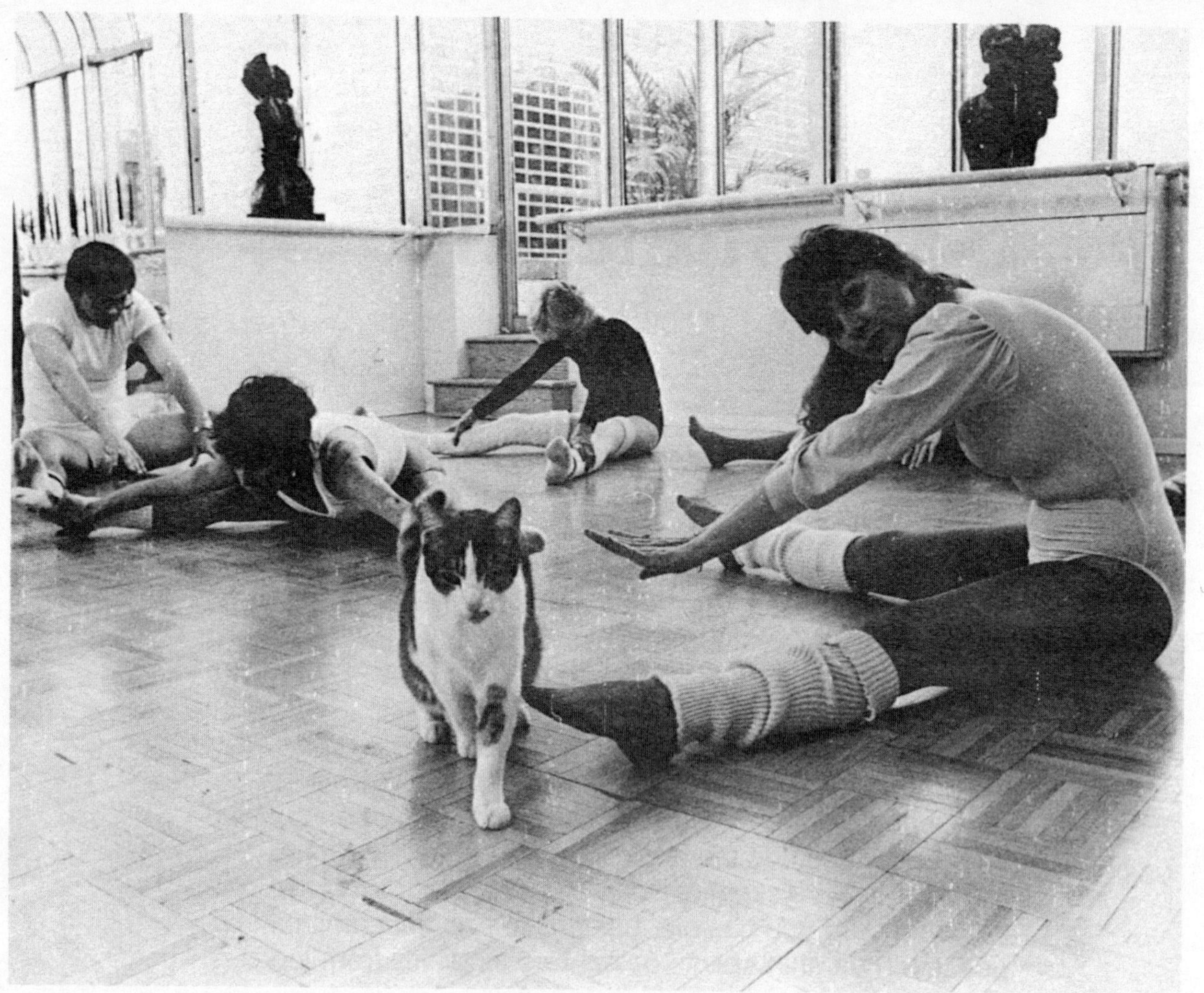

Keeping my students on their toes mentally as well as physically is important to me. The sculptures all around my studio are the works of my friend Edwina Sandys. Every few weeks I borrow different pieces so there is always something new and exciting to interest the eye. Some are sensuous bodies modeled and cast in bronze. Others are clean-cut from Carrara marble. I do this to remind my students that they are also artists, sculpting their own bodies. ▲

trained to work together, you will not be able to determine the extent of stretch the other person has. If he or she is stronger or more stretched than you, or vice versa, someone could be injured. *Never* allow anyone to push your body into position. Only you can know how far your muscles can go.

There is no standard, ideal range of motion for your joints, nor is there a standard or average pattern of muscular stretch. Every body is different, responding with its own non-standard degree of readiness.

I chose a new student who had completed only one class to demonstrate the stretches I teach *specifically* because she has limited stretching ability. Were I to have an advanced student in the photos, who is as limber as a willow, those of you who are not stretched out, or who are unable to reach or stretch as far as she, would be totally intimidated.

The model, Ellen, is a thirty-two-year-old massage therapist. Her shoulder and arm muscles are very tight from her daily work on patients. Until she started my classes, she had not been able to find an exercise program that would fit into her busy schedule. Once she masters the exercises, she can do them anywhere, anytime.

During stretching, which could easily be called "joint preparations," you pull the connective tissue (fascia) which surrounds your muscles, as well as your muscles and the tendons themselves. If this tissue is not adequately stretched, it shortens. This not only limits movement, it also causes muscles to look knotty and bulky.

Each section of exercises contains stretches that complement the deep contractions you are doing. This special stretching routine completes the program. Move in TRIPLE slow motion.

Stretching is *not* an activity that stands alone. It must be integrated into the total program, largely because, in its function of relaxation, it provides a balance for your body. It gives your body a break. It contributes absolutely nothing toward aerobic fitness or muscle strengthening. If anyone says you can tighten your figure through yoga, or any other regimen that is 90 percent stretching, laugh and leave. There is no way that would work. It is physically impossible. You need the balance of deep contractions and complete stretches to bring your body into shape.

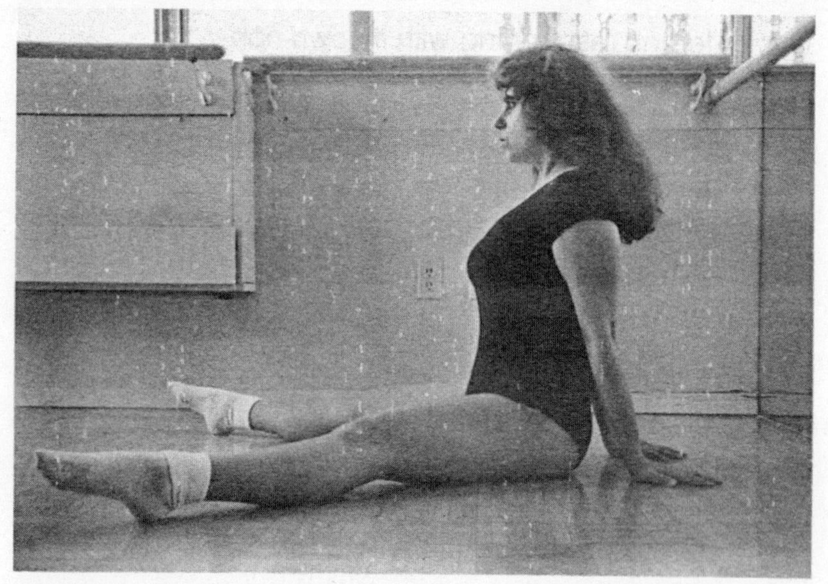

STRETCH #1 *(Stretches inner thighs, hamstrings, lower back, neck, across shoulder blades) (This stretch substitutes for the leg exercises for people with tendency toward sciatica.) Sit on the floor, your legs as far apart as you can take them without upsetting your balance. Place your hands behind your hips, palms down and fingers out. Push your pelvis into the floor and keep your body relaxed. Concentrate on relaxing your legs, putting the energy of the stretch into your pelvis and inner thighs. Don't worry about pointing your toes. Keep your feet and toes relaxed at first.* ◀

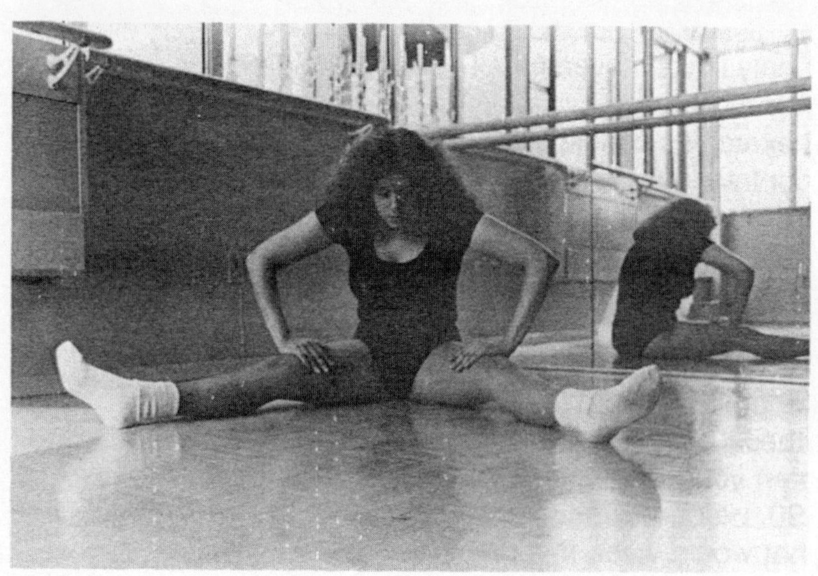

Continuing this stretch to the front, rest the palms of your hands on the tops of your thighs to keep the lower back relaxed. Keep your pelvis pushed into the floor. Round your shoulders and push your elbows out to the sides. Lean forward as far as you can and hold that position for 30 seconds, then gently move a quarter of an inch to an inch further, depending upon your flexibility. Move back and forth from that position very slowly and very gently 50 times. If you are doing this for your legs, do 100. If you are very stretched in the back and shoulders, you may be able to start this movement with your hands below your knees or gently on the floor way out in front of you between your legs. Do not grab your ankles or legs *or you may* pull *yourself over too far instead of encouraging your muscles to stretch at their own level.* ◀

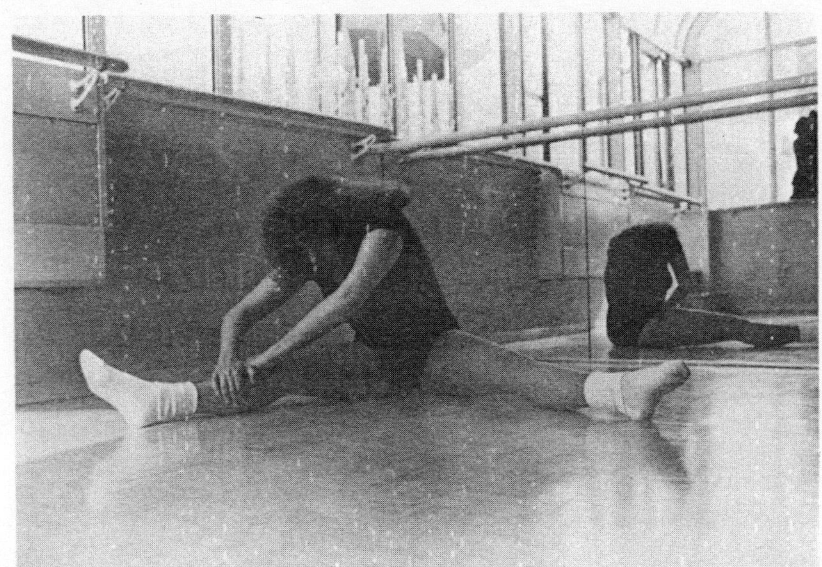

STRETCH #2 *(Stretches inner thighs, spine, hamstrings, shoulder blades, and back and sides of torso) Starting as you would for the first stretch, remembering to keep your pelvis pushed into the floor, turn your body to one side from the waist. Your chin should be facing your foot. Reach down your leg, placing your hands across the leg as close to your ankle as you can. Round your shoulders and push your elbows out to each side. Your goal: to take your forehead to your knee. Hold for 30 seconds, then move a quarter of an inch to an inch further. Move back and forth from that position 50 times. Return to an upright position and then gently turn to the opposite side and repeat.* ▲

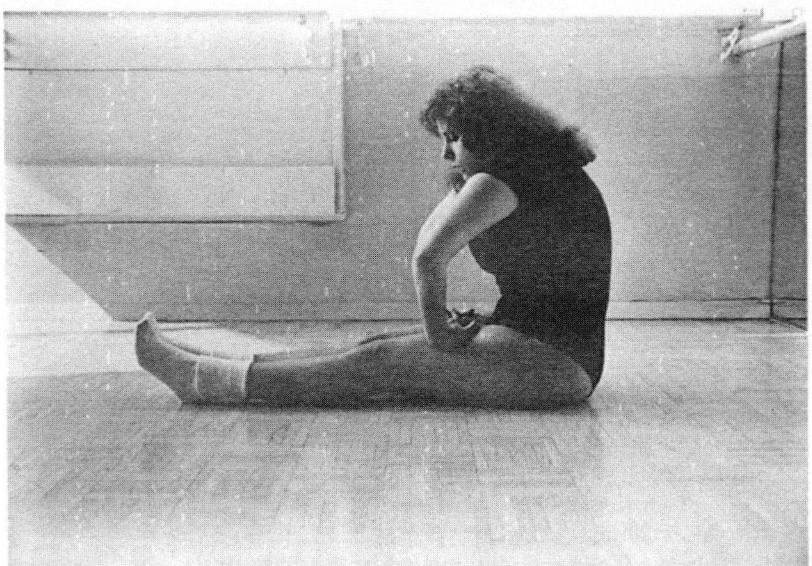

STRETCH #3 *(Stretches the spine, shoulder blades, hamstrings, calves) Sitting upright with your feet and legs together in front of you, relax your legs so that your feet are in a neutral but upright position. Do not lock your knees or push them into the floor. Round your shoulders and place your hands across your legs as low as you can reach. (Do not put your hands across your knees as this could force them downward and may damage the joints.) Your goal is to touch your head to your knees. Stretch over as far as you can. Hold for 30 seconds and, once again, move a quarter of an inch to an inch further. Move back and forth from there 50 times. If you lean your head forward, chin to chest, you will also benefit from a well-stretched neck.* ▲

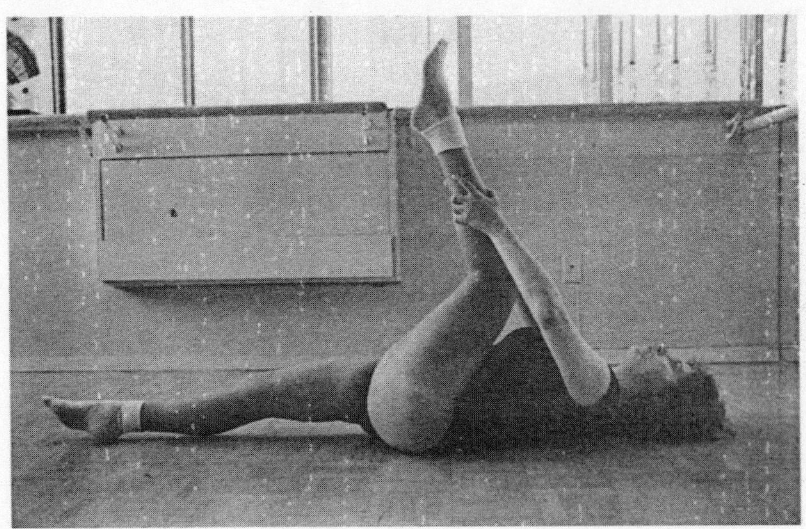

STRETCH #4 *(Stretches the hamstrings, spine, neck, and across shoulder blades) Lie flat on the floor on your back. Straighten your neck and lift your chin toward the ceiling. Concentrate on relaxing your shoulders. Bring your left leg up and grab the back of your knee or calf, whichever is more comfortable. Do not force your raised leg to straighten. Bend your elbows out to the sides and hold this position for 30 seconds. Gently ease your raised leg toward your chest a half inch to an inch closer and move back and forth in a delicate, slow movement. Do 50 and repeat with the other leg.* ▲

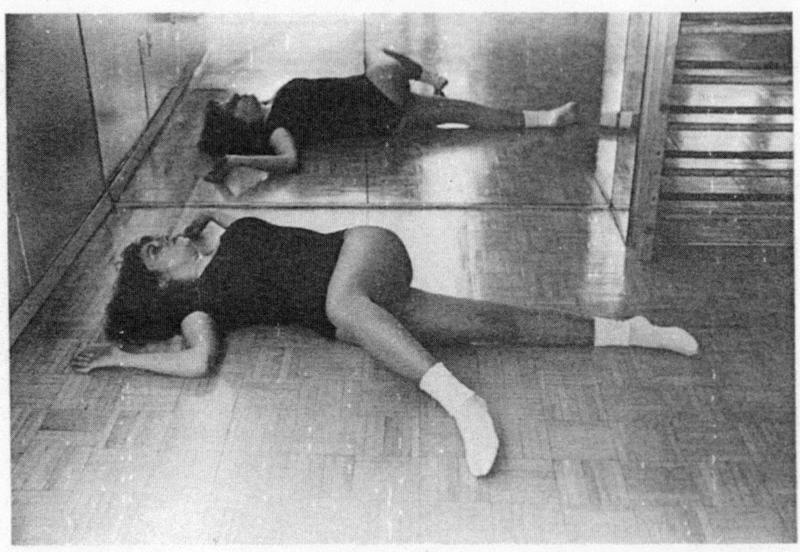

STRETCH #5 (Note: *This is a wonderful stretch for the lower back. Stretches spine, upper back, between the shoulder blades, pectorals, behind, hips, outer thighs, and lower back) Lie flat on your back, legs together, arms out at shoulder level with your elbows bent at right angles. Bend your left leg at the knee and bring it over your right leg, keeping legs relaxed and elbows on the floor. Gently try to bring your left knee to the floor, as close to your right elbow as you can go. Switch sides. Do 50 on one side and 50 on the other. During Ellen's first class, she could not touch the floor with her foot. During this photo session she could, and her knee was much lower to the floor than before. I always do this stretching exercise after I have worn heels, even half-inch heels, to untwist my body and even up my hips.* ▲

STRETCH #6 *(Stretches the calves, hamstrings, inner thighs, and spine—when done correctly) Stand facing a wall or* barre, *an arm's length away, and place your hands on it at*

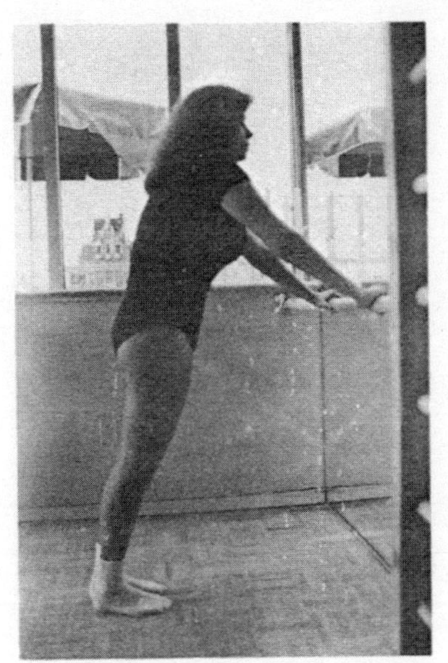

waist level, if possible, but no higher than shoulder level. Step back 1 foot. Keep your feet together, facing the wall. Relax your shoulders and arms and keep your elbows straight. ◄

Without moving your left leg, lift your right knee to a height midway between the groin and knee of your left leg. Push your left heel into the floor. Tighten your behind and tip your pelvis upward. Gently move your pelvis and hips forward as a unit, keeping your elbows straight but not locked. Do not stick behind out. The lower part of your right leg and your foot should be relaxed. (Gravity will pull them toward the floor.) Do not jerk or bounce your body or force your body weight into the wall. *Do 50, then repeat, standing on your right leg with your left leg raised. The result is*

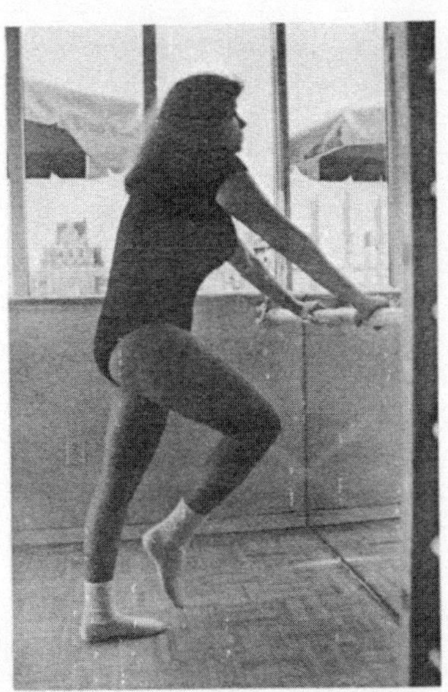

a thorough, balanced stretch with no damage to the shoulders, elbows, or wrists. A variation of this stretching exercise is done on steps or a curb. I used to teach it that way, but decided that the foot-on-the-floor method is superior because it not only stretches the calves, but also gets to the inner thighs and complete spine as well.

Stretches, like all the exercises I have included in my program, must be done precisely and gently. I can always tell if someone has taken aerobic dancing—they are maniacs with their bodies. ◄

CHAPTER THIRTEEN

For the Pelvis

If you have ever watched a Middle Eastern dancer perform, you will know right away where this series of exercises comes from. I learned them from a belly dancer!

From these people I discovered that anyone, even someone with back problems such as mine, can have a limber, flexible spine and a loose, sensuous pelvis.

In the fifties, when the Hula-Hoop was the rage, thousands of people suffered from many different kinds of disc problems, all stemming from twisting and turning their bodies like maniacs. However, for *centuries,* Middle Eastern dancers—men and women alike—have circled their hips in endless, sultry sweeps without harm. These two movements are basically the same. How, then, did the swivel-hipped fiends of the fifties hurt themselves so hideously?

It was common sense to me: Those elegant, exotic dancers who move like Salome discarding her seven veils, control and coordinate every click, twist, and swirl of their bodies with deliberate, precise grace. They know what they are doing . . . and why. Every little move has a reason. It is a very *powerful* feeling to have control over this part of your body in this way.

To learn these movements, concentrate on your pelvis. Isolate the muscles in that area. Slowly and deliberately, rotate your pelvis in a full, glorious circle. Don't stick out your stomach and then poke your behind in the opposite direction, or simply move your hips from side to side. Visualize a circle. Picture having complete control over your body as you move in a circle.

As you practice the movement patterns outlined in the following chapter, you will realize that subtle movements like these strengthen the back. But the real payoff comes from the development of the inner thighs and pelvic muscles, which will enhance your sexual enjoyment. ▶

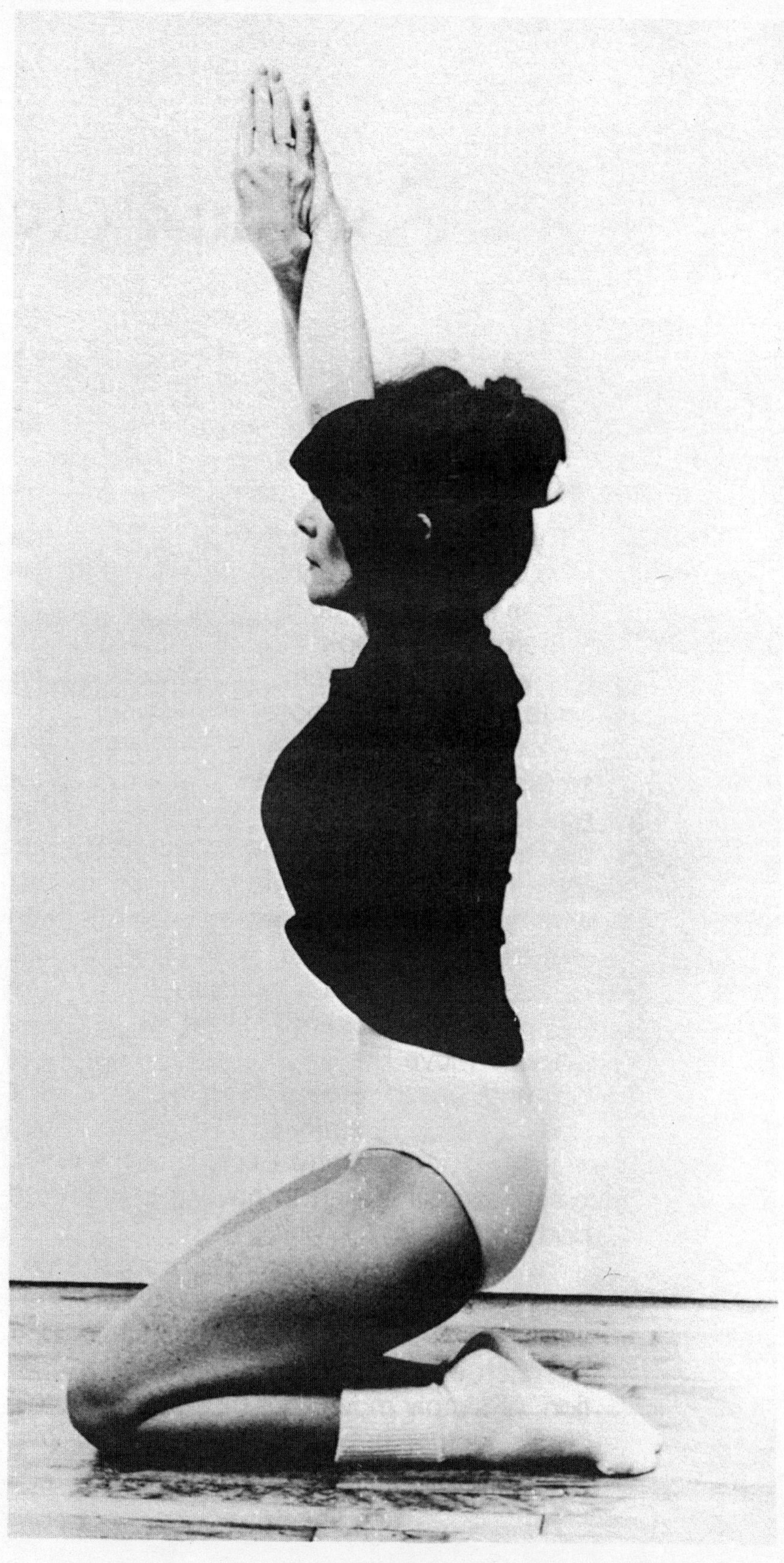

In no time your pelvis will flow with graceful, soft movements. Of all the exercises I teach, these are the ones that both men and women put their hearts and souls into. They learn them quickly and enthusiastically, and tell me that they practice them at home.

This series of exercises works on the behind, thighs, inner thighs, lower back, and the stomach. The Pelvic Rotations stretch your thighs completely, while the Pelvic Scoop contracts them totally. The final stretch works on the thighs and stomach to complete the sequence.

Do these exercises in front of a mirror, even if you must kneel on the bed to see yourself. Try it. Watch how your body moves.

If your calves hurt at first, you need to stretch them more. You may have been wearing high heels and using your calves when you walk. To ease this ache and add stretch to your calves, simply bring your arms in front of your body, rounding your back, as you do the movements.

Hold your head high. Stretch your arms over your head or hold them out to each side. You may even want to put them on your hips. Do whatever makes you feel wonderful.

Once you have perfected the basic movements and are able to perform them with ease, you may want to turn on some sensuous music and move your body in time with it. Now, *you* will be in control of what your pelvis is doing. You'll be surprised at how much strength you have.

Anna, who demonstrates the exercises in this section, is a New York businesswoman in her early forties. When she took her first series of classes with me several years ago, she was under treatment for tachycardia (sudden attacks of rapid heartbeats). She had a nice, but flabby body. Because of her heart condition, I would not let Anna do more than five minutes at her first class. At the second class, she did ten minutes. We increased the time five minutes per class until, as her strength improved, she was able to do the entire routine.

After Anna shaped up, she stopped classes. She resumed classes two years later and had completed two sessions when we took these photos. She was so strong, her body grew noticeably tighter by the hour.

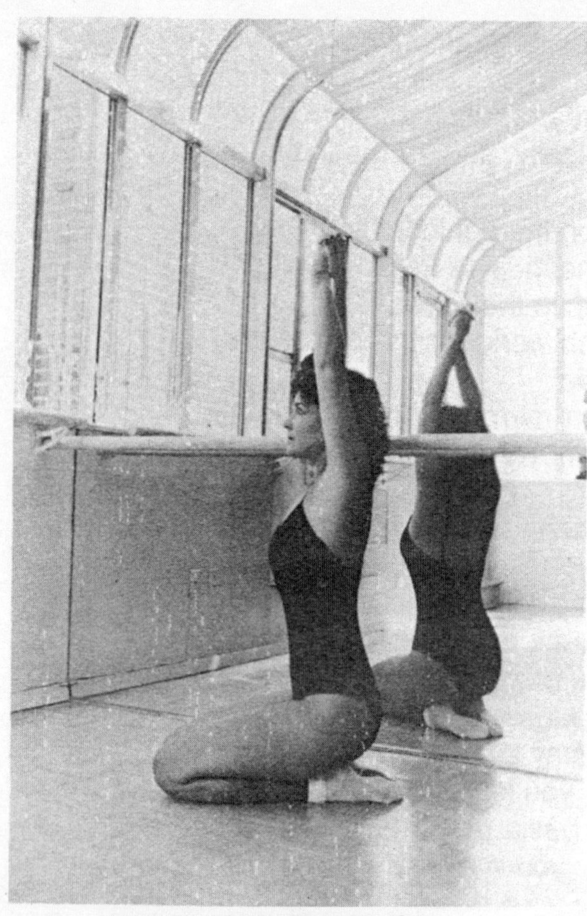

PELVIC ROTATIONS *Sit back on your heels. Stretch your arms over your head. Lift your head and torso high, stretching upward so that you feel you are 2 inches taller than you really are. Feel your abdomen stretch. To protect your knees, kneel on a pillow or cushion that is large enough to pad both feet and knees.* ▲

Raise your body 3 inches off your heels. Stretch straight up. Then take your hip to the right as far as you can, while maintaining your stretched position. Your arms and head should be held high. ▼

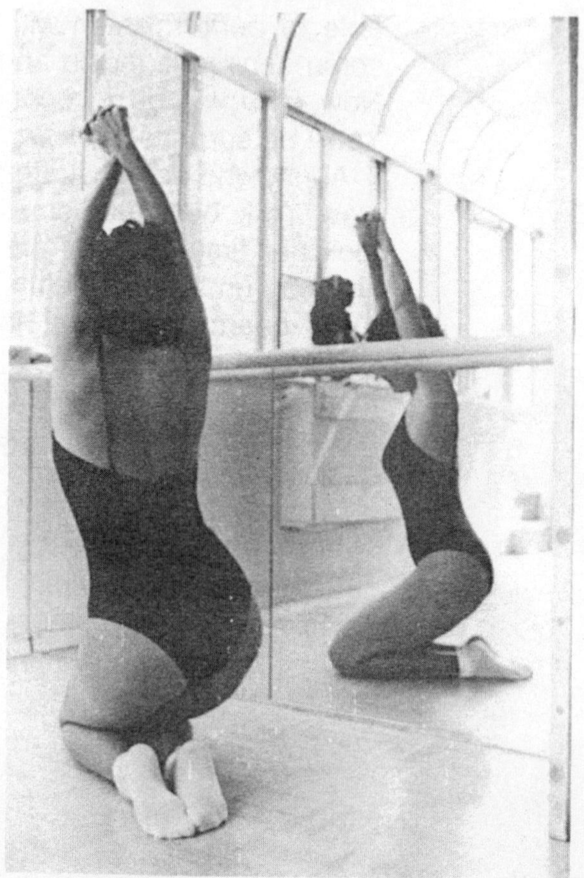

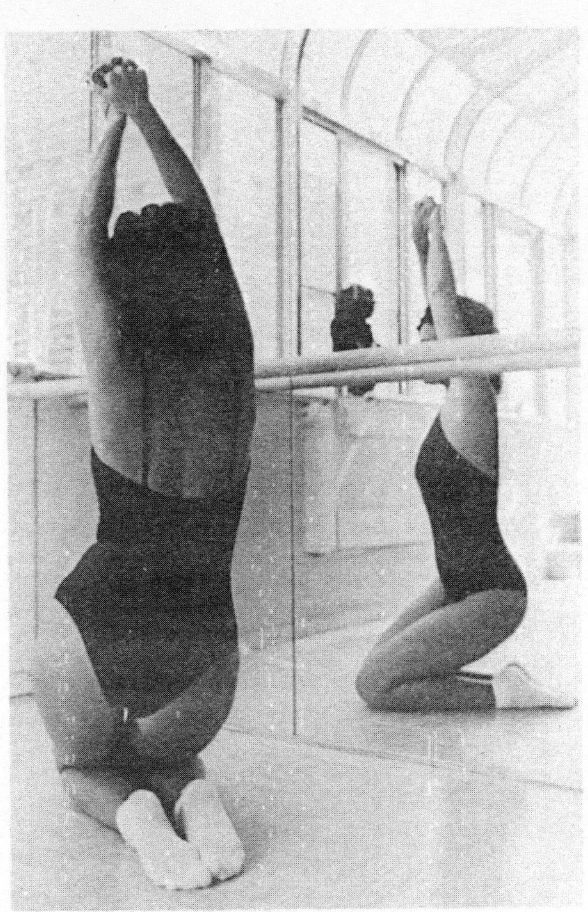

Continue to slowly move your pelvis to the front in a circular motion. Pretend you are stirring a pot of soup with your pelvis. Your body will be farther off your heels than when you started with your pelvis tipped to the front. ▼

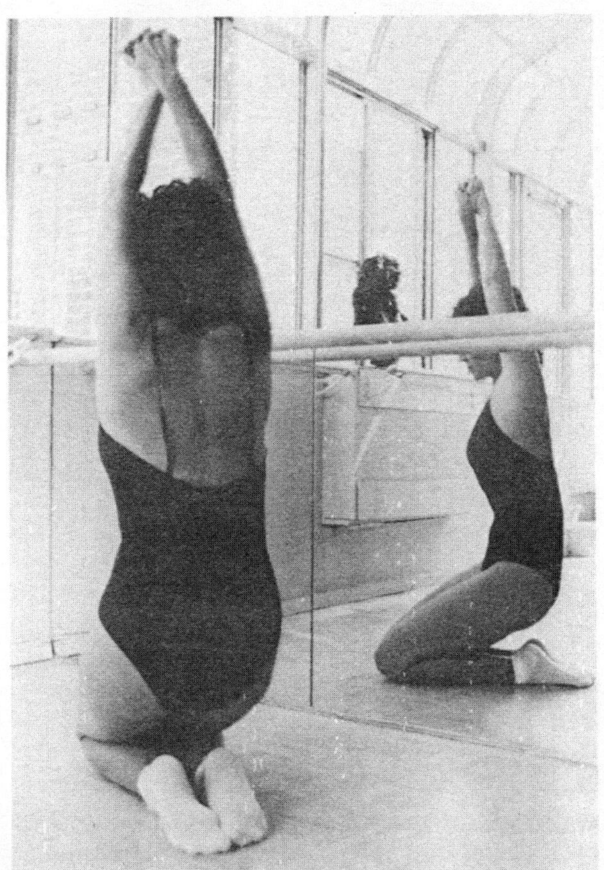

Still stretching your body upward, move your pelvis to the left side as far as possible. Keep your knees together and hips even. Now, take your behind to the back, your buttocks over your heels, to complete the circle. Complete 5 circles to the right and reverse. (You can also do 10 Figure 8 rotations.) This loosens your pelvic girdle and stretches your thighs. ▲

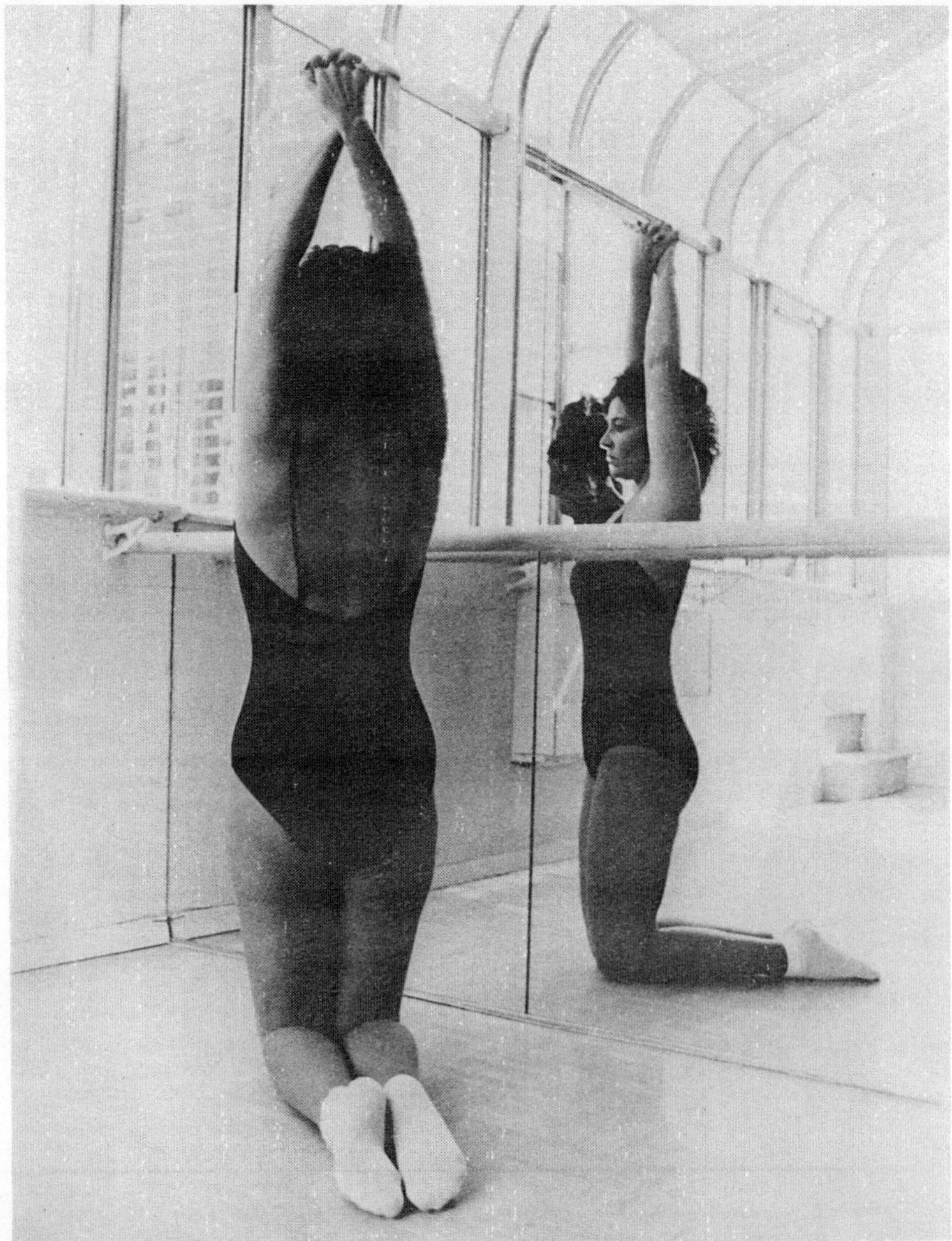

THE PELVIC SCOOP
Kneeling, knees and feet together and arms crossed high over your head, stretch your torso up as far as you can. If you have pressure on your calves, round shoulders and stretch arms forward. (Pretend you are diving into a pool.) ▲

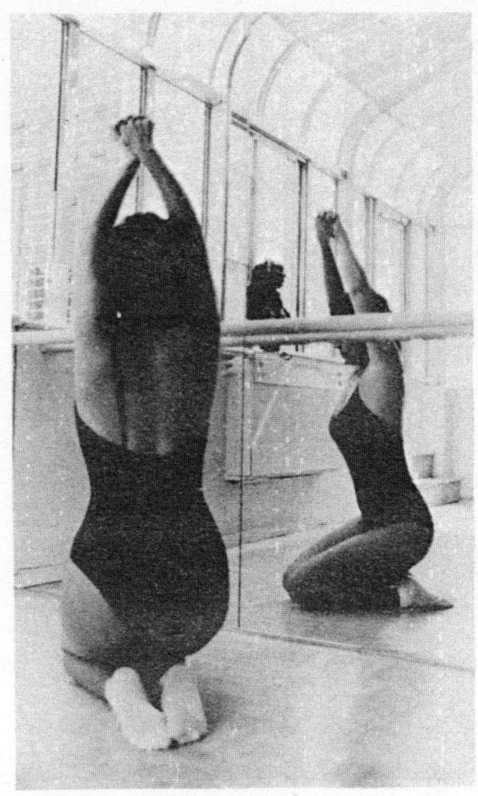

Keep your body straight. Your arms are stretched over your head or, if you prefer, on your hips. Lower your behind in slow motion, aiming it toward your heels. As you feel your behind brush your heels, tighten your behind muscles and slowly tip your pelvis up. Hold for 2 seconds, keeping your pelvis up. ▶

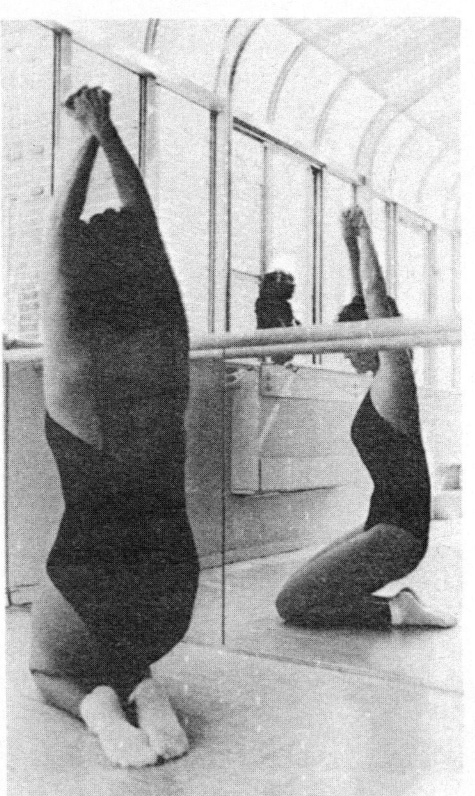

Keeping your knees together and pelvis tipped upward, gently scoop *your pelvis up, lifting your body with the strength of your inner thighs and pelvis, to the original kneeling position. Remember to keep stretching your torso. All movements are slow and graceful. Do 10.* ◀

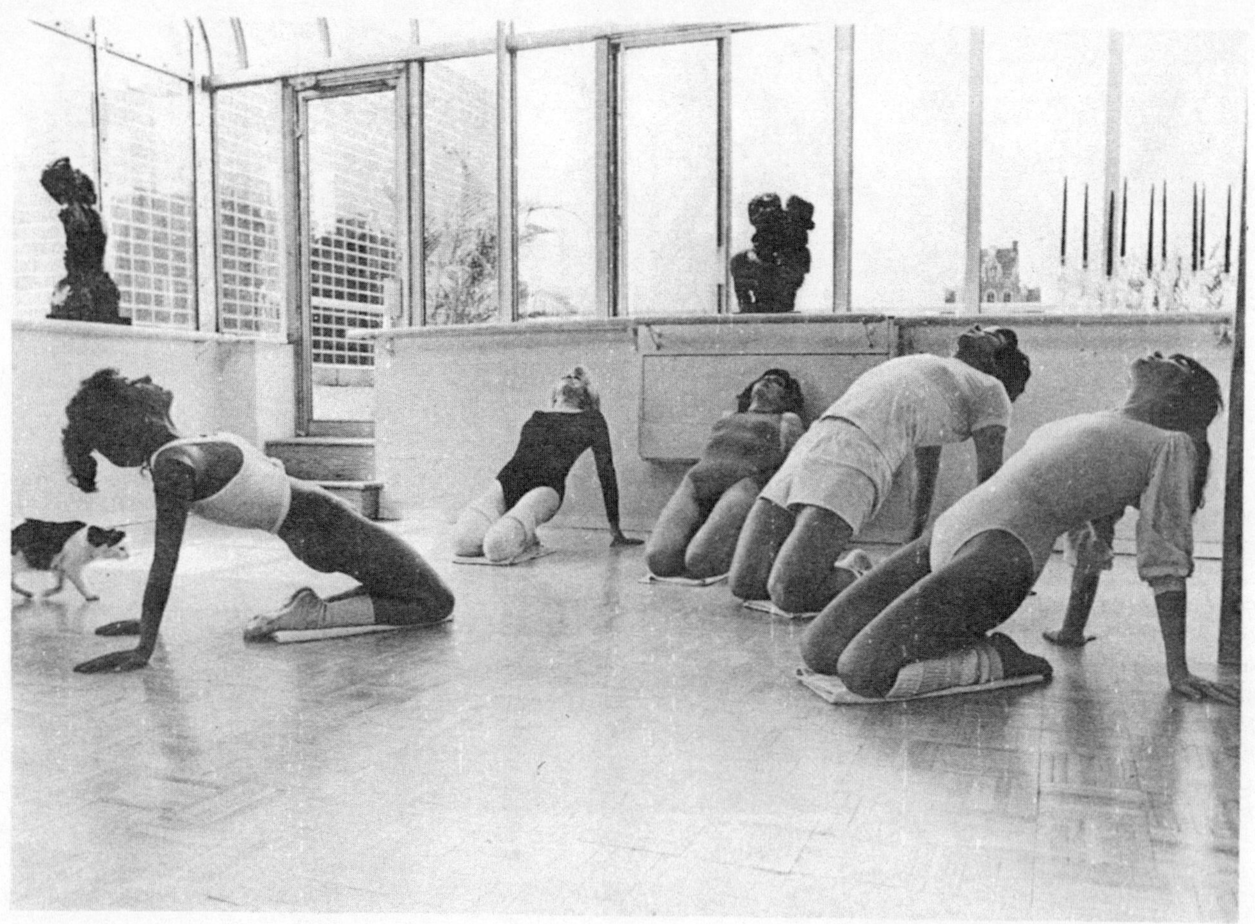

THE THIGH STRETCH
Kneeling with your knees and feet together, put your palms on the floor either beside or behind your toes. Tighten your behind and stomach. Slowly tip your pelvis up as high as you can go. Hold for a count of 10, trying to go higher at each count, then relax. Do 10 times. This also stretches your neck, pectoral muscles, spine, and stomach, as well as your thighs. This stretch does not *tighten the behind.* ▲

CHAPTER FOURTEEN

Inner Thigh Squeeze

If your legs look wonderful but your inner thighs jiggle when you walk, you are not alone. Inner thighs and underarms are the most difficult areas of the human body to firm up.

I cringe at the very thought of the time and energy wasted on exercises that are supposed to tighten the inner thighs and don't. Especially since I've found an exercise that works. In fact, it works so well I wouldn't teach anything else.

Pay special attention to this area of the upper leg because, as the *outer* thigh becomes tighter, the *inner* thigh will appear to be flabbier and fleshier than ever before.

My primary objection to other inner thigh exercises is that they are incomplete. Most are stretches without the all-important balancing action of a contraction. Unless your muscles are contracted, you will have well-stretched legs with mushy, dangling inner thighs.

This is a peaceful exercise—a perfect way to end an exercise session. It can be done wherever you can sit on the floor, spread your legs out straight in front of you, and squeeze the sides of a chair, table, or ladder—whatever you have handy. Just make sure it's not your great-grandmother's Queen Anne lady's desk chair or anything else that is fragile. Many chair legs have been broken by inner thighs so strong that the deep contraction crushes the furniture.

When deciding what you should squeeze, look for a chair or table with legs between twelve and thirty-six inches apart. The distance does not really matter, but this span is most comfortable.

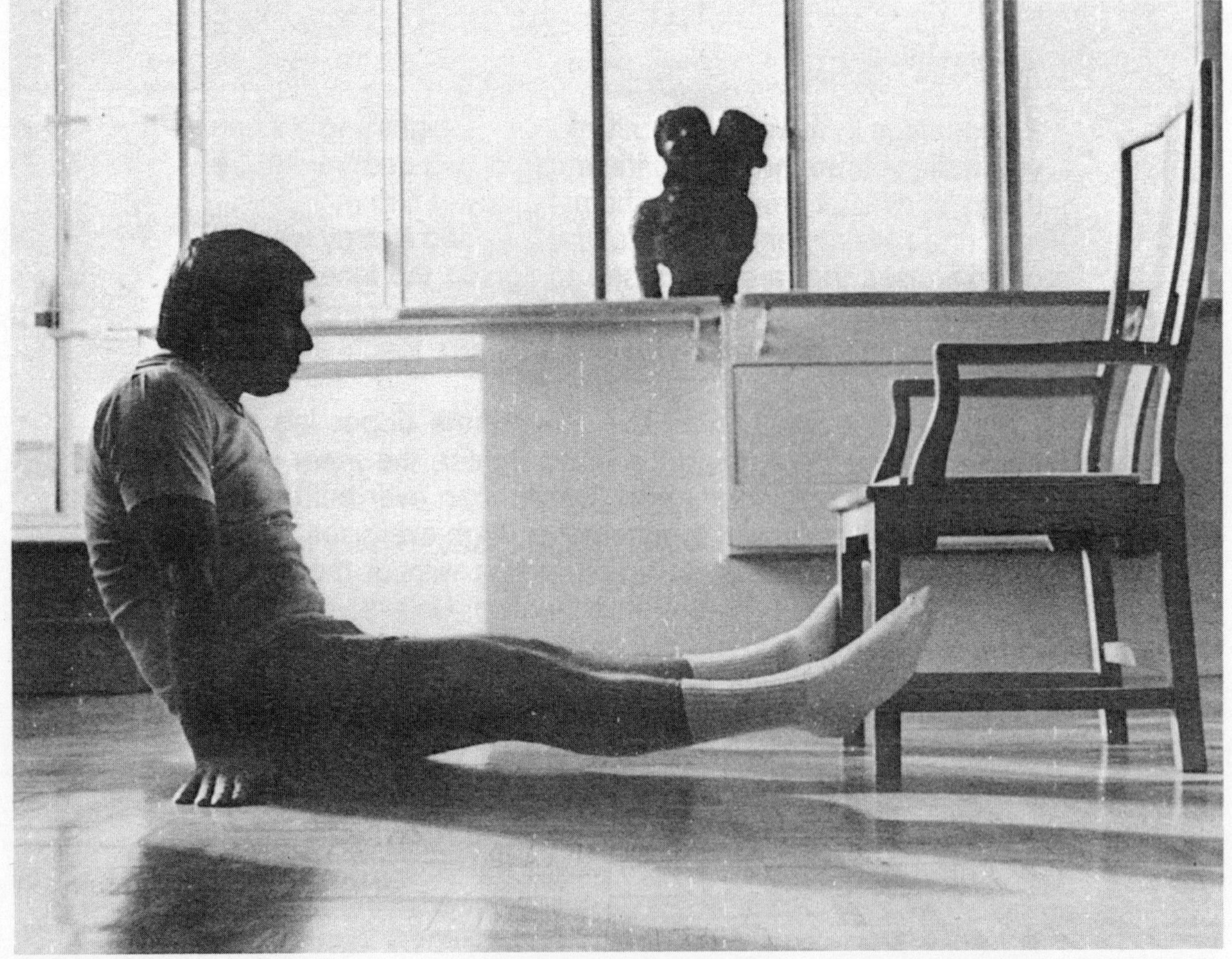

THE MAIN SQUEEZE *Sit on the floor in front of a chair, legs out in front of you. Place the arch of each foot on the outside of the chair legs, pointing your toes as though trying to crush the chair legs together with your feet. Place hands gently on the floor beside your hips or slightly forward. Relax the top of your body and let your head and shoulders fall forward so as not to put pressure on your lower back. Squeeze your feet and legs together around the chair legs, tightening your inner thighs as much as you can for a slow count of 100. Hold steadily; do not squeeze and release. When you first start this exercise, you may feel the muscles in the calves and inner knee areas working. This is because your inner thighs are lazy. They've never worked this hard before, and will let anything do their work for them. Very soon you will only feel it in your inner thighs.* ▲

Harvey, who had been to two classes when these pictures were taken, demonstrates two ways to do this very valuable exercise.

As you can see, we women are not alone in wanting our legs to be firm and fit all over—including our inner thighs.

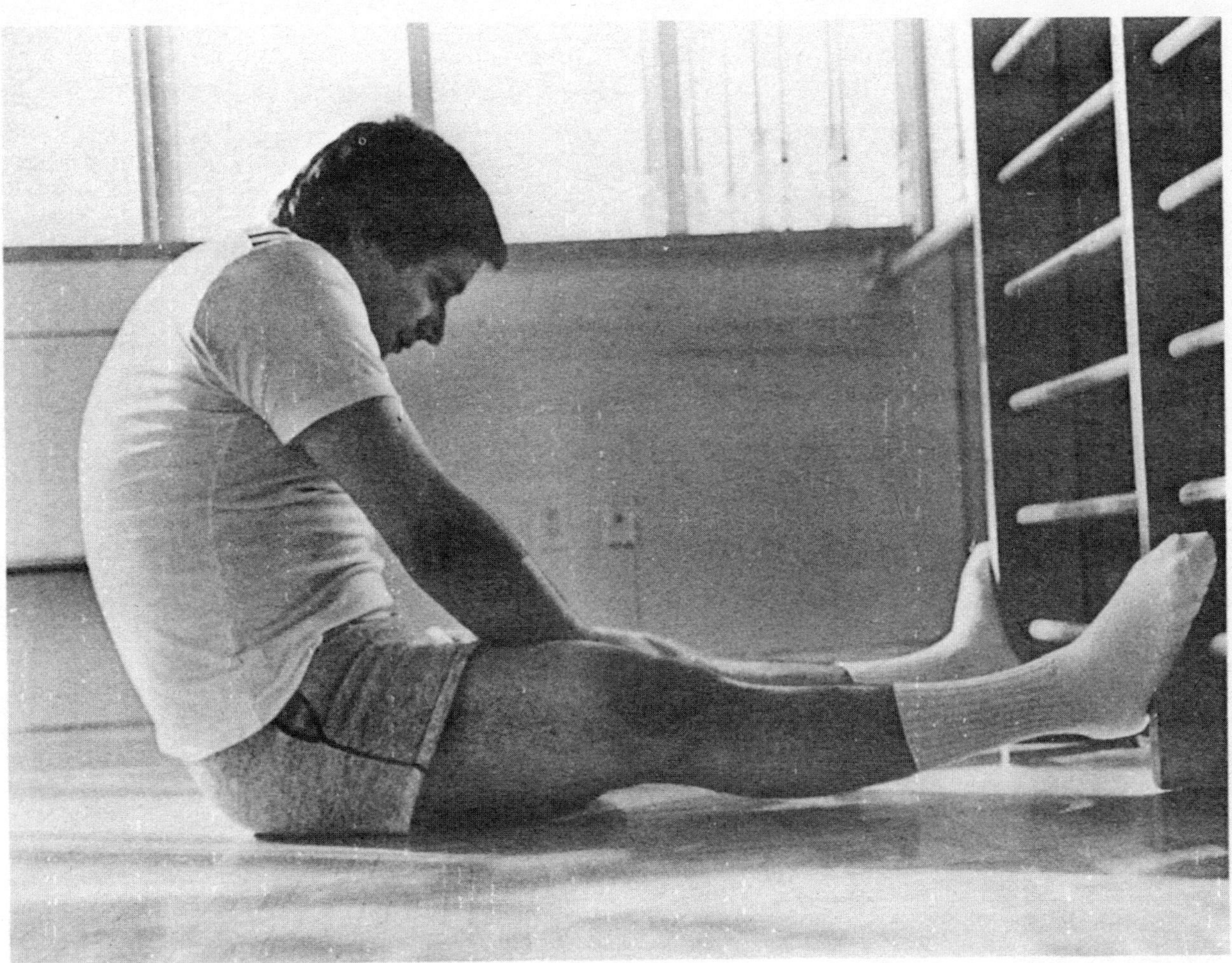

A VARIATION ON THE MAIN SQUEEZE *The difference here is in the placement of the hands and arms to release your lower back more. Rest your hands gently on the floor between your legs, rounding your shoulders forward so that your hands are even with your knees. Whenever you do this powerful exercise, relax your neck, arms, lower back, shoulders—everything* but *your inner thighs—and think peaceful, positive thoughts. This will make you even more aware that you do not have to put pressure on your lower back. At about the count of 50, you will feel the shift and your inner thigh muscles will take over. By your third session, you will be counting to 300 before stopping this relaxing squeeze. To accomplish this, count to 100, release, and repeat by 100s.* ▲

CHAPTER FIFTEEN

The One-Hour Program—A Summary

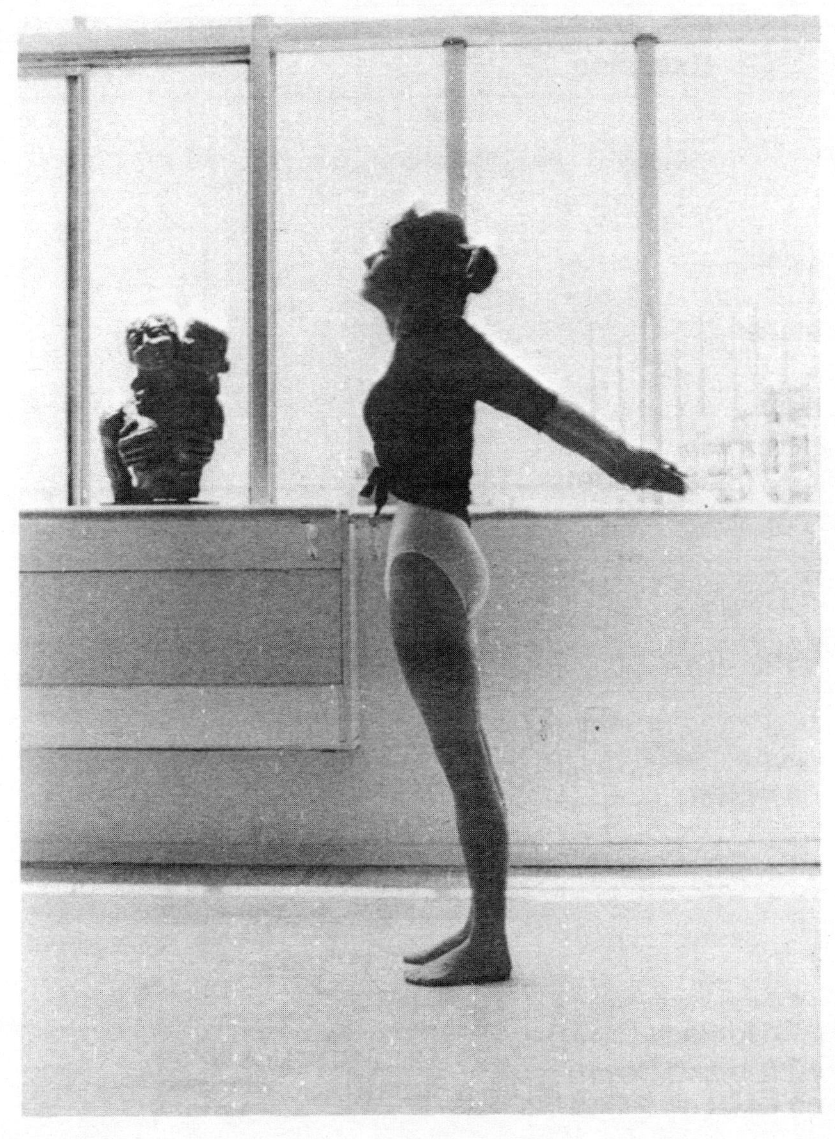

INSTRUCTIONS

This chart can provide you with the cues you need to guide you through the One-Hour Program. Use the column at the right to pencil in the number of repetitions you need to do, or make little sketches that will tickle your memory about the position you should be in.

Exercise	Progress / Notes
WARMING UP Warm-up # 1 (Hanging) Warm-up # 2 (Up and Down) Underarm Tightener Waist Stretch Hamstring Stretch Neck Exercise #1 (Roll) Neck Exercise #2 (Side to Side)	
FOR THE STOMACH For the Stomach #1 (Knees Bent) For the Stomach #2 (One Leg Up) For the Stomach #3 (Both Legs Up)	
FOR THE LEGS For the Legs #1 (Up-Back-Down) For the Legs #2 (Up and Down) For the Legs #3 (Heel on *Barre*) For the Legs #4 (Arch on *Barre*)	

Exercise	Progress / Notes
FOR THE BEHIND AND HIPS For the Behind and Hips #1 (Seated, Leg Bent) For the Behind and Hips #2 (Seated, Leg Straight) For the Behind and Hips #3 (Kneeling, Leg Bent) For the Behind and Hips #4 (Kneeling, Leg Straight)	
OPEN & CLOSE	
STRETCHING Stretch #1 (Legs Apart) Stretch #2 (To the Sides) Stretch #3 (Legs Together) Stretch #4 (Hamstring Stretch) Stretch #5 (Leg Over) Stretch #6 (Calves)	
FOR THE PELVIS Pelvic Rotations Pelvic Scoop Thigh Stretch	
INNER THIGH SQUEEZE The Main Squeeze Variation on Main Squeeze	

CHAPTER SIXTEEN

The 15-Minute Maintenance Plan

When I hear someone say they exercise an hour every day to try to get a beautiful figure, I find it difficult not to laugh. If a beautiful body is what they want, these people have the wrong idea about exercise. I don't spend an hour a day on my own body, and exercise is my profession!

Most people don't have the time to exercise for an hour each and every day, or even three times a week, as many people recommend. It is not realistic, especially for busy people who have families to take care of and normal, nine-to-five jobs.

The truth is this: An hour a day does not necessarily keep the flab away.

To promise yourself that you will make this unrealistic demand on your time and your body is setting yourself up for failure. This is especially true if you are doing exercises that do not produce rapid results. Nine times out of ten you will quit exercising altogether if you are unable to maintain this one hour per day regimen for yourself without seeing dramatic and rapid improvements in your body. I've seen it happen too often.

This 15-Minute Maintenance Plan is my answer to the time problems facing today's busy person. I first designed it for my students who travel and don't have time for one-hour workouts. Once students have completed a program of classes and have their bodies looking the way they want them to, they often adopt this as a daily routine.

Do not expect to discontinue the One-Hour Program in favor of this 15-Minute Maintenance Plan until you com-

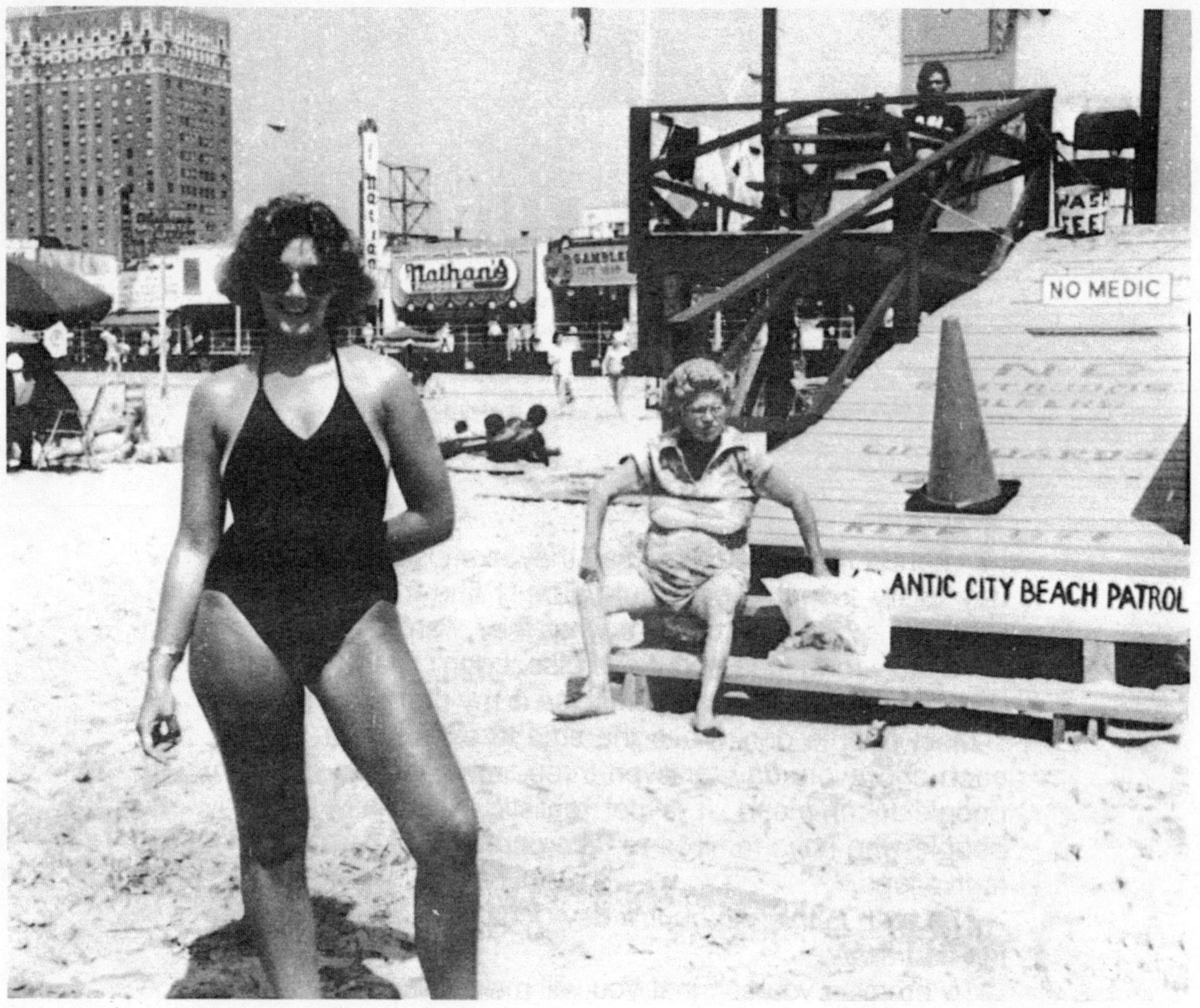

Before she tightened up her body so much that she no longer wore large-size clothes, Kelle Kerr was a busy model for the larger woman. This snapshot will give you an idea of how hefty she was at her prime as a model. ▲

pletely understand the movements and want to maintain your fitness level. This is *not* a program for beginners. I cannot stress this warning enough.

The 15-Minute Maintenance Plan is an abbreviated version of the One-Hour Program. It is the basics, timed to take fifteen minutes from start to finish.

Should you want to concentrate on a specific part of the body that is not emphasized in this short session, feel free. Add whatever exercises from the One-Hour Program that you feel you should, but also add to your schedule the amount of time that you will need to do them. *Do not* eliminate any exercise simply to allow yourself time to do another exercise within the fifteen-minute time period.

This program is balanced to work on the parts of the body that generally need the most work. To omit one exercise in favor of something else, or something you find easier or more comfortable to do, would upset this balance. You won't get the rapid results you desire.

Break down the 15-Minute Maintenance Plan even further, interspersing your exercises with your daily schedule. One young mother I know works a full-time job. She does five minutes of the exercises in the morning, before she wakes the children for nursery school, and then works in five minutes more at her office, instead of having coffee and danish on her morning break. She completes her program before bedtime, after her little ones have gone to sleep.

One might think she could get enough exercise with her busy schedule, but she can't. By dividing the fifteen-minute program to fit her time requirements, she now has the time to take care of her body *and* do everything else on her daily agenda.

This student decided to take my advice after she had spent hundreds of dollars joining health clubs and gyms. She reasoned that, since she had paid so much to join, she would *make* time to go and work out, but for no other reason than to get her money's worth. She never had the time, no matter how much she juggled her schedule. Now, she gets in an hour and fifteen minutes of concentrated exercise per five-day work week and feels fabulous for it. She knows that she could have faster results in shaping her body if she interspersed the One-Hour Program with the 15-Minute Maintenance Plan every second or third day, but that *is not* always possible.

Kelle Kerr, who demonstrated these exercises for our photographs, is a model in real life. She was one of the top large-size models in the business when she started coming to my classes to tone up her body. After a very short time, however, she had tightened up so much that she was too small for the job, even though she had not lost any weight.

For a while Kelle was able to continue working with the help of a padded body suit that made her body her pre-exercise size. Before long that didn't work—her neck had become too long and thin, and her legs, too slim and sleek to be in proportion with her padded, larger body.

With her new, voluptuous body, Kelle is getting many new modeling jobs, often more exciting than before.

No matter what other shape-up program Kelle has tried, she invariably comes back to these exercises to keep her body in top form . . . and she doesn't have to take time off from her career to exercise, either.

When you see the exercises in this 15-Minute Maintenance Plan, you may want to refresh your memory with the more detailed instructions in the One-Hour Program.

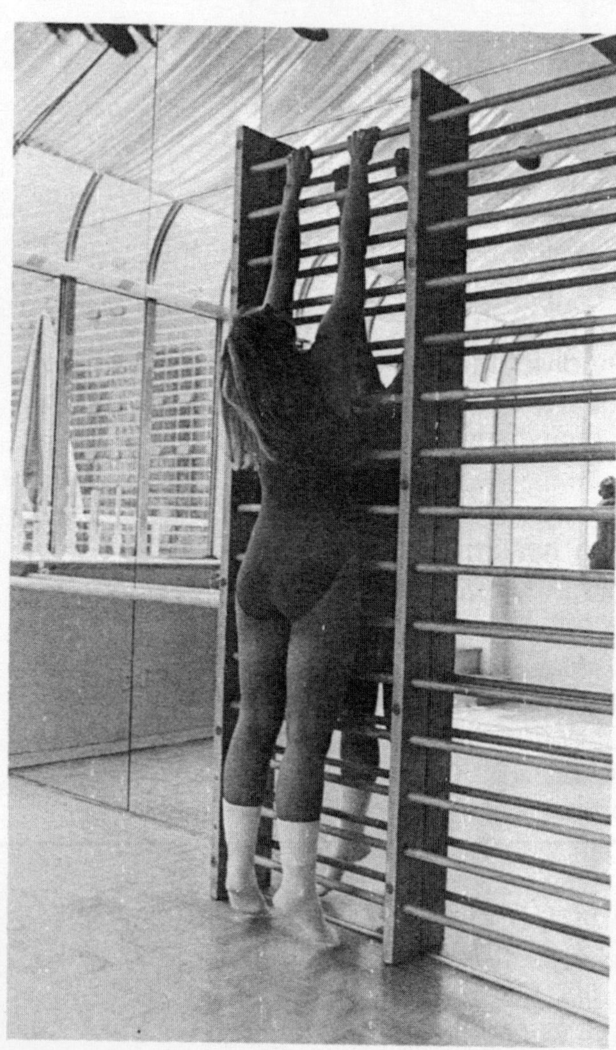

WARMING UP # 1 *Hang from a ladder or door, completely relaxing your body and allowing any tension or stress you may feel to drip like wax to the floor. This stretches the spine and relaxes the body, readying you to begin exercise. Hold for as long as your wrists and arms will allow. The longer you can hang, the stronger your arms and wrists will become and the more your entire body will stretch.* ◀

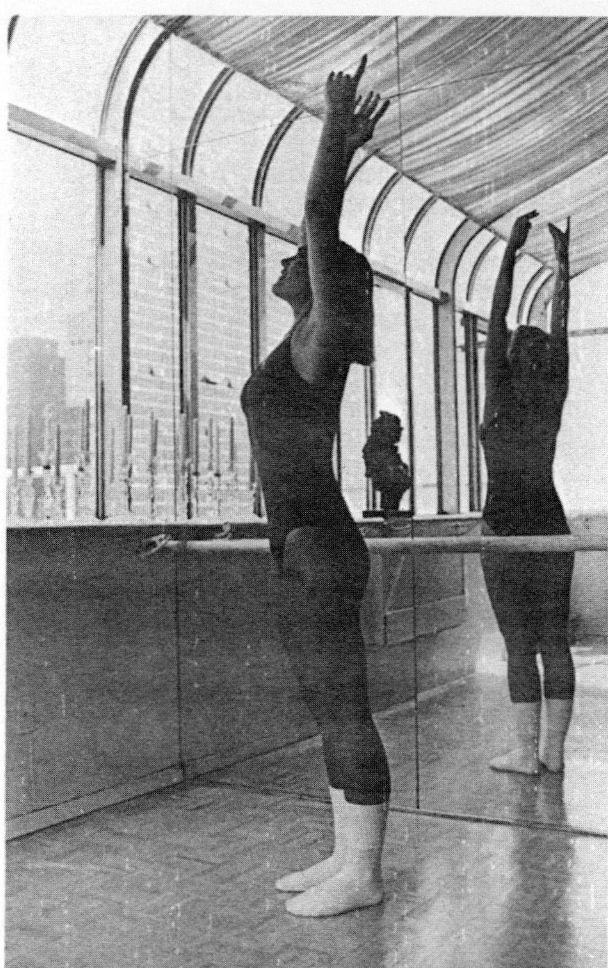

Stand erect, with legs and feet together or no more than a foot apart for balance. Stretch arms up over the head, lifting the torso as high as you can, as if you were trying to make yourself 2 inches taller. ▲

Flex the knees and bend forward, gently moving your arms out in front of you. Be sure to keep stretching out with your torso as you move. Continue to bend your legs and stretch your torso. Hold in your stomach and breathe naturally. Stretch your arms up behind you as far as possible. Do not swing or jerk your arms. Every move must be gentle and precise. Gently move your arms forward again and stretch upward into an erect position. Reach for the sky. Repeat 5 times. ▼

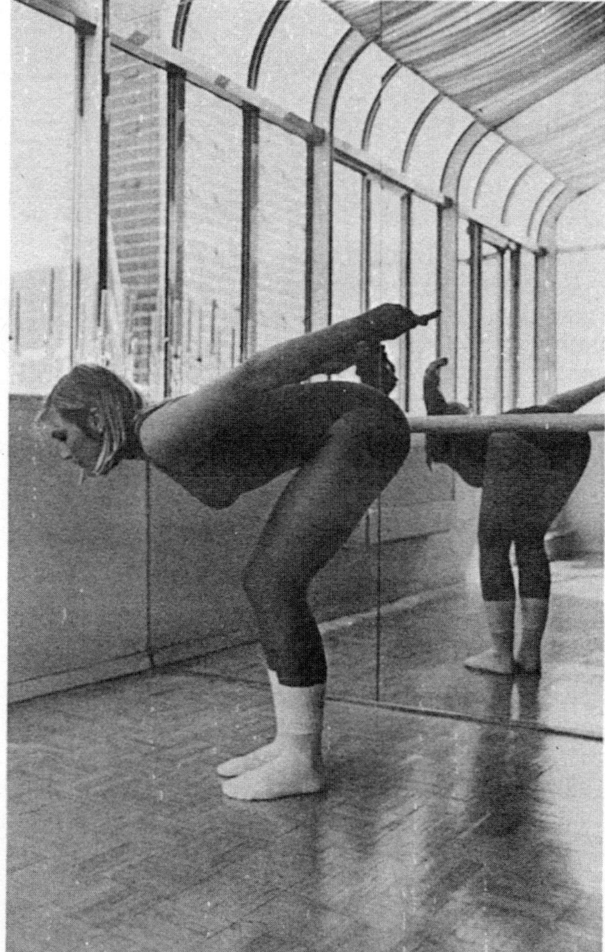

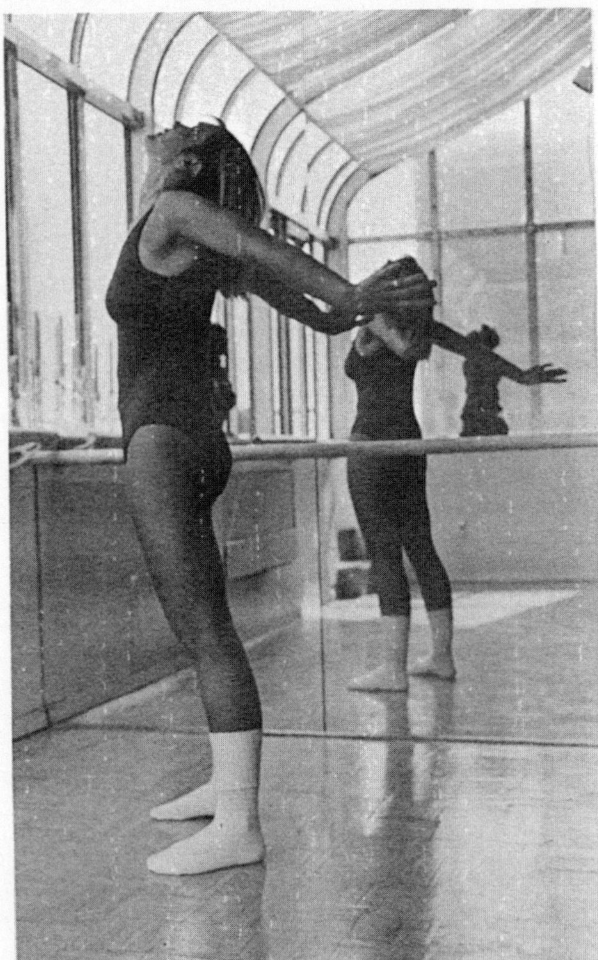

FOR TIGHT UNDERARMS *Stand erect with your arms stretched out straight to the sides at shoulder level. Roll arms forward from the shoulder so that your thumbs face upward. Reach your arms to the back, as though trying to lock thumbs. Hold your head and shoulders back to loosen tightness between your shoulder blades and in your pectorals. Gently move arms back and forth a half inch in each direction. Do 75.* Remember: *Keep your buttocks tight, pelvis tipped up, and hold in your stomach as you do any of these standing exercises.* ▲

WAIST STRETCH *Stand up straight, placing your left hand on the side of your left leg, elbow out. Tighten your behind muscles and tip your pelvis upward. Keep your tummy tight and your hips even. Stretch your body upward. Reach over your head and to the left with your right arm, keeping your elbow straight and stretching out with your fingers as though you were trying to touch something on a table beside you on the left. Reach as far as you can and then reach a half inch farther. Your left arm will bend as it rests on your leg. Relax neck. Do not bounce and do not throw your hip out if at all possible.* Remember: *Bring your upper body and arms around to the front before you straighten up. Do 75 on each side.* ▼

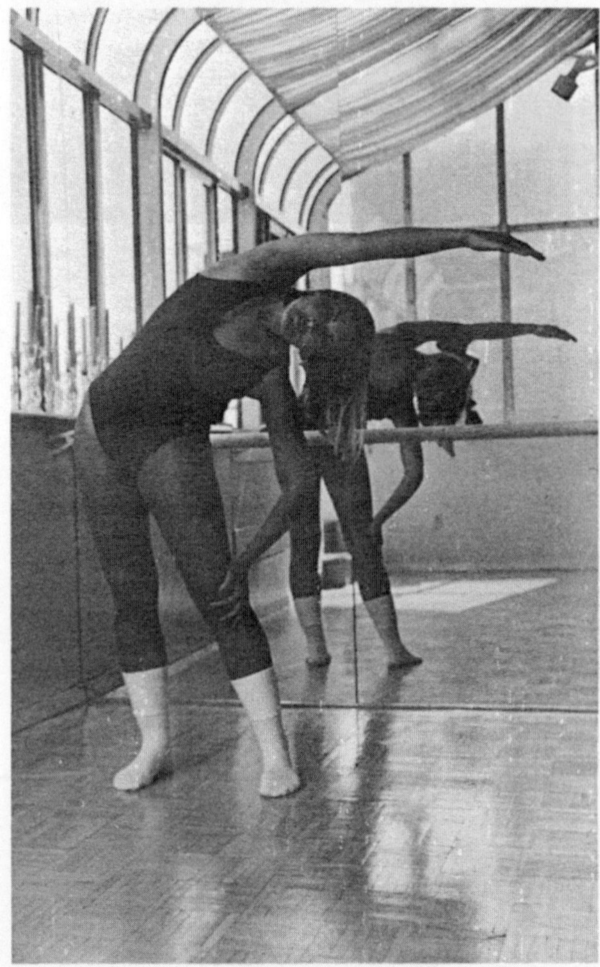

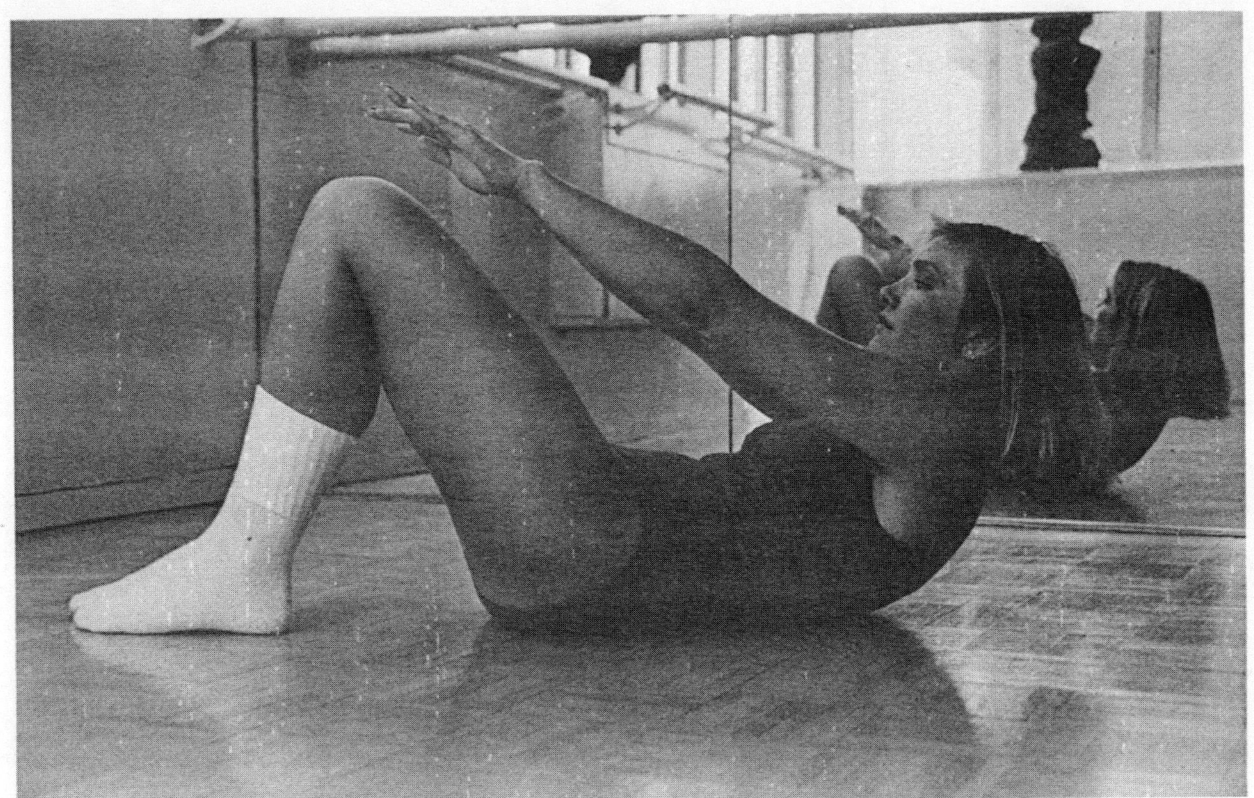

FOR THE STOMACH #1 *Lie on your back with your knees bent and feet flat on the floor. Push the small of your back into the floor. Grab your inner thighs, elbows out, and gently pull your upper body up as far as you can. Keep your shoulders rounded and relaxed. Raise your arms parallel with your thighs without letting your head and shoulders drop back to the floor. Reach forward from this point a half inch to an inch further. Do not do this exercise by moving your head. Reach with your arms, shoulders, and upper body—rounding upward from just under your bust—as one gentle movement. The behind and legs do not move. Keep them relaxed. Repeat 75 times.* ▲

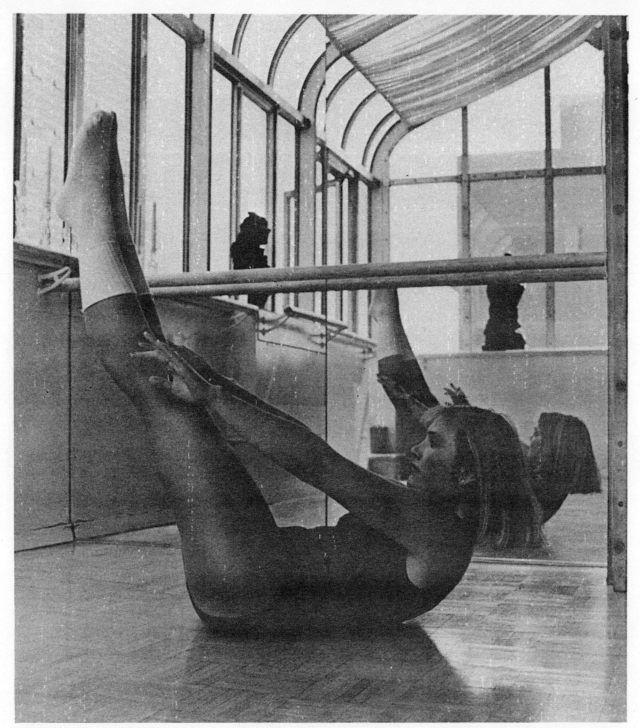

FOR THE STOMACH #2 *Lie flat on your back, pressing the small of your back into the floor, and raise your legs straight upward to at least a 60-degree angle with the floor. Grasp your outer legs as close to your knees as you can reach. Extending your elbows out to each side, round your shoulders, and pull the top of your body upward toward your legs. Without dropping your legs and arms or your upper body, release hold on your legs. Reach arms upward, as if you were trying to touch your toes. Move the top of your body up and down a half inch to an inch in each direction. Repeat 75 times. Return to starting position.* ▲

FOR THE LEGS #1 *Stand on your toes, facing the* barre, *with your heels together, knees and toes turned out to the sides, back erect and stomach in. Relax your shoulders and arms as you gently grasp the* barre *with both hands. Lift your head high. Imagine you are being seated in a chair. Do not stick out your behind—tighten your buttocks and tilt your pelvis upward. Let your pelvis go back to the starting position. Lower your body not more than an inch, keeping your legs as relaxed as possible and your knees bent, heels touching.* ▼

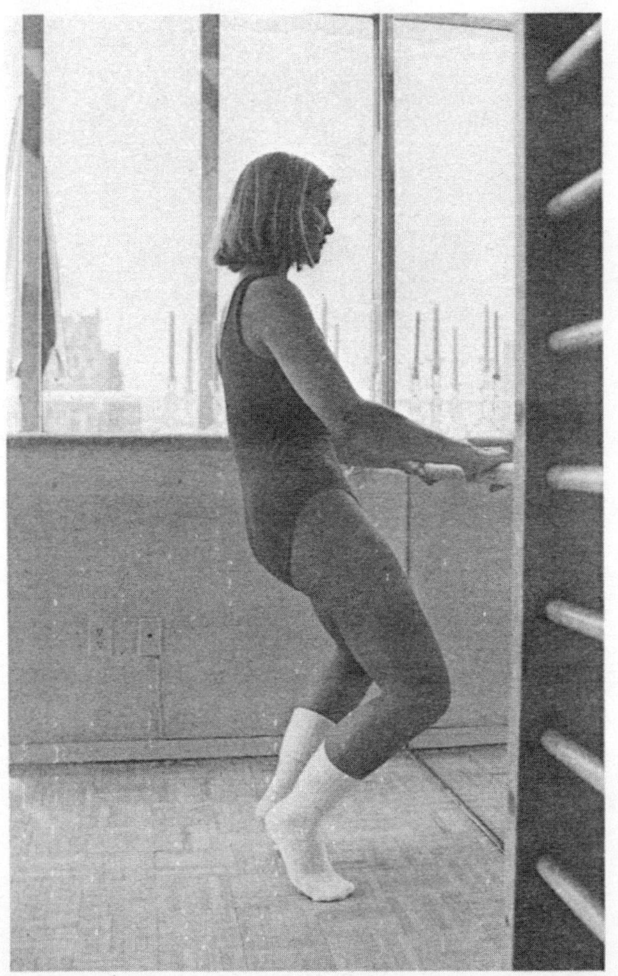

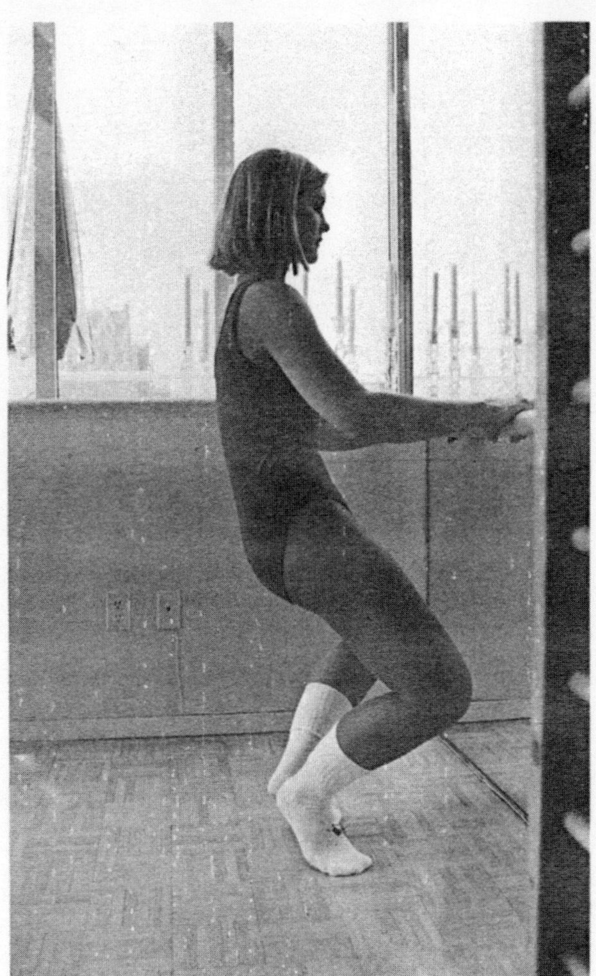

Tilt your pelvis up again and then return to the straightened position, 1 inch lower than when you started this exercise. Lower your body another inch. Repeat this combination 1 more time, lowering your body another inch, and then return to a standing position by reversing the process—tip pelvis upward, back, and then raise your body 1 inch higher, continuing the process until you are at the original starting position. Do 5. Do not let heels go down when reversing the process. ▲

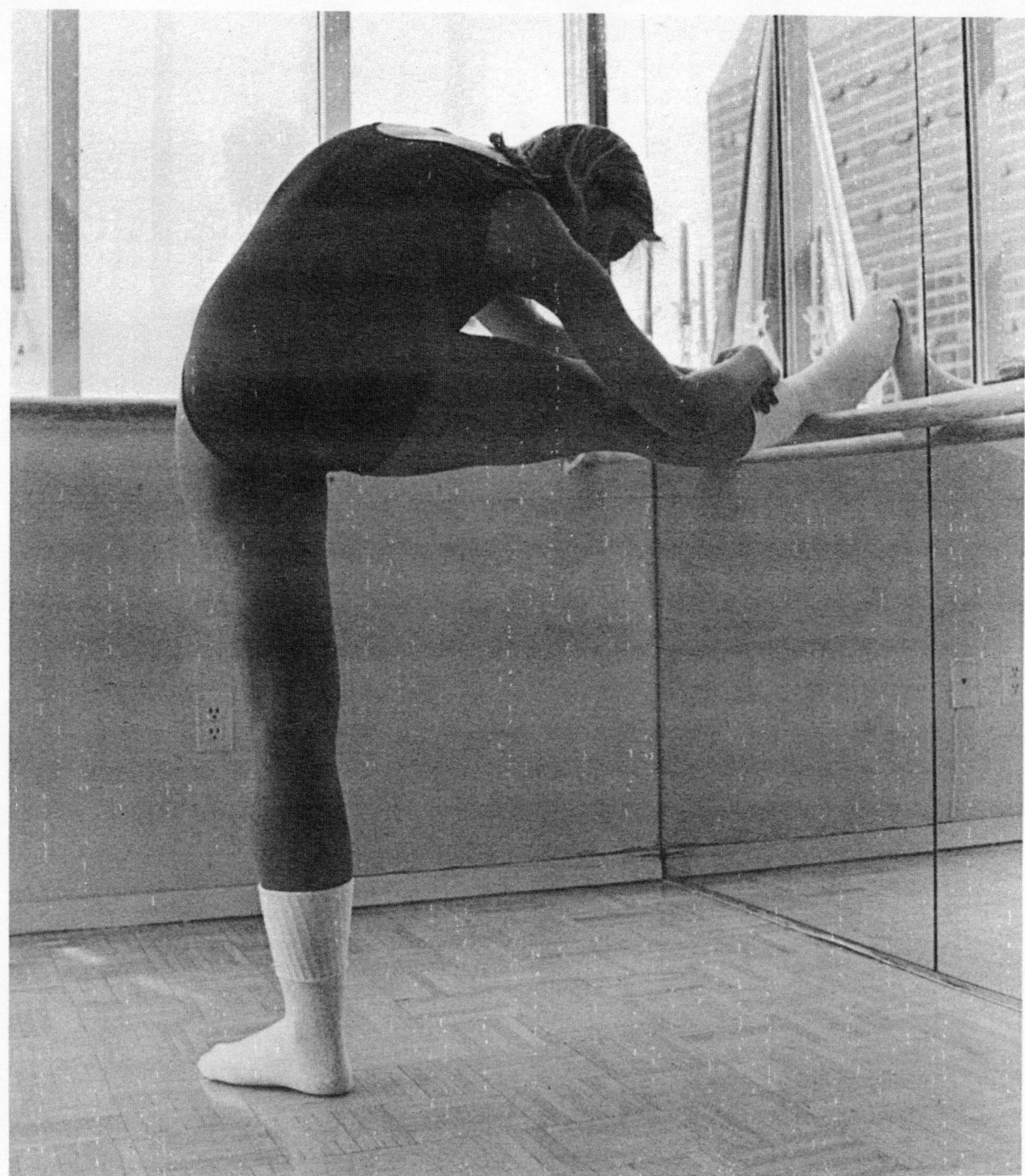

FOR THE LEGS #2 *Stand erect with 1 foot resting gently on the* barre. *Raise your arms high over your head, stretching your entire body upward. When you put 1 foot up on the* barre, *you must not lock the knee of the leg you are standing on. Turn your torso forward, bending your body over your raised leg, and stretch your arms gently toward your ankle. Fold your hands across your raised leg, as close to the ankle as possible. Gently lean forward over your leg, holding that position or moving the upper body back and forth, a half inch in each direction, 25 times. Do not jerk. Make slow, precise motions. Change legs and repeat.* Remember: *People with a tendency toward the sciatica syndrome should ask their physician or chiropractor if they should do this exercise.* ▲

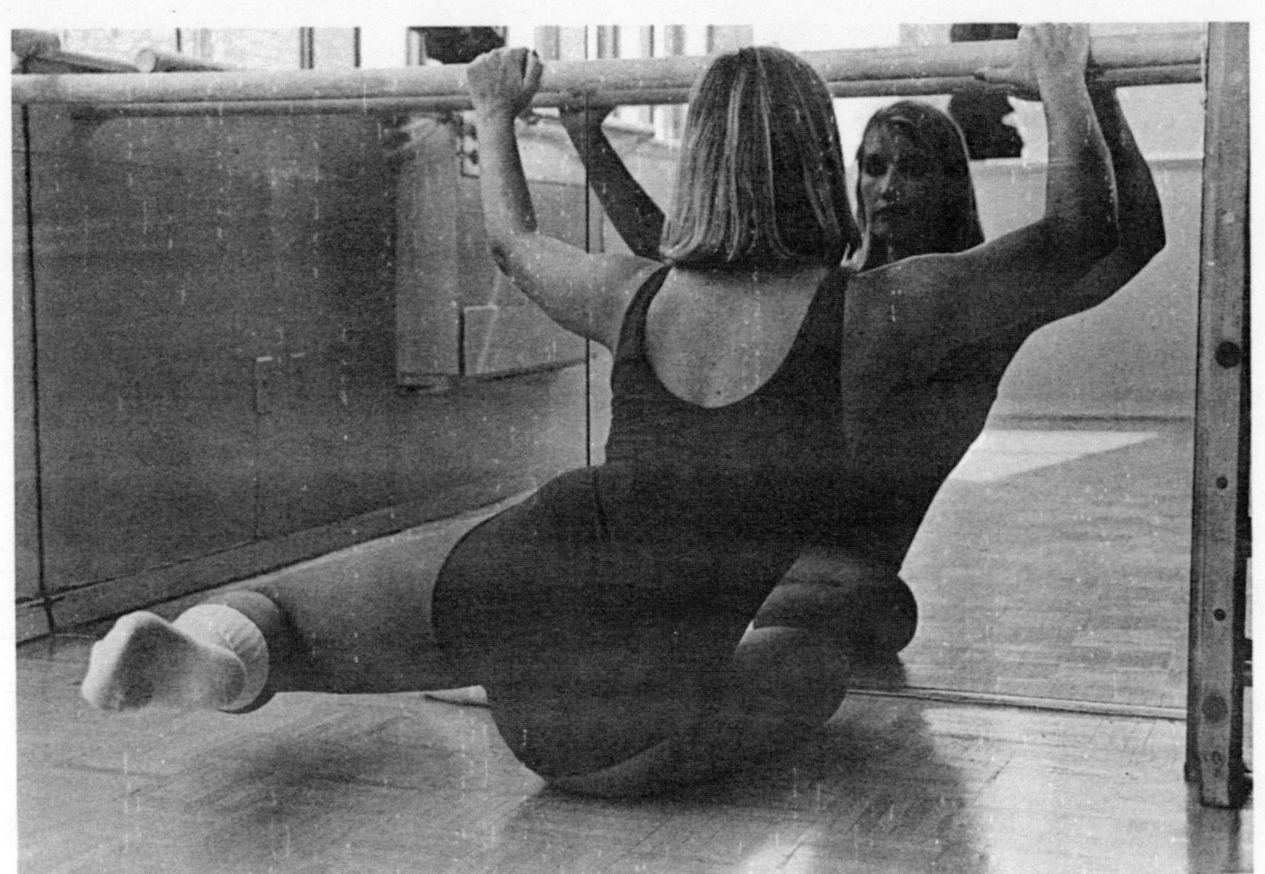

FOR TIGHTENING THE BEHIND AND HIPS #1 *Sit on the floor, facing the* barre*—or whatever you're using as a* barre*—with the right leg bent in front of the body and the left leg extended to the side, knee bent so that foot is behind body. Clasp the* barre *with both hands. Roll left hip forward, allowing the left foot to come off the floor. The foot should be turned upward, higher than the left knee. Tighten behind, and tip pelvis up. Lift knee 2 inches off the floor. Move left leg gently back 1 inch, keeping left hip rolled forward so that both hips are even. Return leg forward 1 inch. Repeat 75 times on each side.* Reminder: *Do not bring knee in front of hips.* ▲

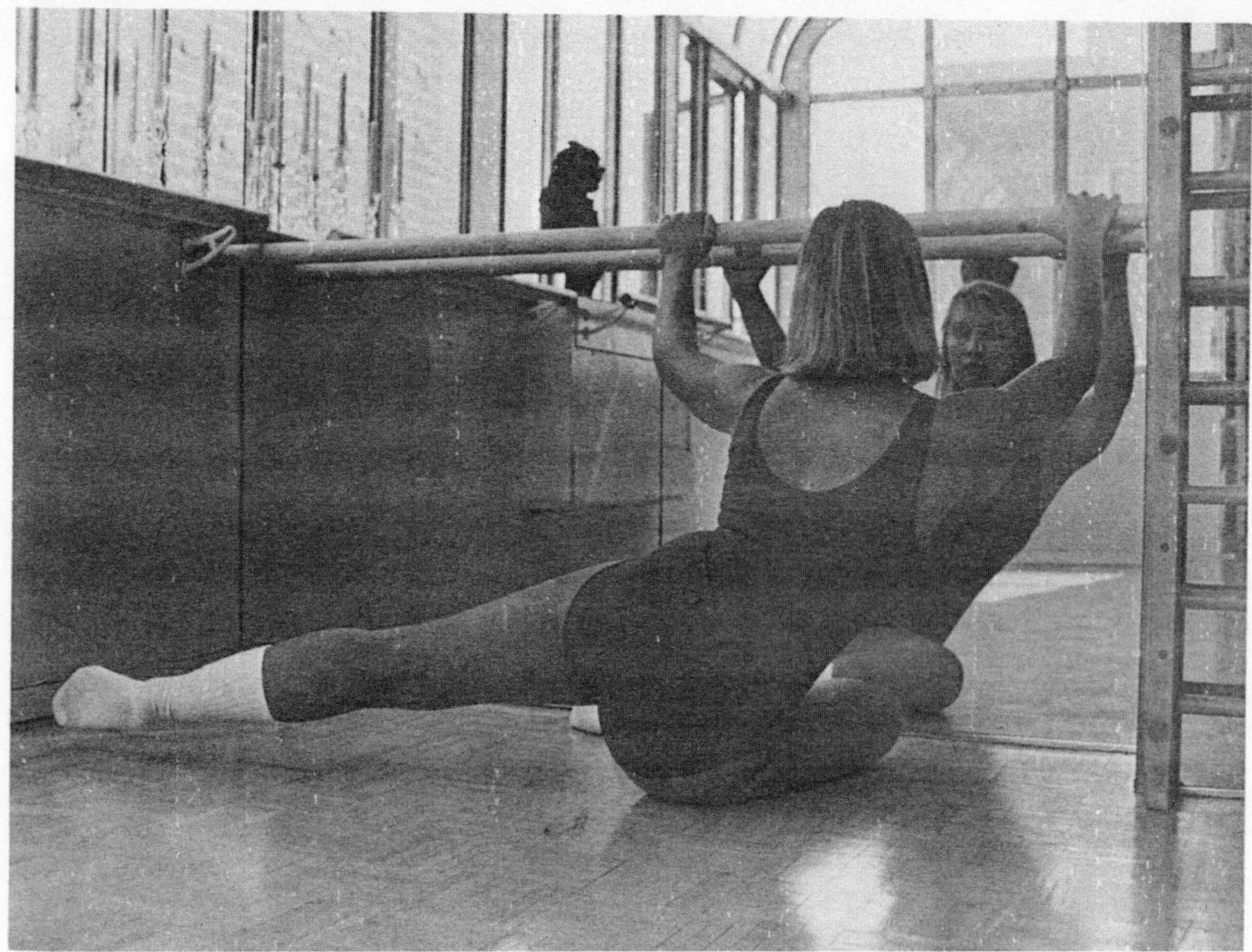

FOR TIGHTENING BEHIND AND HIPS #2 *Sit on the floor, facing the* barre, *in the same position—the left leg stretched out straight to the left side. If you completed the preceding exercise with your left leg working, start this exercise with your left leg bent in front and your right leg out to give the muscles on your left side a breather. Clasp the* barre *with both hands. Roll the left hip toward the* barre *and tip pelvis up. Try to turn the top of the left foot toward the floor. Raise left leg 1½ to 2 inches off the floor, keeping the leg straight and the left hip rolled forward.* Remember: *If you can raise your leg more than 2 inches off the floor, you are throwing your hip out and not keeping it even. This transfers contractions to your front thigh muscles. Repeat 75 times on each side.* ▲

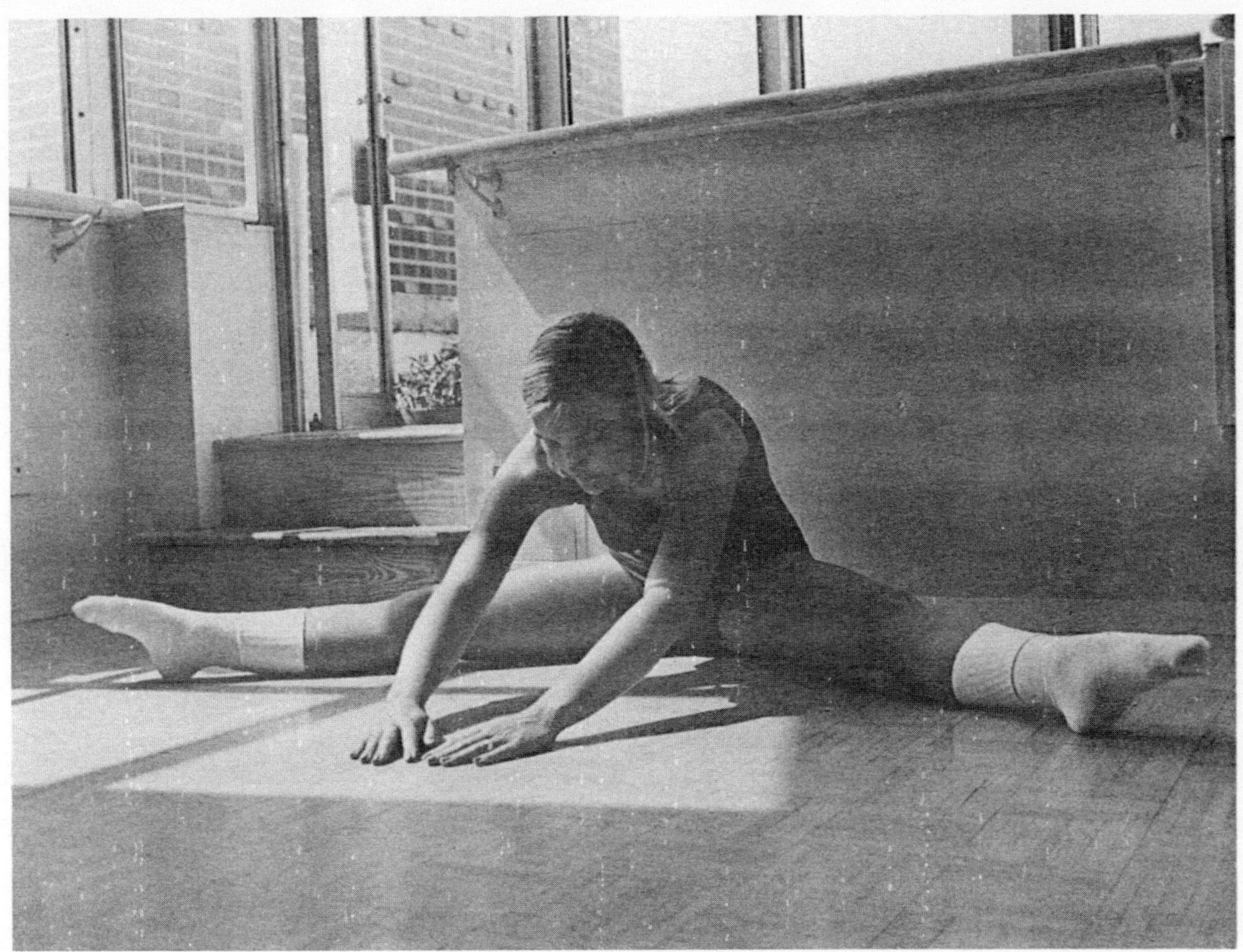

STRETCHING #1 *Sit firmly on the floor, legs spread out to each side. Reach both arms out in front of your body and gently stretch as far forward as you can from that position. Rest hands on floor. Move torso back and forth a half inch in each direction 25 times. Do not jerk or bounce. Remember to curve your shoulders forward to stretch your spine more. Don't worry if you still can't touch the floor with both hands. Keep them on your thighs. Some people stretch easier than others.* ▲

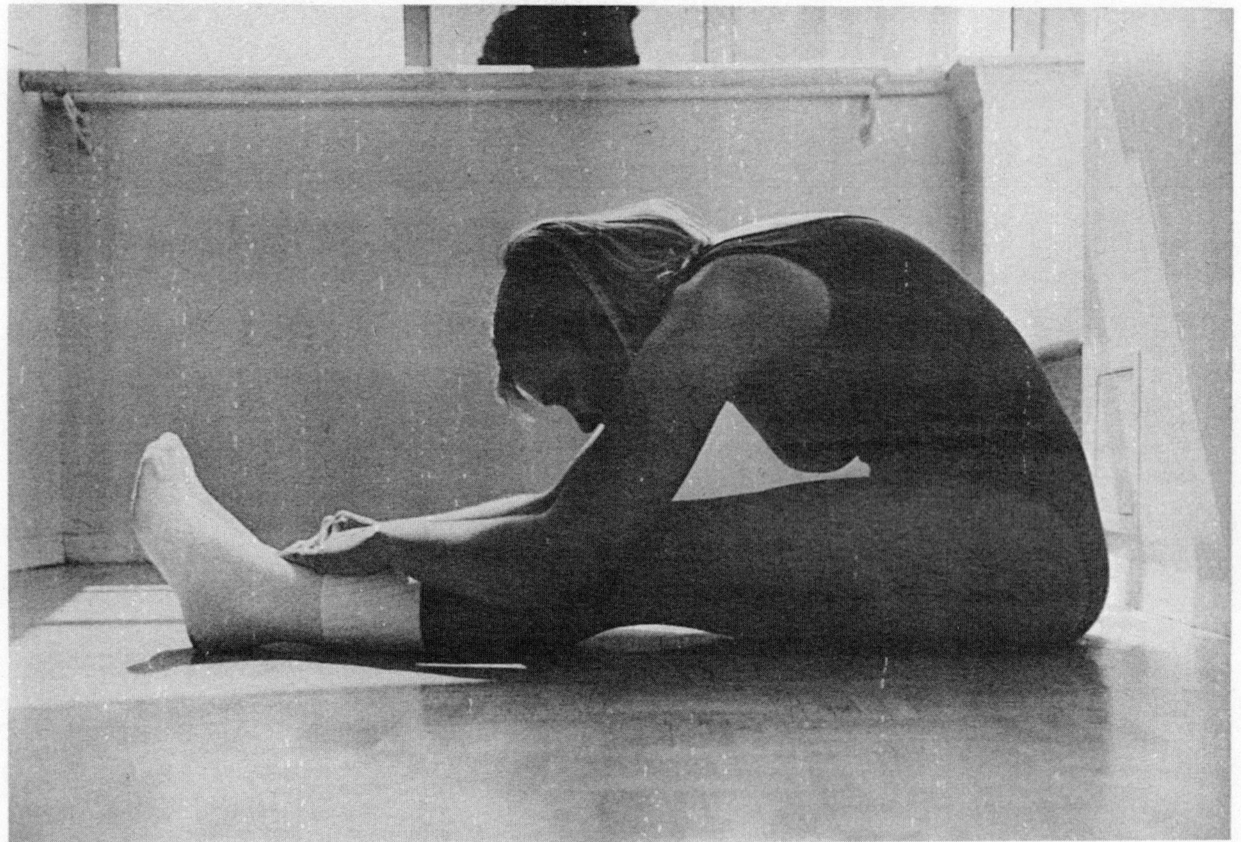

STRETCHING #2 *Stretch your legs out in front of you, knees and feet together. Curl your shoulders forward and stretch your entire torso forward gently, as if you were trying to touch your knees with your forehead. Resting your wrists across your shins for balance, stretch your body as far as you can for a slow, gentle count of 25.* Remember: *The straighter you have your legs, the more intense the stretch. This is not a stretch to be lackadaisical about.* Warning: *No jerking and no fast movements.* ▲

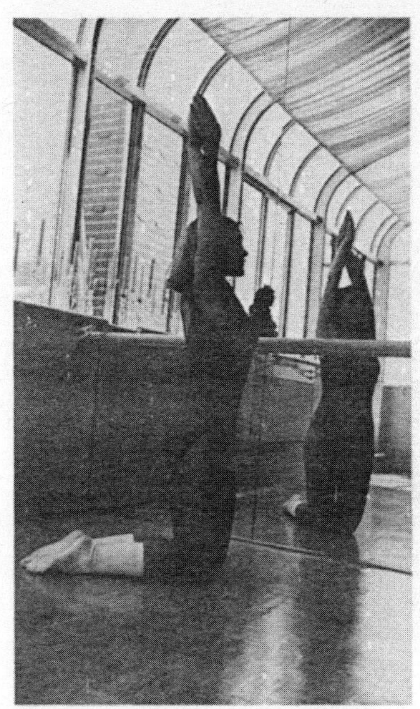

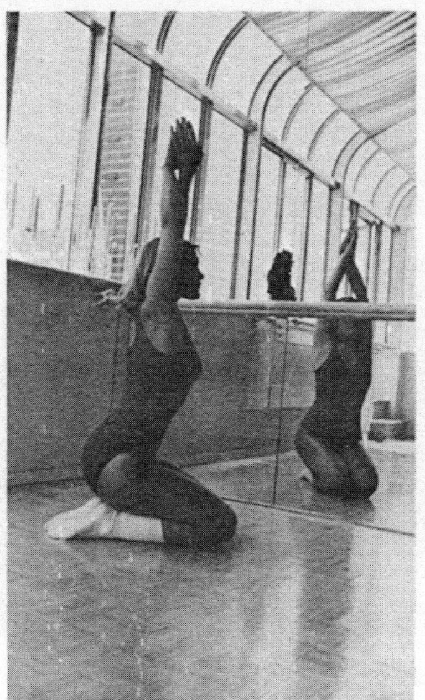

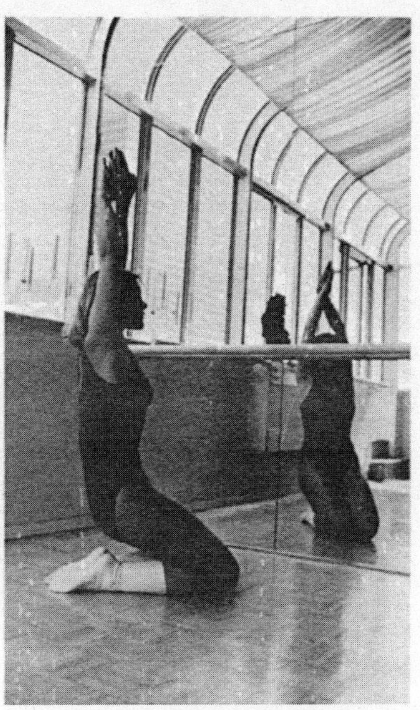

THE PELVIC SCOOP *Kneel on a pad, knees and feet together. Stretch your body upward, lifting your arms high over your head. Do not arch your back. Relax as you do this exercise. From this position, slowly aim your behind down toward your heels. Make sure to keep your torso upright, reaching your arms over your head. When you feel your behind brush your heels, tighten your behind muscles and slowly tip your pelvis upward, as you "scoop" your pelvis up from this low position to your upright starting point. Move delicately, carefully, and do not jerk your body upward. Do 8.* ▲

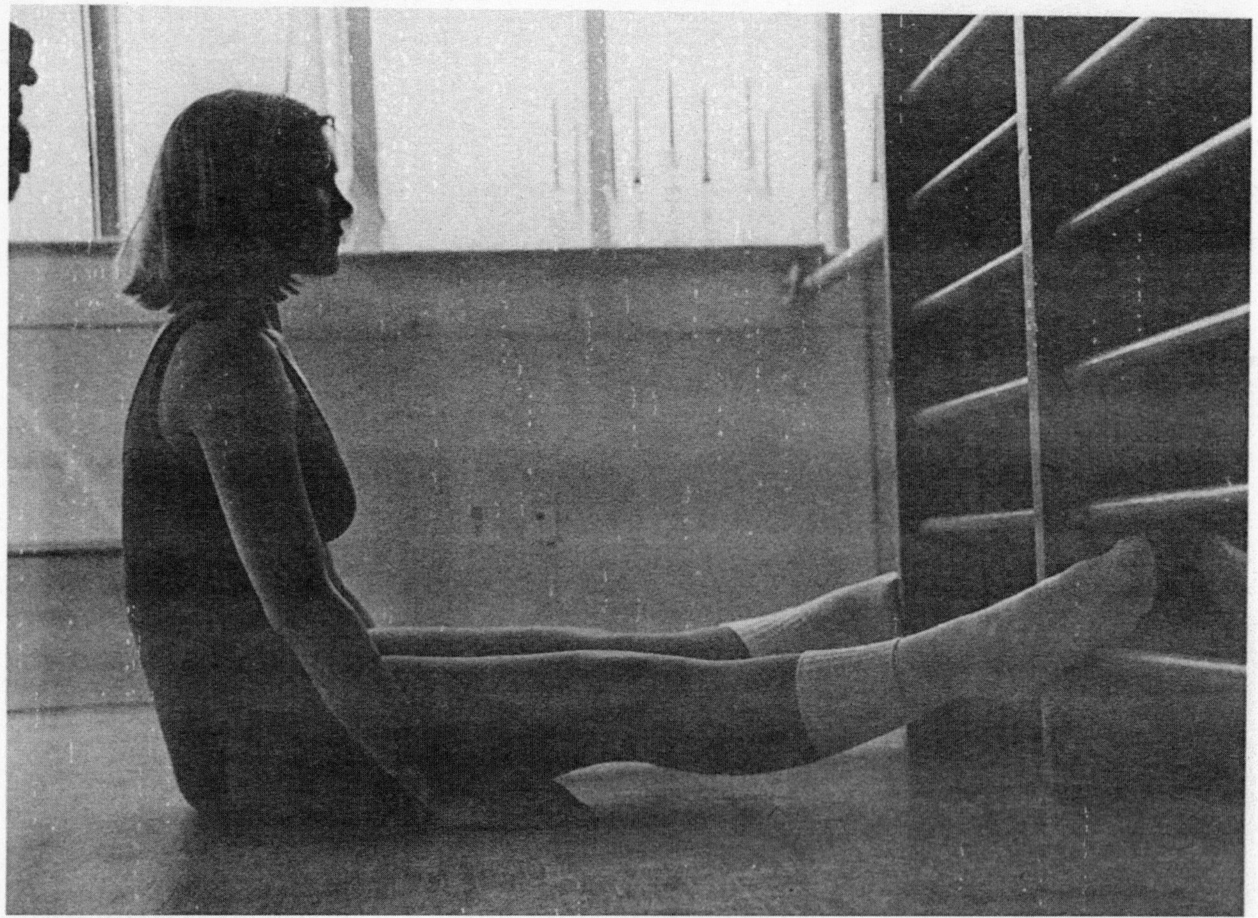

THE INNER THIGH SQUEEZE *Sit on the floor in front of a chair, legs out in front of you. Place the arch of each foot on the outside of the chair legs, pointing your toes as though trying to crush the chair legs together with your feet. Place hands gently on the floor beside your hips or slightly forward. Relax the top of your body and let your head and shoulders fall forward a bit to ease back pressure. Squeeze your feet and legs together around the chair legs, tightening your inner thighs as much as you can for a slow count of 100.* ▲

CHAPTER SEVENTEEN

It's No Wonder My Back Hurt

Being a nomad for the better part of ten years, everything I owned was either stuffed into, or strapped onto, a rucksack that I carried on my back. For a while I even carried a three-by-five-foot Persian rug with me; at another point, a large African tribal drum.

Often walking great distances between towns, thumbing rides when and where I could, it was sometimes a three-day wait before any means of transportation came my way.

During this time, my sixty-five-pound rucksack and I traveled by bus, train, camel, mule-drawn wagon, and, best of all, by truck. Trucks were preferred, because one could stretch out and sleep in comparative privacy. If I sensed danger, it was not too difficult to roll my pack off and jump out after it.

Most of the time while roaming the world, I weighed less than eighty pounds—especially after several bouts of dysentery. My fragile condition was exacerbated by the constant pain and pressure on my knees, rubbed raw from supporting a weight almost equal to my own for many miles a day. So, between the knees, scoliosis, disc problems, swayback, and distorted feet, it's no wonder my back hurt.

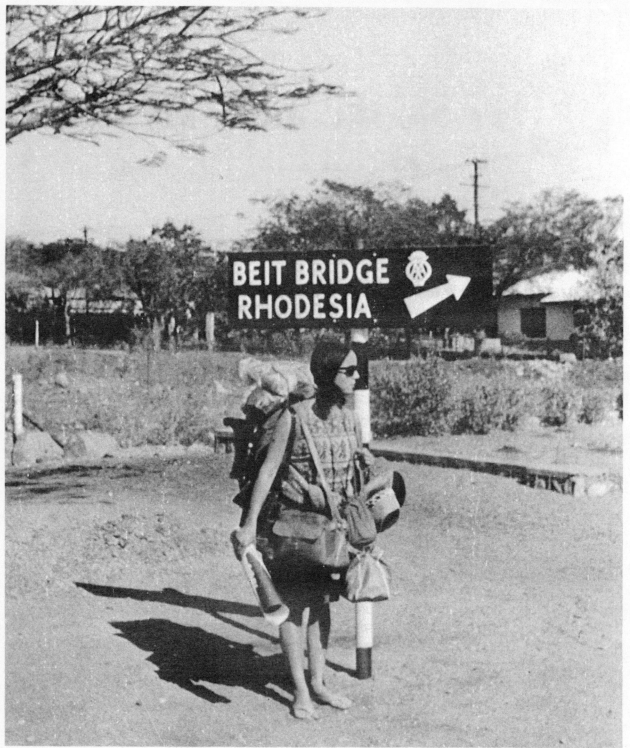

Laden with all my wordly goods, trudging toward Beit Bridge in Rhodesia (now Zimbabwe). I made sure I was clean and tidy so my parents could remember me that way in case I was maimed, raped, or killed—if not all three at once. ▲

CHAPTER EIGHTEEN

Take Care of Your Back

If you have trouble with your back, either from birth defect, stress, illness, or injury, exercise can be your best friend or your worst enemy.

If you do the right exercises, you can improve mobility and minimize pain; if not, you can be in trouble.

Simple stretching exercises, for example, can relax tension in the muscles along the spine. Other exercises can strengthen the abdominal and behind muscles, among others, to provide your spine with additional support.

"Back trouble" is a rather broad term for many very specific problems—a tear or pull of muscle or ligament, a muscle in spasm, compression or degeneration of a disc, degeneration of bone, a curvature of the spine, and even tension. You may even have an infection in some other part of the body that produces what is called a referred pain along the back.

Many of these troubles can be eased considerably, if not reversed, simply by adjusting the way we move. Chronic lower back pain, for example, usually can be alleviated by (1) losing weight, (2) exercising to strengthen the muscles of the pelvic girdle to provide support for this region of the spine, (3) improving posture, and (4) controlling stress instead of letting stress control you.

Who gets back pain is a puzzle. Many people constantly complain of aches and pains, while others live to a ripe old age with scarcely a twinge. It is a bizarre lottery that gives pain to some and none to others.

The way we live almost guarantees that we will have difficulty recovering if we do injure our backs. Our sitting habits, shoes, furniture, the hard pavement of city sidewalks, sports, even emotional stress, come into play, making it practically impossible for us to give our backs time to heal. Everyday tension can put some people into muscle spasms. That's a painful price for the fast pace we live today.

Even in the midst of our ever-growing fitness craze, we lay ourselves open to back injury by some of the very exercises we do to strengthen and stretch our bodies. A certain amount of exercise—besides walking to the kitchen or car—is essential to maintaining muscle tone and cardiovascular fitness, not to mention burning off calories.

The most prevalent problem lies in selecting the most beneficial exercises suitable for people with back problems, or potential back problems. Each of the exercises in this chapter, as well as in the One-Hour Program, come from my own experience. Tobi, the student demonstrating these exercises, is a thirty-four-year-old mother with a seven-year-old son. She has scoliosis—which you can detect in the stretch she does from the chair—and a slight swayback. She is so strong, however, from these exercises, that she is now almost completely into the regular program, with few of the modifications you will see in this chapter. It took her only three classes of special exercise before she was able to move into the regular routine.

Scoliosis is a lateral curvature of the spine creating asymmetry and an "S" or a "C" curve that is visible from behind. Lordosis (swayback) is, simply explained, a "C" curve of the spine when viewed from the side, which forces the stomach forward, no matter how thin a person is.

Parents can check for the signs of scoliosis in their children at an early age—the best time to treat the condition. Have your child bend as if ready to dive into a swimming pool. The back should be bare, so that the spine is visible. Look for a lack of symmetry, such as a twist to one side or the other, a protruding muscle or shoulder blade, or one hip, shoulder, or shoulder blade higher than the other. Females appear at higher risk, but males are far from exempt from the problem.

Detected early, spinal defects such as these can be treated with exercise. This may avert the damage the disorder once caused and avoids crippling in the later years.

Doctors admit that they do not know exactly what causes this problem, but they are finding that the earlier it is detected, the more problems can be averted. Much of the time, exercises that strengthen the muscles along the sides of the spine will be enough to halt the formation of the curvature.

If you detect any problems in your children, see your pediatrician. Ask for a recommendation to an orthopedist who specializes in pediatric bone problems. The progress made in the field is so vast that, detected early, long-range problems can be eliminated. Even people who require surgery, something that is becoming increasingly less frequent, are able to lead active lives whereas in the past they were limited in mobility and flexibility.

The most important part of caring for the back is self-awareness. Pay attention to the signals your body gives you with regard to movement and use. If you detect a pattern of activity followed by pain, consult a physician.

If your physician talks about surgery, ask for and get a second opinion—preferably from someone who is neither a surgeon nor an associate of the first doctor. What you may need is not an operation but, instead, special braces or even a set of stretching and strengthening exercises to free you from the specter of back pain.

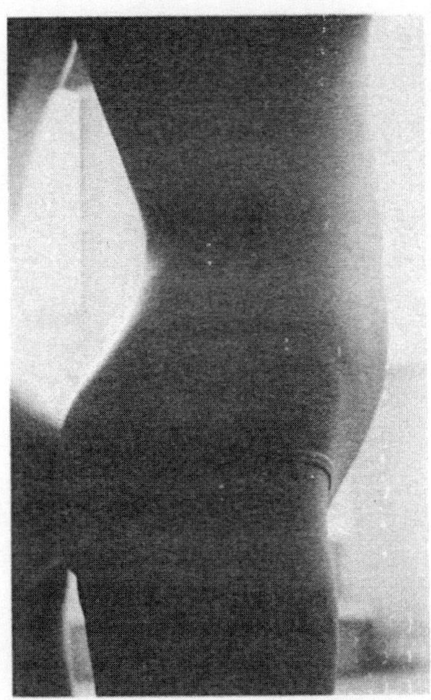

When my students see my stomach pushed out, they know I am reverting to my old posture and am not standing correctly. It is impossible for me to stand with my spine straight against the wall. If I press the small of my back to the wall, I must curl my shoulders forward and move my feet out almost a foot. The normal position of the human spine is a relatively straight column with four slight curves: the cervical, at the neck; the thoracic, through the chest; the lumbar, the five vertebrae in the region of the loins; and the sacrum, the bottom of the spine, where the five sacral vertebrae have become united into a single bone. For me to appear to have a normal posture, I must stand erect, shoulders back, and tighten my behind while tipping my pelvis up. This way, no one will ever know. ◄

Note: All body movements should be done in triple slow motion. Jerking and fast movements can irritate back problems. Key word: gentleness.

EXERCISES I HAVE FOUND TO BE SAFE FOR PEOPLE WITH BAD BACKS

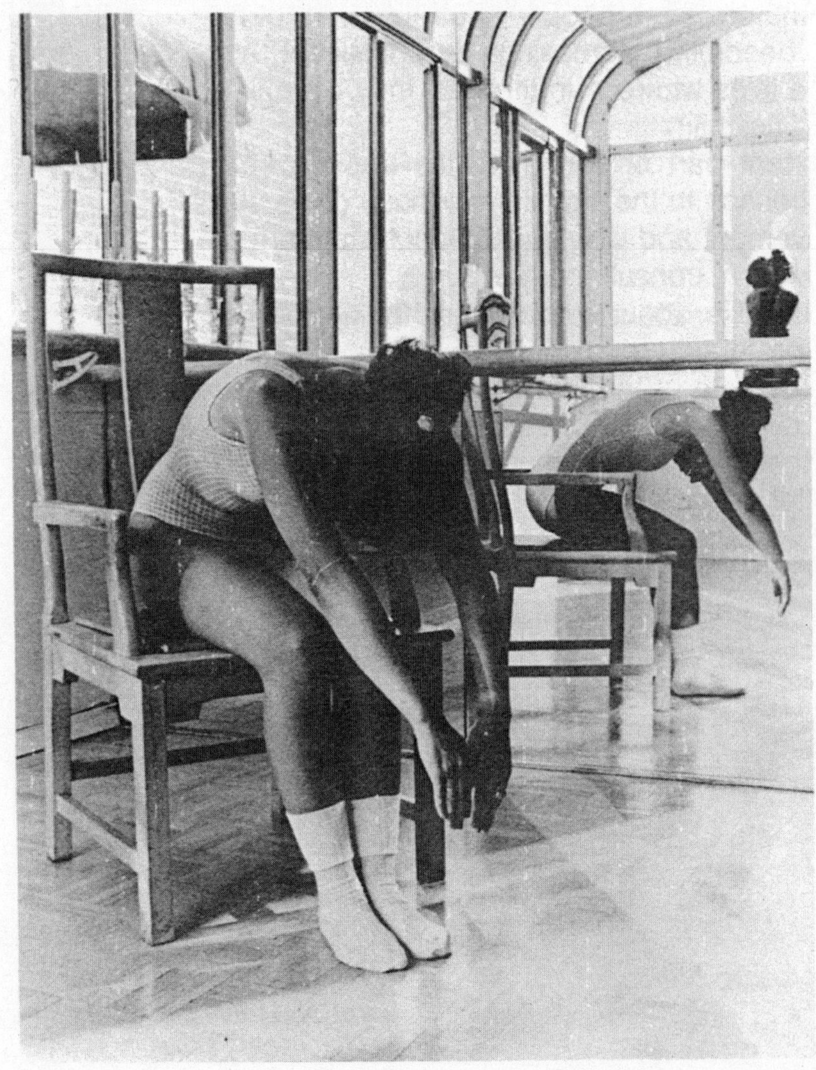

To stretch the spine, sit in a chair and lean over with rounded shoulders. This loosens the muscles around the spine just enough to begin other warming-up exercises. ◀

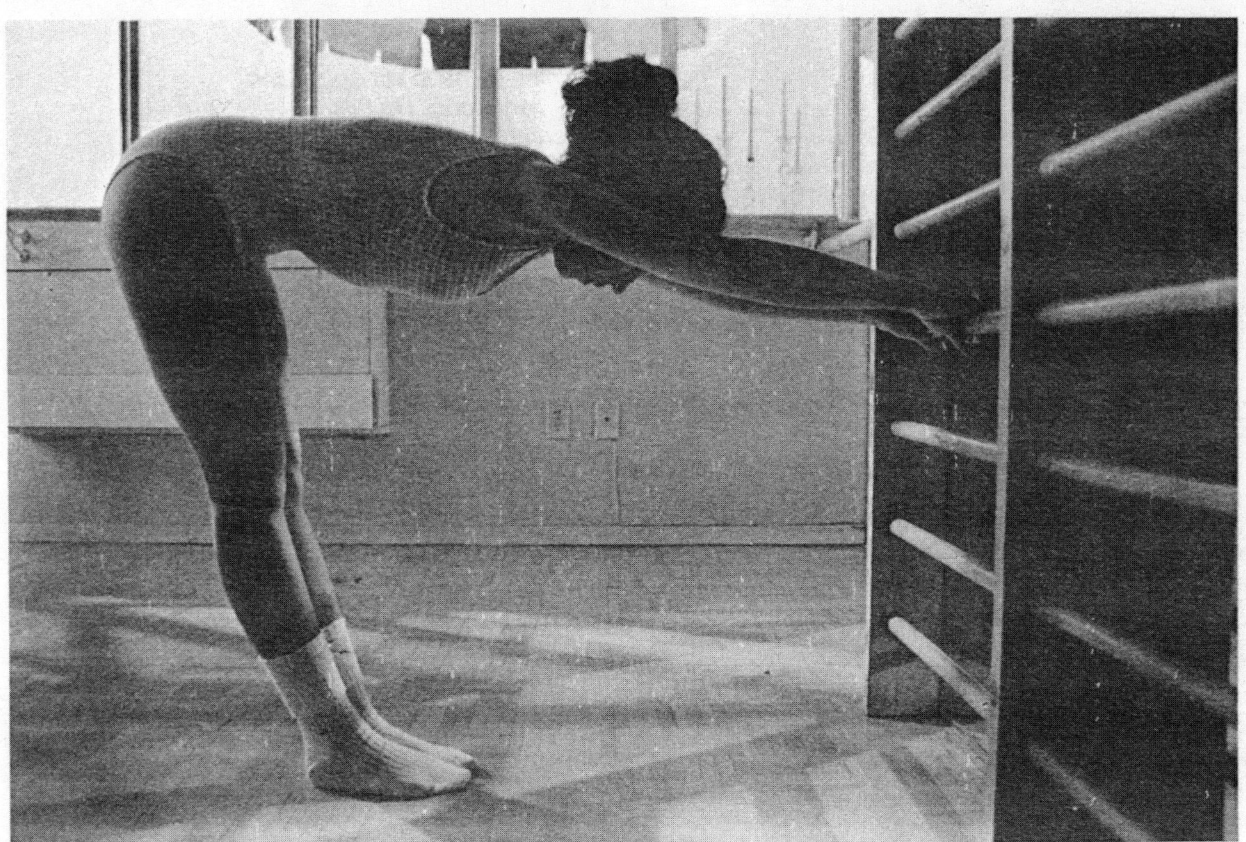

For this spinal stretch, Tobi leans toward a low barre *with her feet far enough from the wall to force her to lean forward to hold on. Hold arms straight and relax both arms and legs. Lean back so that the back is completely straight and parallel with the floor. Feet can be apart or together, whichever is more comfortable. Stretch your body away from the* barre *and hold for a slow count of 25.* ▲

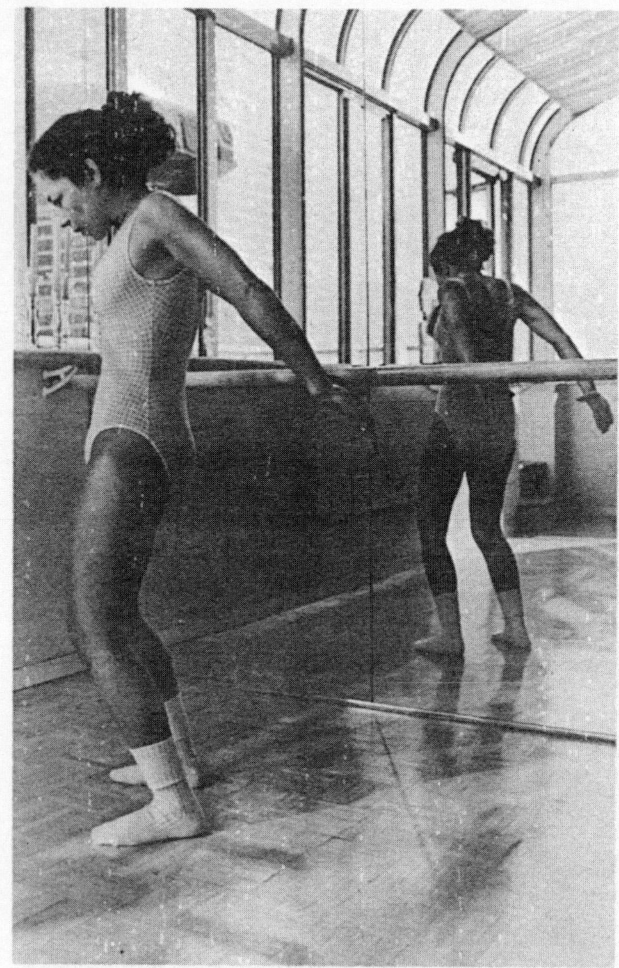

The difference in the way most people do the underarm exercise and the way I ask Tobi to do it is simple. Knees are bent and feet about a foot apart. The pelvis is tipped up and the behind is tight, helping stretch the spine as well. Lean the head forward, neck relaxed, unless this is uncomfortable; otherwise, hold head straight. Move arms behind body as far as possible, palms up and thumbs as high as possible. Move arms slowly back and forth a half inch. Start with 50 and build to 100. ▲

This is a version of the waist stretch found in the One-Hour Program. It pulls the side muscles in the lower spine and feels very good. Do this extremely gently and move slowly to the side without jerking up and down. Don't take the body directly to the side. Instead, bend slightly forward. Tighten the behind and tip the pelvis up. Keep the knees relaxed and slightly bent. Rest your right arm, elbow bent, on the upper right thigh. Do 50, building up to 100, on each side. ▼

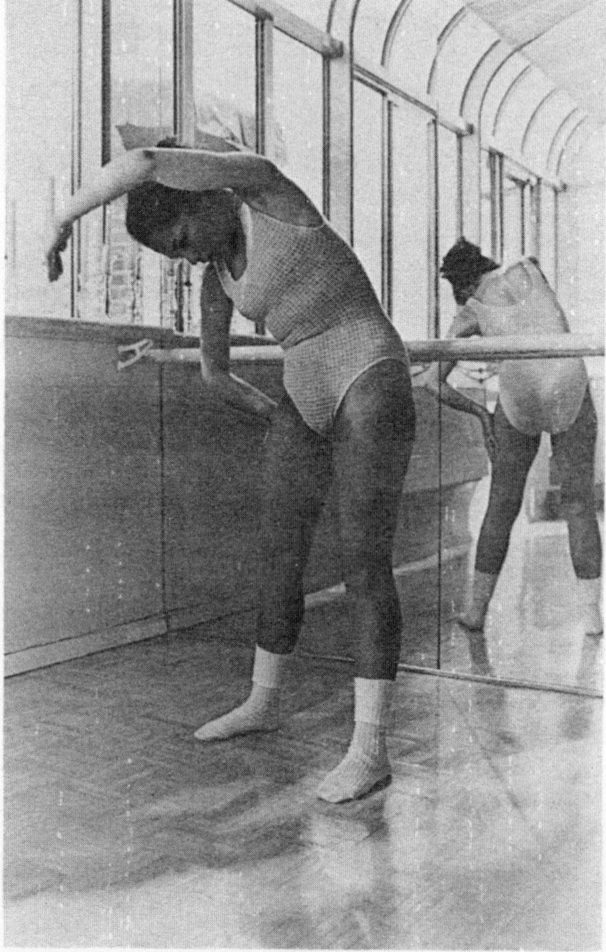

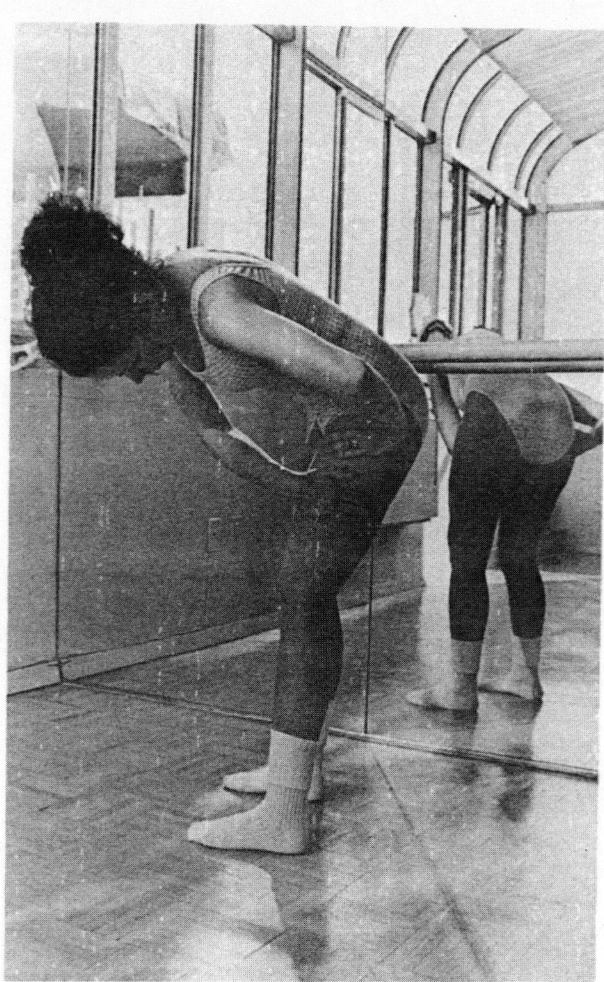

Begin the hamstring stretch from the One-Hour Program with knees bent, feet about a foot apart. Stretch your arms forward and round your back a little. Tighten your behind and tip your pelvis forward. Relax your legs and neck. Still stretching the spine, bring arms down, dangling them toward the floor. Move the torso up and down a quarter of an inch in each direction or, if that is uncomfortable, just hold. Do 20 without standing up. ▼

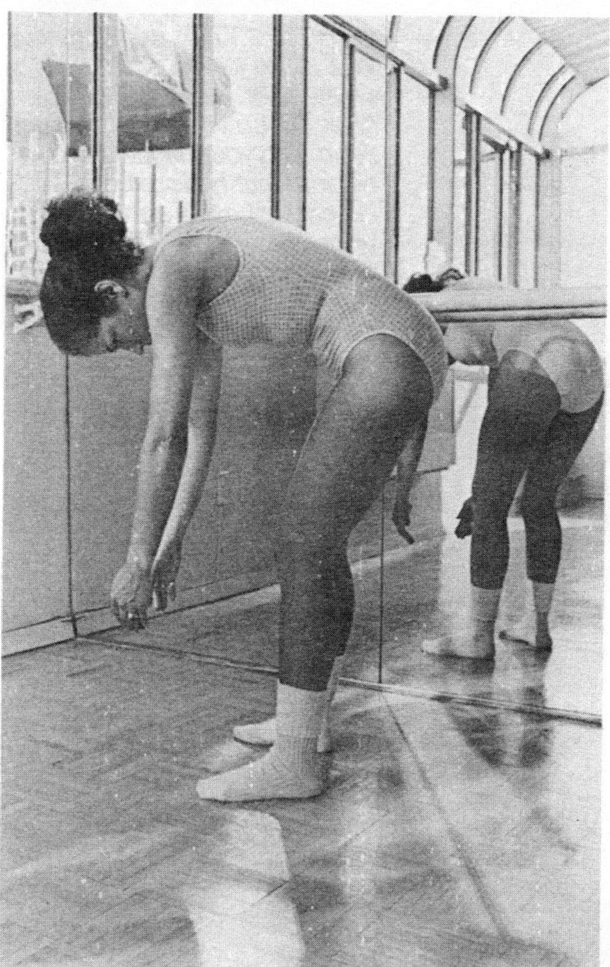

Keeping the hips even, turn the upper torso to one side. Bend over and place hands on the upper outer thighs. Then move torso up and down, again moving only a quarter of an inch in each direction. Hold this position if you prefer, or do 20 on each side. When switching sides, do not stretch torso upward again; simply move slowly and gently to the other side. ▲

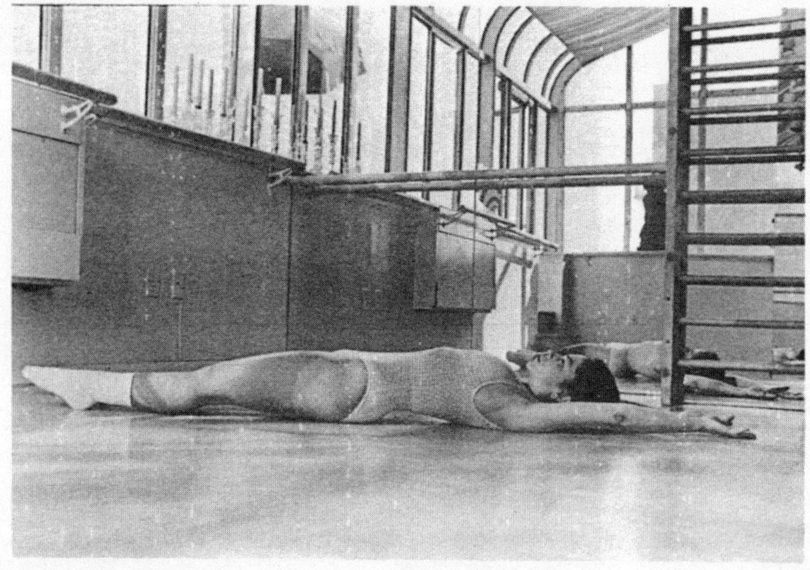

Lie flat on your back and stretch your arms over your head and your legs straight out as though trying to make your body feel 2 inches longer. In this picture, you can see how Tobi's spine is curved. ◄

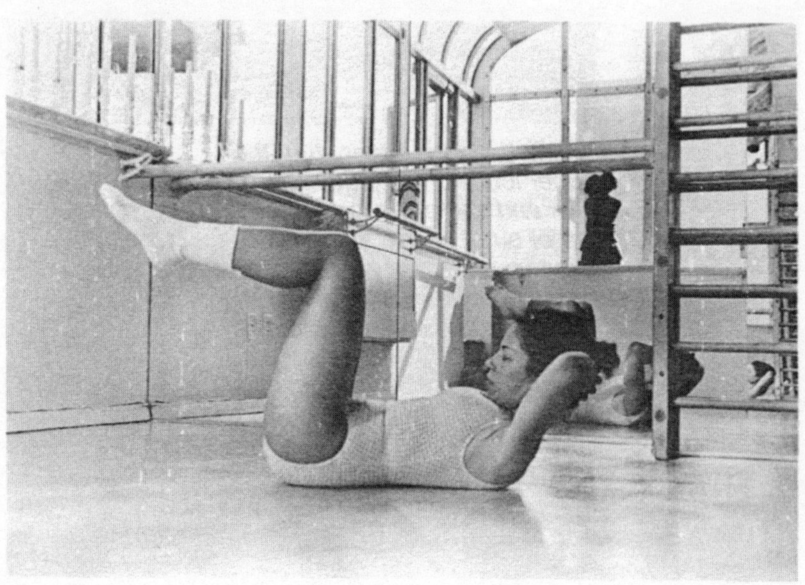

Lie on your back, bending your legs at the knees, shoulders flat on the floor. Raise feet off the floor. Lift up your shoulders and head with your hands clasped behind your head, elbows out. Do not tense any part of your upper body as you move your chin toward your chest. Gently lift head and shoulders up a quarter inch and down a quarter inch. Move only from under the bust as you move up and back. Do not jerk. Do not move your head. Also, do not move your behind back and forth. All movements must be in triple slow motion. Do 20 to 50. If your legs feel too heavy and you have no control over them, put your feet up on a chair and lift shoulders up and back in quarter-inch movements. ◄

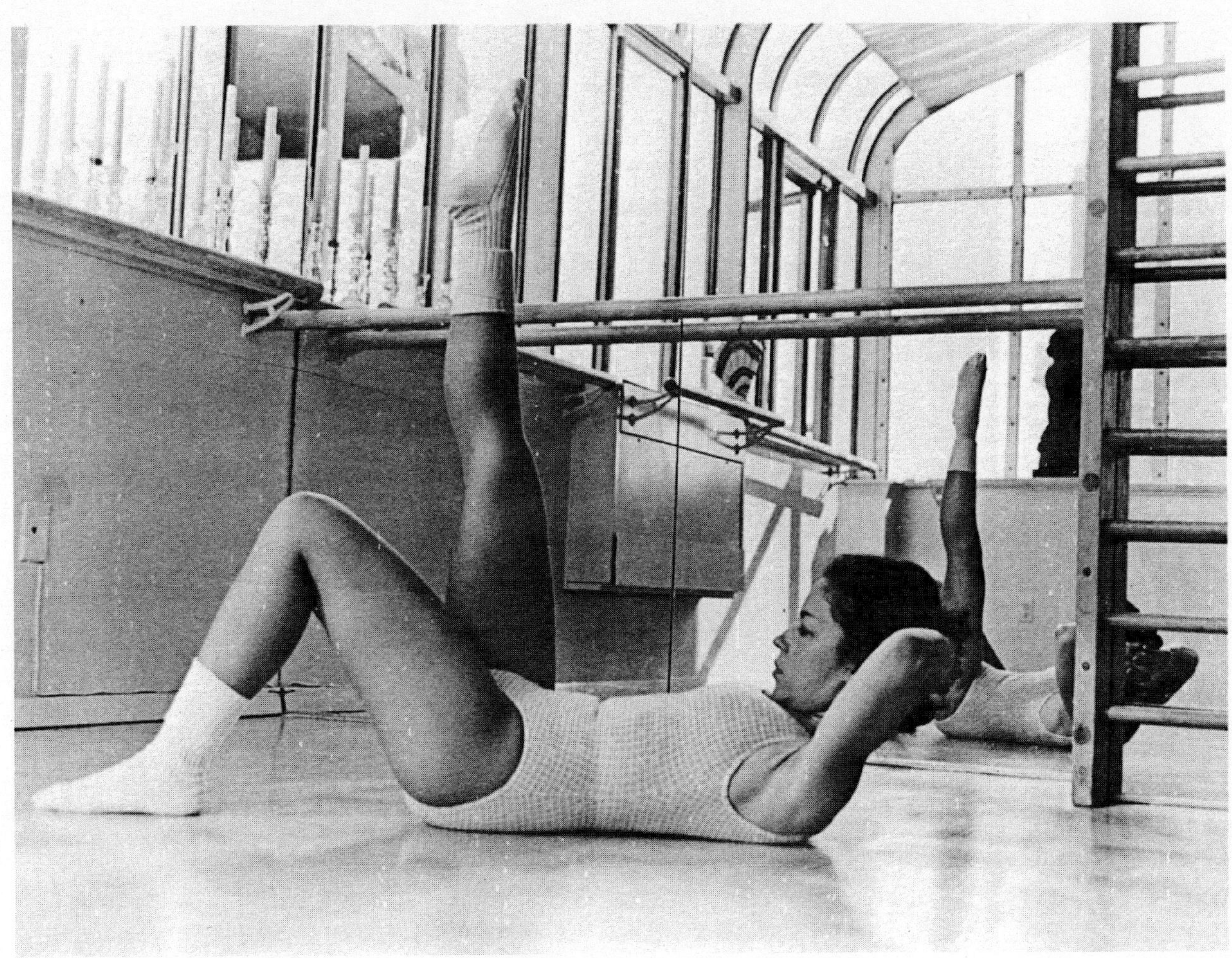

This variation of the preceding exercise for the stomach calls for you to bend your left leg and place your foot flat on the floor. Stretch your right leg up. Clasp your hands behind your head. Round your shoulders and hold your elbows out to the sides. Raise your head and shoulders off the floor. Move your upper torso up and down a quarter of an inch in each direction, making sure that every movement is gentle and easy. You may bend your raised leg if you wish. Do 20 to 50 on each side. ▲

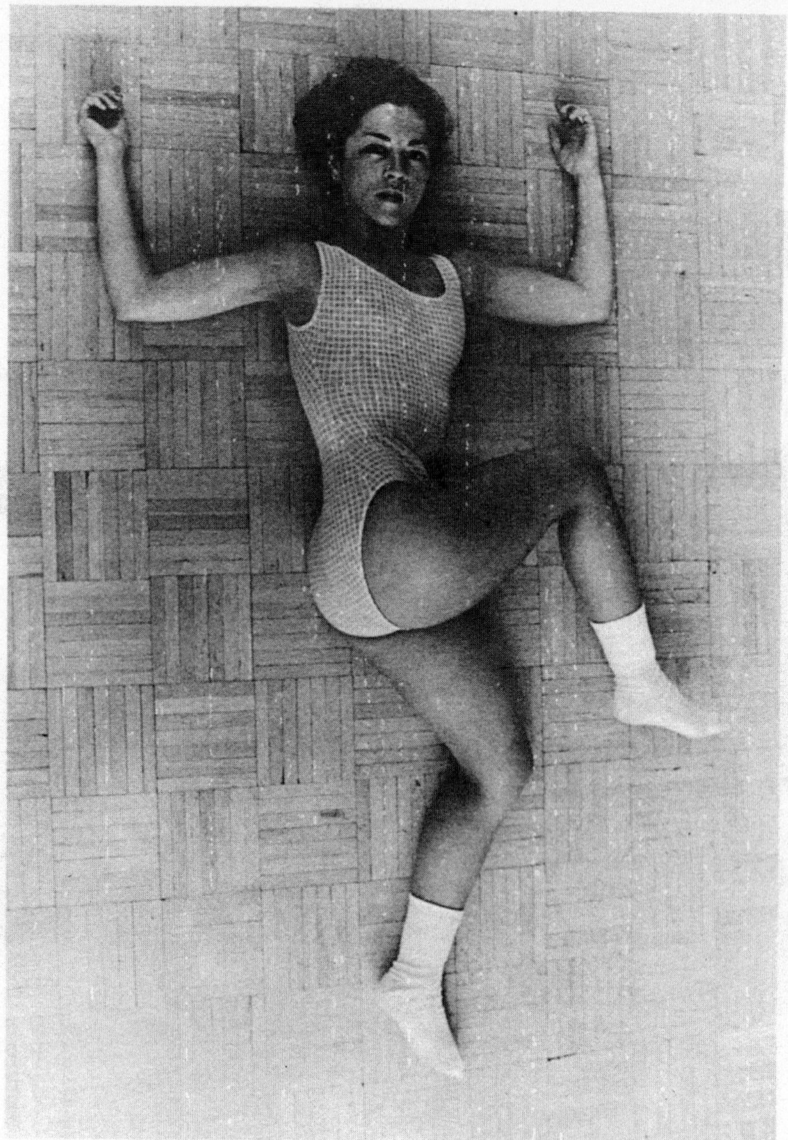

I consider this to be one of the best back stretches in the world. Lie face up on the floor. Bend arms out at shoulder level, elbows flat on the floor. Bending your right knee, bring it up and over your left leg, as though trying to put your right knee to the floor. If that is impossible, just hold the position, then move your right knee a quarter of an inch farther. Your knee will go lower when it's ready. Do not let your elbows and shoulders come off the floor, if at all possible. Slowly change sides. Do 25 each side. ▲

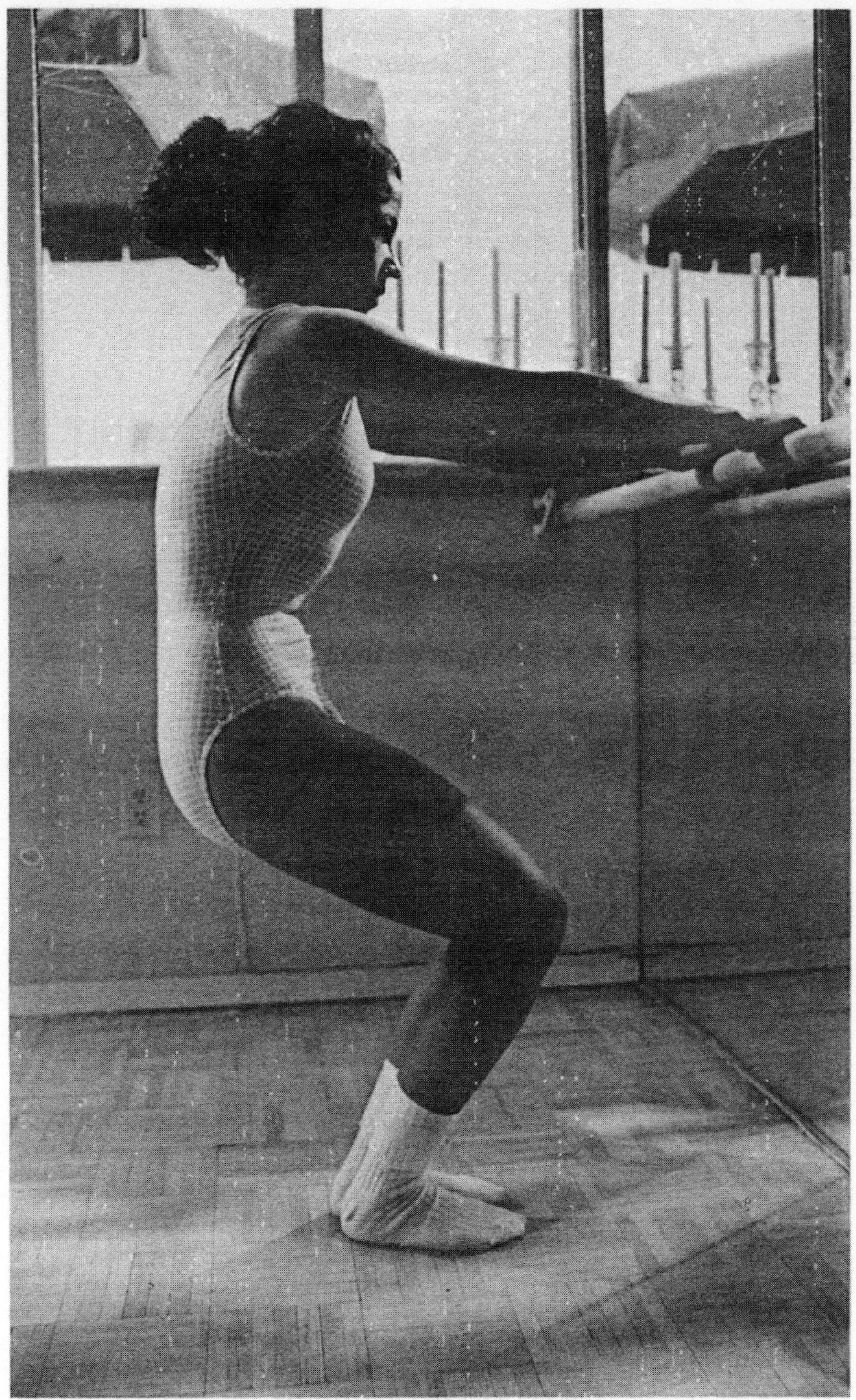

This is for the legs and pelvis and, as a bonus, strengthens the feet and ankles. Stand straight at the barre, *clasping it with your hands at shoulder width. Feet are together or as much as 6 inches apart. Tighten behind and tip pelvis upward. Round shoulders and keep your elbows straight. Move pelvis back and forth slowly and gently 10 times. Do not stick behind out. Once you are strong enough, you will be able to go to the exercises in the One-Hour Program.* ▲

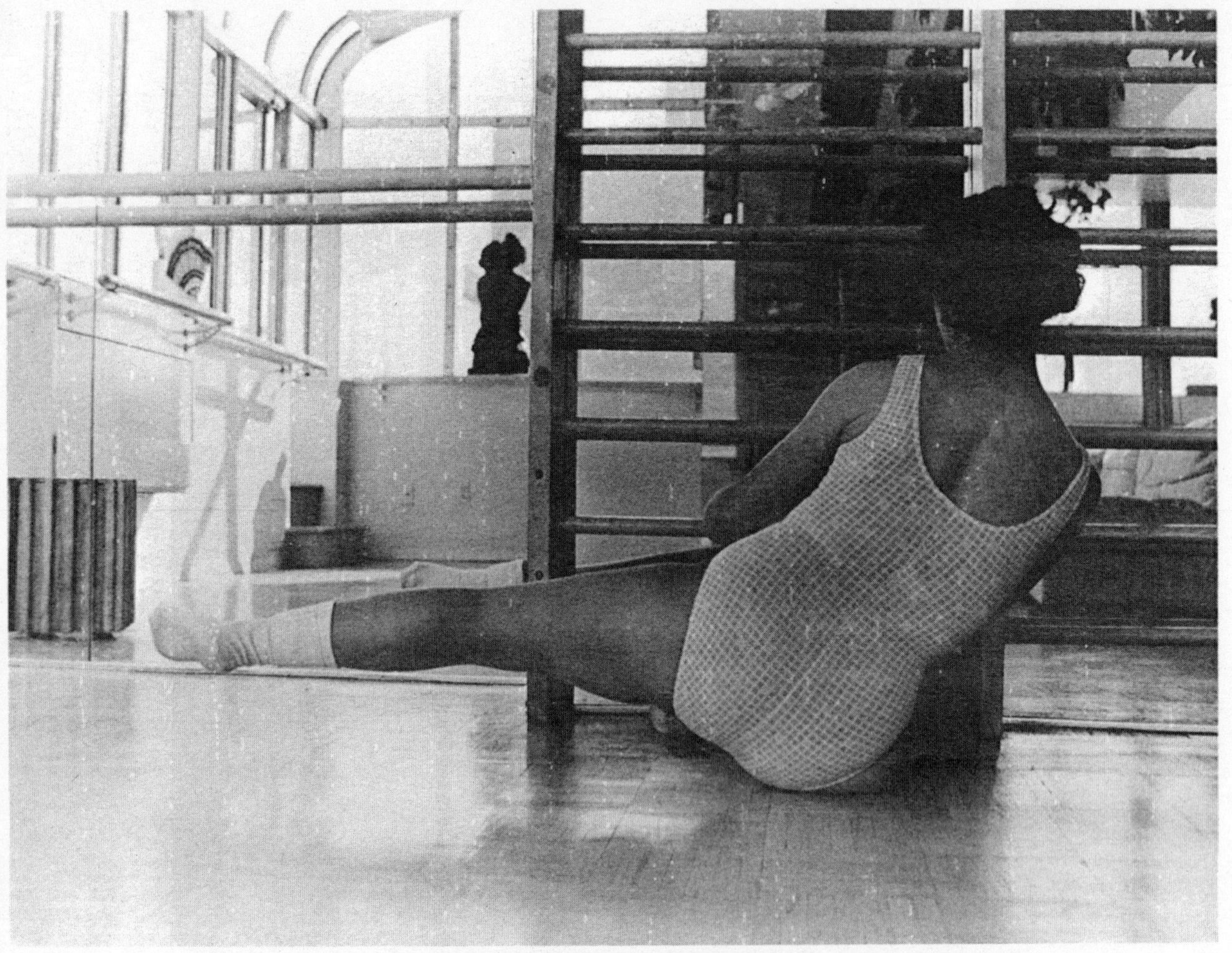

Because of back problems, it is advisable to sit in front of a sturdy chair or low table, with your right leg bent in front of you. Clasp the barre *with both hands at waist or chest level. Stretch your left leg out straight to the side. Keep hips even. Raise and lower your leg very slowly not more than 2 inches off the floor. Do 20 on each side, taking your time, building up to 100. It's all right to lean your shoulders to the right to maintain your balance. Concentrate on keeping your behind tight and your pelvis tipped forward and up. As you build strength, you should be able to do the behind and hip exercises from the One-Hour Program.* ▲

Kneel on a pad, knees and feet as close together as possible, with your hands on the sides of your waist. Relax your shoulders and hold your elbows out to each side. Slowly aim the behind to your heels, stretching your back without sticking out your behind or arching your back. When you feel your behind touch your heels, gently tighten your behind, tip your pelvis upward very slowly, and scoop upward, returning to the kneeling position. Do 5. If you have any aching in your calves, you can lean forward with your arms, head, and shoulders extended in front, as if you were diving into water. See the Pelvic Scoop in Chapter 13. ▼

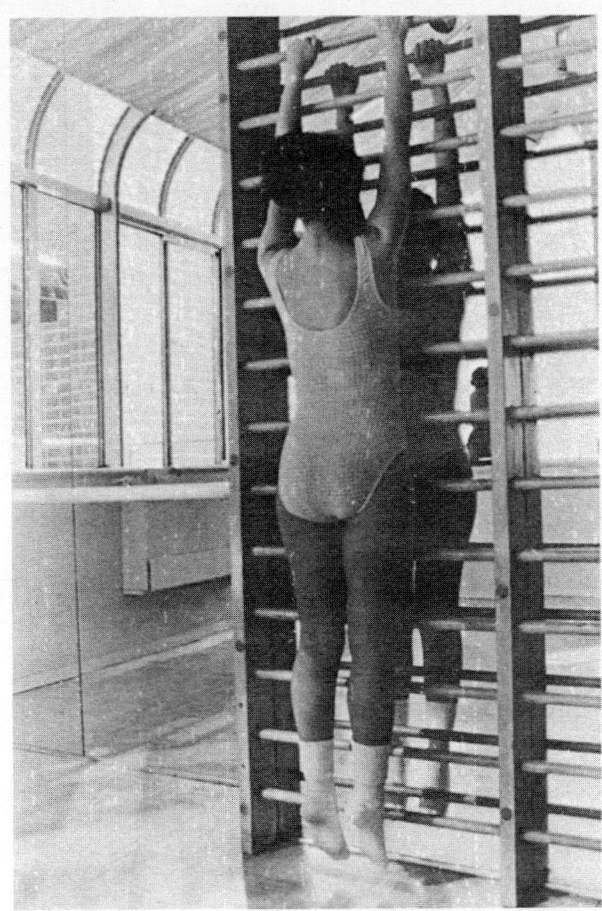

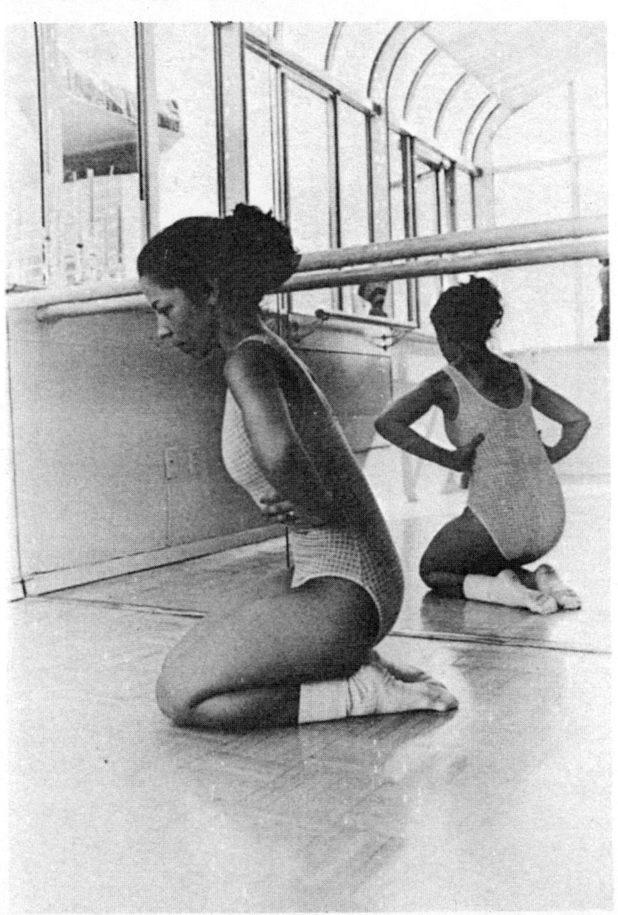

Attempt this only if you have access to a high barre. *For people with bad backs, hanging comes as the* completion *to the exercise program. The muscles are warm and stretched, therefore there is no risk of your becoming too tense—a tendency people have when hanging. As a result of your prior exercises, your back will stretch more fully at the end of the program. If you do this, relax the lower back and pretend your body is like melting wax dripping onto the floor.* ▲

CHAPTER NINETEEN

You're Never Too Old to Have a Fabulous Figure

Youth and fitness do not necessarily go hand in hand. However, fitness is definitely a key to having a youthful body, regardless of your age.

Look at Margaret, the student demonstrating the exercises in this chapter. Who would believe she is in her mid-seventies? What is even harder to believe is that she exercises every day—despite the fact that four vertebrae in her neck were surgically fused ten years ago, using bone and tissue taken from her hip, and she has arthritis in her shoulders and back.

"I'm afraid *not* to exercise," she explains. "If I miss one day, I feel intense muscle pain down my spine and I start to stoop over. It sets me back a week."

Despite teasing from her husband and friends, Margaret wears her leotard around the house while doing her housework. "Every time someone calls me I'm on the floor exercising. They think I'm silly, doing this at my age, but I feel great."

She must be in great condition, too. A week before these pictures were taken, she slipped and slid down four carpeted steps, hit a newel-post and fell three feet to the hardwood floor. Her only injury was a massive bruise on her hip and leg, where she landed. You can see it in some of the photos. That is why she is wearing leg warmers.

Falling is one of Margaret's greatest fears, since further injury might break the cervical fusion. Had she settled for a sedentary, overly careful life, doing little physical activity, she would have become a crippled old woman ages ago. Instead, she has worked with her body, starting as soon as she was physically able—about six months after her sur-

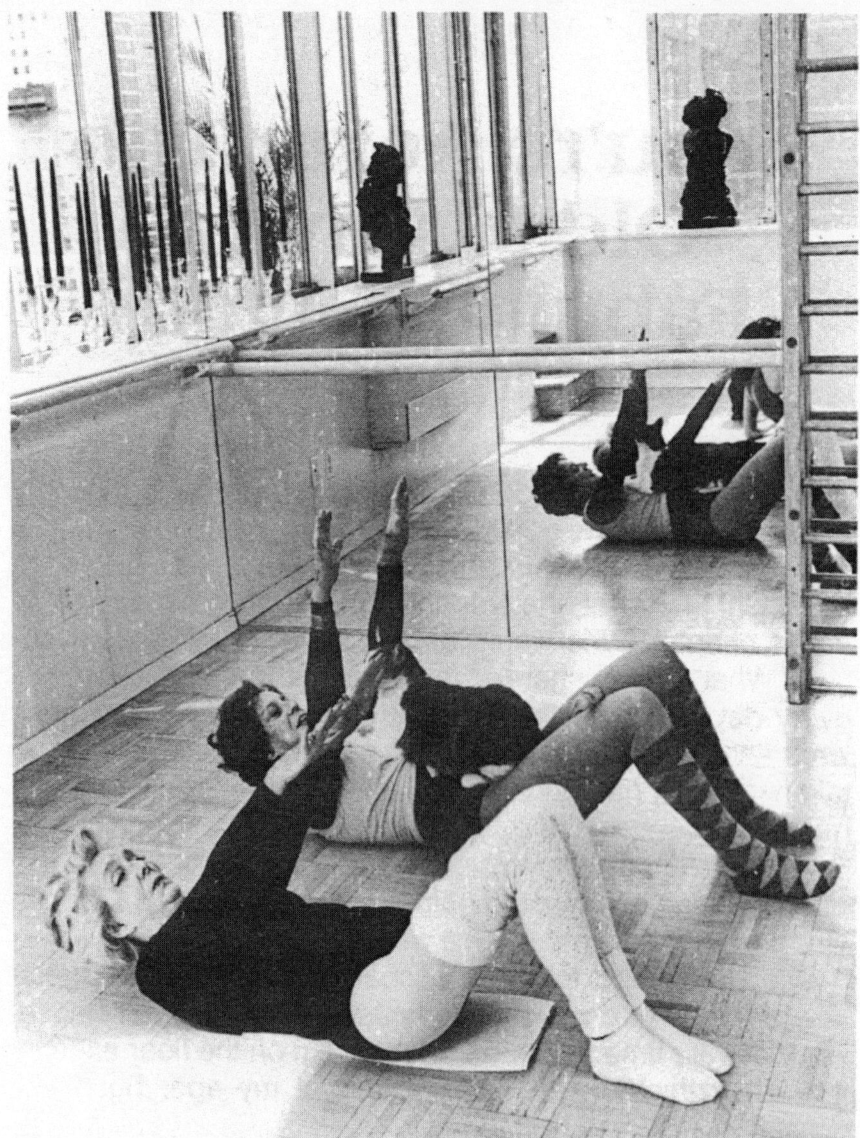

Because of the fusion of the vertebrae in her neck, Margaret cannot do the regular stomach exercises. I have taught her to protect her neck, so that now she is so attuned to her body, she is able to do far more than one might expect and occasionally she will do one of the regular stomach exercises. As soon as she feels pressure on her neck, she adjusts her position or stops. Sixty or so years ago, IdaMay, seen here with Scarlet, was an Earl Carroll's Vanities *showgirl. Still fit and in her mid-eighties, she works at her own pace and completes the class with everyone else.* ▲

gery—doing only what she could. Little by little she restored her body to good health. If she had been stiff and creaky and totally out of condition, she might have been severely injured by this recent fall.

"These exercises are saving my life," she swears. "I am strong and I'm flexible. I see people my age, even younger, deteriorating before my eyes. They have stooped shoulders and stumble and shuffle about, taking hesitant steps. I'm terrified of becoming that way. If I don't keep exercising, I know I will hunch over like a little old lady."

There is medical data to substantiate her observation about her own body. Inactivity does indeed speed the aging process. Often the limited movements and halting, painful steps of old age result from abuse or disuse begun in youth.

A dowager's hump and feeble posture are *not* the inevitable badges assigned by fate to women as they pass through middle age and beyond. In many ways, old age really *is* a state of mind. If you eat correctly and live and think like a young person, it stands to reason that you will look and feel young. You will move and walk with youthful ease. Some people are old and crotchety in their twenties; others are *never* old, despite what the calendar says.

The truth is that we all begin to age the moment we are born. Consequently, our bodies are ever aging. By the time we reach our forties, we begin to detect some real differences, most noticeably in our hair and skin, which change in color and texture. As our body chemistries change, we may notice some alteration in muscle tone, stiffness in our joints, and aches and pains in places we have never felt them before.

There is no need for a long explanation about cholesterol, triglycerides, and low-density/high-density lipoproteins, atherosclerotic plaques, arteriosclerosis, or even osteoporosis and calcium deficiencies, basal metabolism and cardiovascular fitness. You can keep abreast of the latest in medical data through current women's magazines and newspapers and, most important, by asking your doctor specific, candid questions about your feelings and about your body's changes.

Don't settle for a pat on the head and a "that's-a-good-girl" attitude from your family physician. Despite the natural changes our bodies experience—including the cessation of the menses and subsequent loss of estrogen in a woman's body—it is *not* normal or natural to creak through life after middle age.

The bottom line is this: The stooped, aching, feeble movements associated with the elderly can be avoided in most cases if we take care of our bodies while we are young. I am still paying the price for carrying around a heavy rucksack on my back for so long. If I don't exercise, I am in trouble.

There are some changes we must be aware of. Our eyesight often loses acuity. Bones often become brittle, making it all the more important that we keep our muscles in shape. Who wants to take a spill and break a hipbone? That can happen if one is out of shape and does not know *how* to fall.

Regular exercise is essential to maintaining minimim fitness, even more in the elderly than in the young. It is not enough to walk to the car or do your housework or gardening or play a round of golf or even tennis once a week. Make exercise a habit to forestall problems. As you exercise, you increase your energy level and, naturally, your body's potential. My older students can do as many as the younger students. I believe the older you get the more exercise your body needs.

The exercises Margaret does come from the same basic program I give to my younger students. As with anyone I teach, movements are adapted to what she can do. Sometimes she is able to do more, sometimes less. Because of her neck and back, I do not allow her to do the basic stomach exercises. Instead, she has devised her own version, using a pillow to raise her head and shoulders. Because of this, I refer you to the exercises for people with bad backs for your stomach exercises (see Chapter 17). As a rule, I do not give these to my older students until after their third class. If you have a pacemaker, they may be too strenuous for you.

For the sake of pictures, I had to insist that Margaret not show off. She does the exercises in the One-Hour Program usually better than women half her age. She can raise her leg to the *barre,* but since most people her age won't be able to do this, she is photographed using a lower ladder. I did not want her to intimidate someone less fit than she! I asked her to demonstrate this chapter because at her age and with her medical problems, she is more than aware of how gentle one must be with the body. This is the way she did the program before she built up her strength.

"I feel terrible if I don't exercise," she says. "The important thing is to stay active. Don't let yourself get past the point of no return, where your body can no longer move. So many people over fifty need a stick of dynamite to get them moving."

When someone seventy or so arrives in my class, the red carpet is laid out. Usually, they are mothers of my younger students. Most of them come to me demanding, very shyly, the same results as their children. I require that they tell me everything they are feeling, with every little movement. They are adorable! A sparkle comes to their eyes, especially after about the third hour, when they are beginning to keep up with the rest of the class and starting to see their skin becoming tight.

The stiffer a student is when I start working with her, the more I enjoy my work. Her body becomes very straight in an amazingly short amount of time. Eventually she walks very erect, and puts some teenagers to shame!

Older people are fun. They laugh a lot, and they are so gracious. It is very inspiring for everyone around them to see them work at their own pace, take a breather, and then keep on going. It doesn't bother me to see someone staring at herself in the mirror for five or ten minutes before getting back into the routine, because I know that it is just a matter of time before she will be able to keep up with the class and complete the entire hour's program without interruption.

The exercises photographed for this section are modifications of the One-Hour Program that everyone does. I see no reason to separate the age groups any more than the sexes! Study these pictures and read through the One-Hour Program, as well as the exercises for people with bad backs.

Work at your own pace, doing *what* you can, *when* you can, for as long as you can, until you are able to complete a program. Trust your body. It will let you know what you can and cannot do. When you feel you are ready, go to the One-Hour Program if you wish.

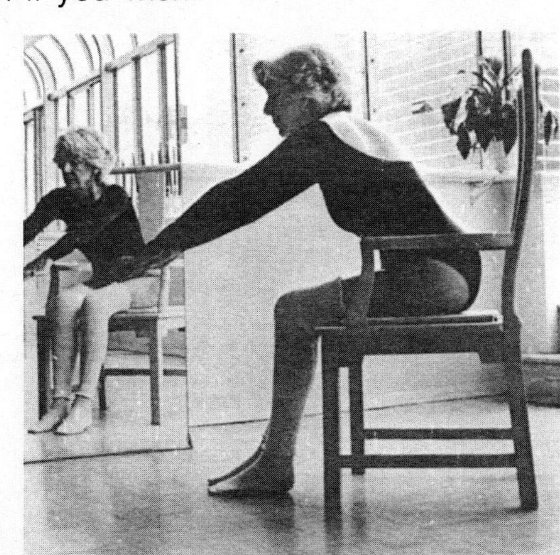

Note: *No jerking, no forcing. Every movement should be done in triple slow motion. Key word: gentleness.*
This is preparation for the warm-ups—stretching the spine. Sitting in a chair, you should lean your torso forward and stretch your arms out in front of you. Relax your body. ▸

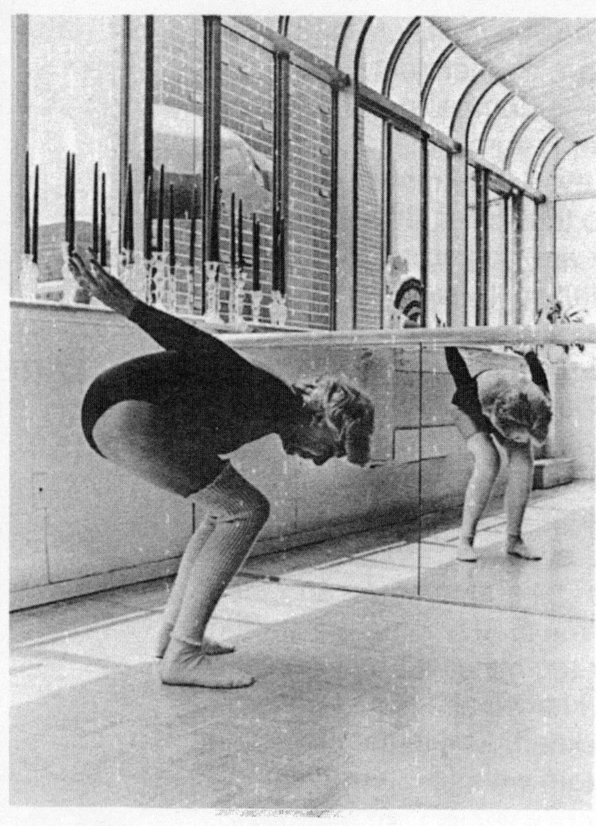

This basic warm-up is taken from the One-Hour Program. Stretch your arms up to the ceiling. Make your body feel 2 inches taller. Gently bend your knees. Keep your feet about a foot apart. Lower your arms, moving them high behind you. Return them to the side of your body and reach to the ceiling. Do 5. ▲

To stretch the waist, stand erect with your legs a foot to a foot-and-a-half apart. Put your left hand on your left hip, elbow bent. Tighten your behind and tip your pelvis upward as you reach your right arm high over your head. Gently bend your torso to the left with your right arm straight. Keep your behind tight and your pelvis upward. Keep your feet and hips even. Only bend over as far as you can to maintain proper balance. Gently move your torso back and forth a quarter of an inch. Start with 30 and build up to 50 on each side. ▼

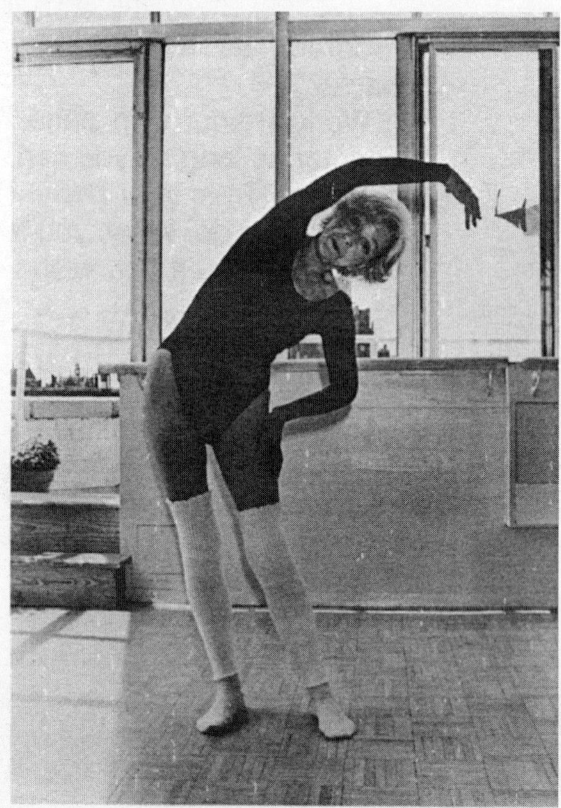

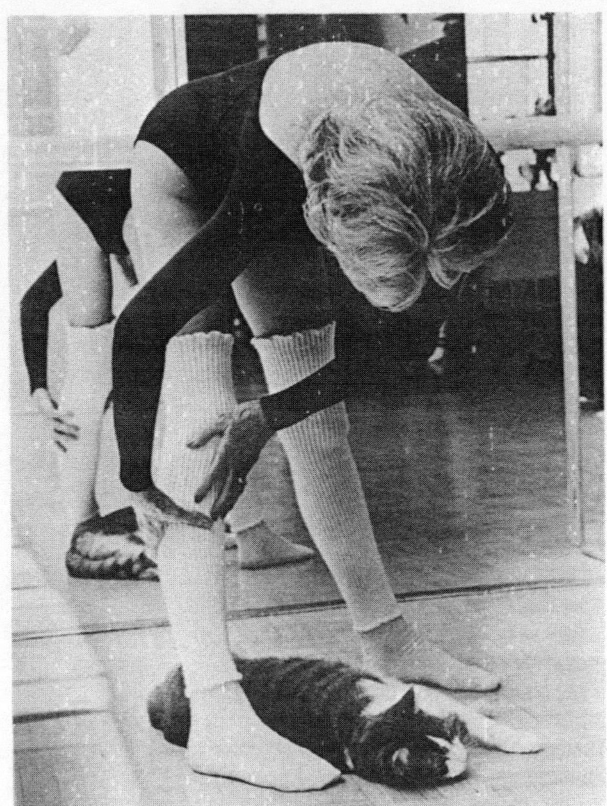

Be very conscious of your body while doing this stretch for the spine and backs of the legs. With your feet a foot and a half apart, bend your body over toward the floor. Keep knees bent and put your hands above your knees for support. This way, your weight rests on your hands and thighs. Hold this position for a count of 20. Then move back up a quarter of an inch and down a quarter of an inch. Do 15 movements up and down. Never jerk or bounce. Do not move your torso more than a quarter of an inch. Without standing up, grab your inner knees with your hands. Gently move your body as if you are trying to push your head between your knees. Move a quarter of an inch at a time. Relax your legs and keep your knees flexed. Do 15 quarter-inch movements. ▼

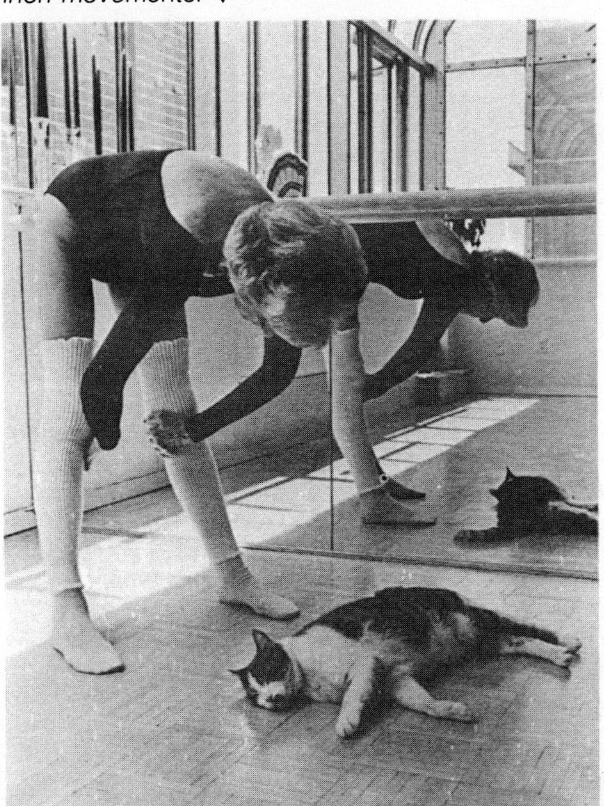

Again, without straightening torso, gently take both hands to outside of the right knee. Make quarter-inch movements down with your head, shoulders, and upper body as though trying to put your head between your arms and your knee. Keep your legs relaxed and knees bent. Do 10 movements to the right, stretch torso out to the front, and then over to the left to do 10 on the left side. Then stand by rolling your spine upward until you are erect, using triple slow motion. ▲

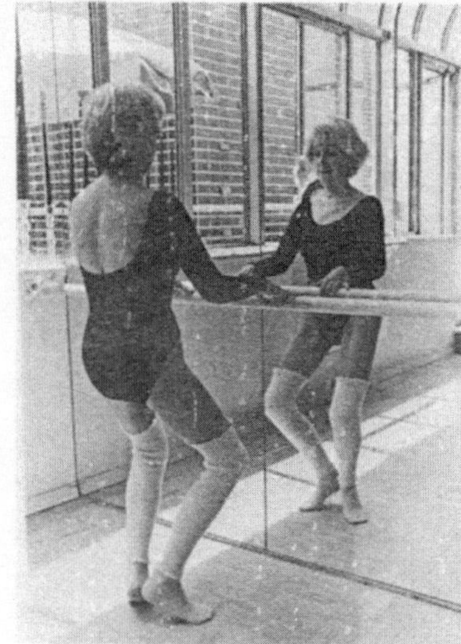

If you do not have a barre, *use the back of a sofa or sturdy chair, or even the kitchen counter. Use your imagination. The height of the* barre *is not important. Stand facing your* barre, *holding it with your hands at shoulder width. Stand on the balls of your feet with your heels together. Slightly bend your knees out to each side. Lower your body 1 or 2 inches and then return to the original position. Do not go lower. Do 10. Margaret is so fit that I had to hold her back for these pictures. Most older people have not worked their knees for quite a while, so special attention must be paid not to damage them. If you go lower than 2 inches, you will be putting too much pressure on the knee-joint complex at first. Hold on to the* barre *as much as you wish. Do 10. This works on your thighs, calves, ankles, and feet, building flexibility and strength.* ▲

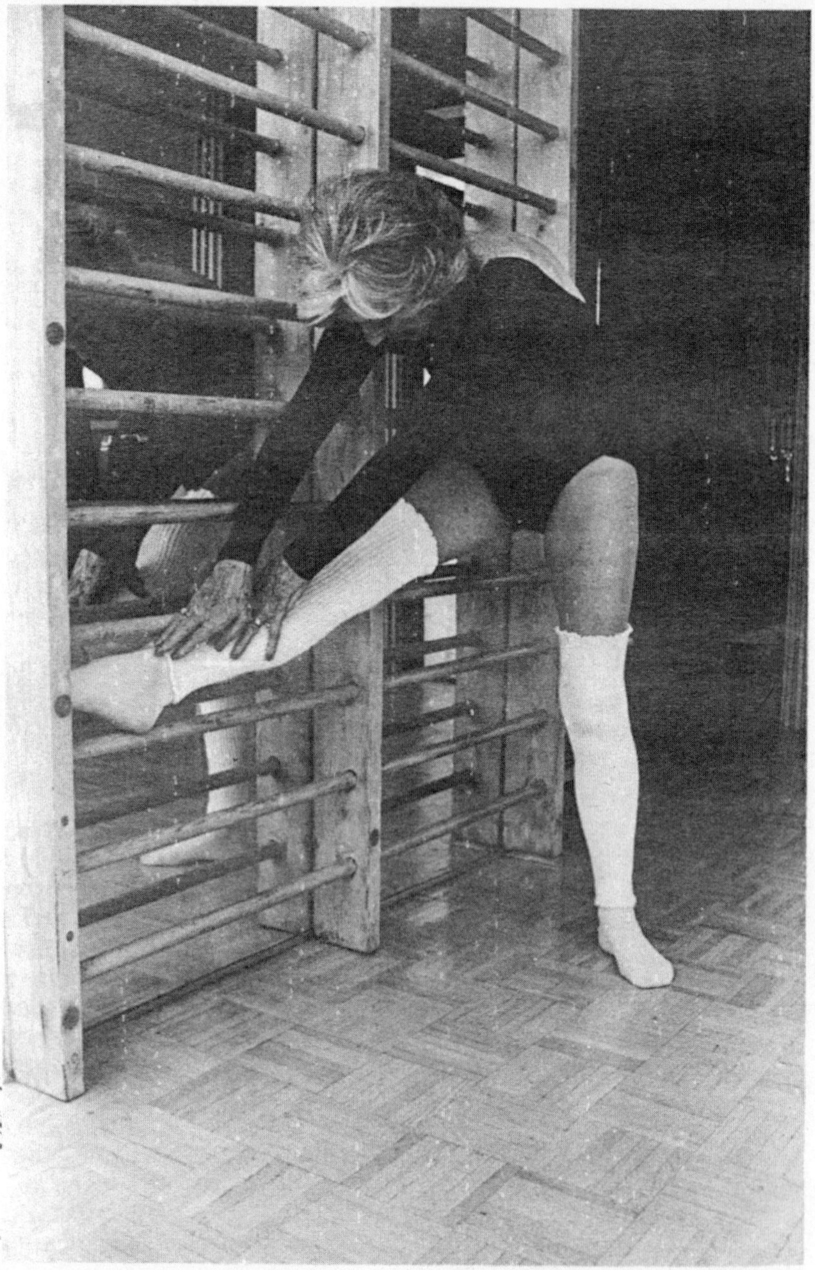

For this hamstring stretch, put your heel on a low table or chair, padding the table surface to protect your heel if necessary. Gently position your hands on any part of the leg except the knees. Move your torso a quarter inch toward your foot. Do not force. The body and legs should be relaxed, especially through the knees. Move torso in triple slow motion up and down a quarter of an inch, if you can. Do 20. Switch legs and repeat. With this, or any of the exercises you see in this chapter, if movement is difficult, don't move at all. Simply hold the position. ▲

Older people can adapt the exercises for the behind and hips that I teach in the One-Hour Program. Sit on the floor on your left cheek (far over on your left hip). Bend your left leg in front of your body and position your right leg on your right side, even with your right hip with the knee bent. Put both hands on the floor to the left of

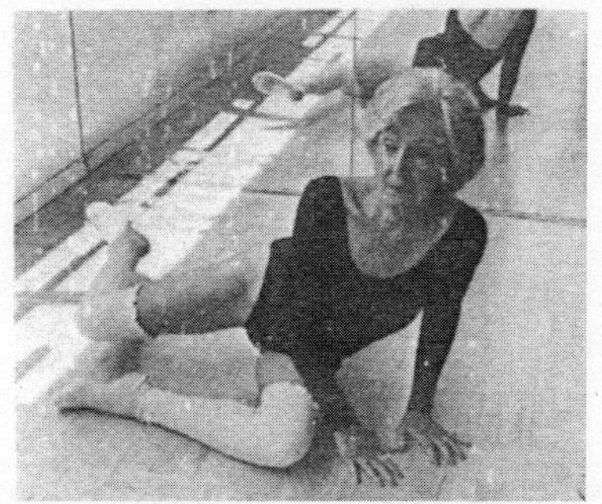

your left knee for balance. Relax your torso. Gently lift your right knee and foot off the floor and with half-inch movements, push the right knee to the back and then return to the original position. Keep hips even. Do 15 to 20 on each side if possible the first time. As you feel stronger, increase to 30, and then to 50. ◄

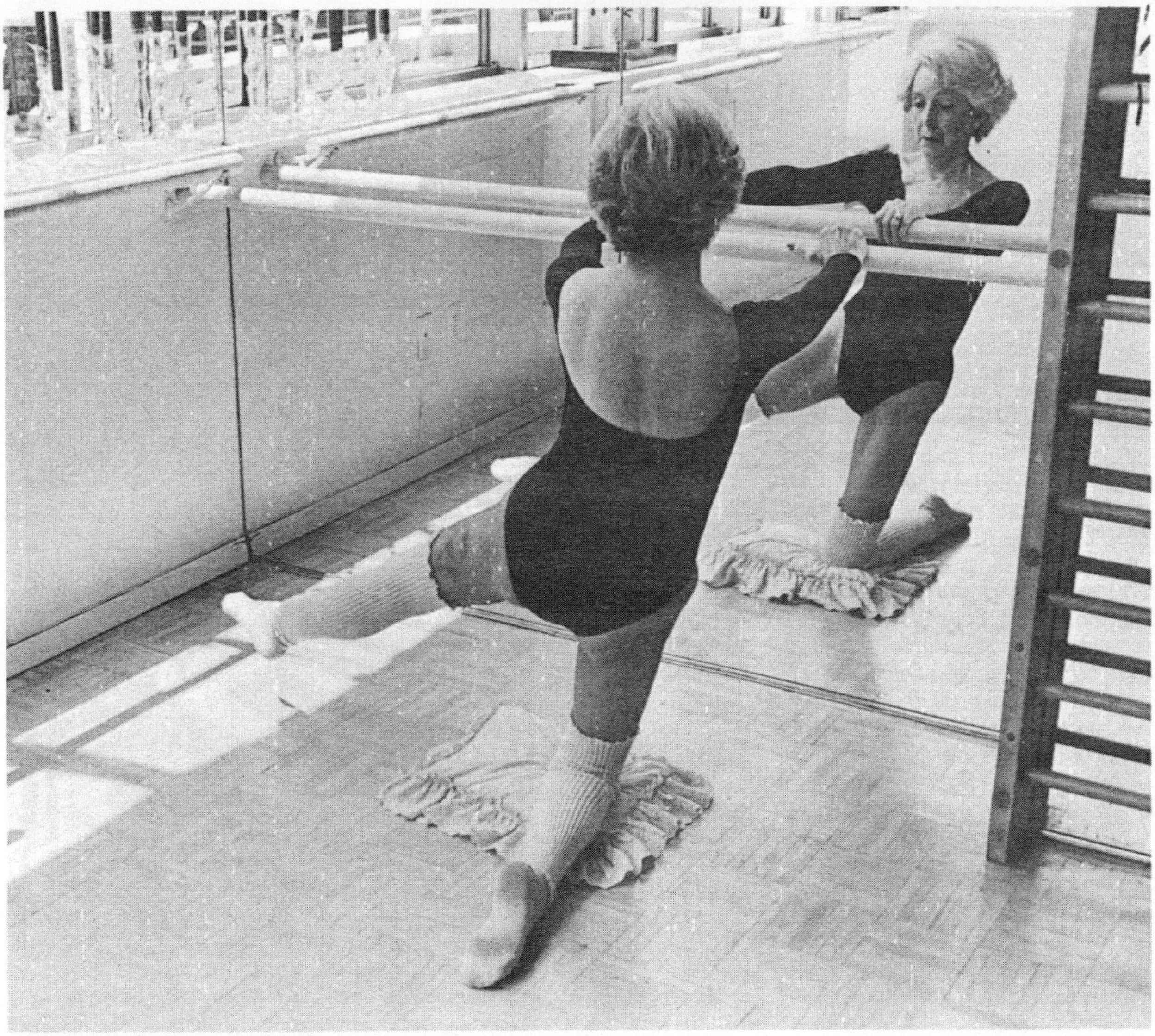

Kneel on a cushion in front of whatever you are using or barre, arms extended outward. Grasp barre at shoulder width and lean back so that your elbows are straight. Keeping your hips even, extend your left leg out to the side. Tighten your behind muscles and tip your pelvis up. Relax and round your shoulders. Gently lift your left leg up and down, moving only 2 inches off the floor. Even if you can't lift your foot, keep trying. Talk to your leg. You'll be able to do it sooner or later. Do 10 on each side. If you have knee problems, ask your doctor if you should do this. You may also try doing it while standing, as long as you bend a little the knee of the leg you are standing on, following same directions. ▲

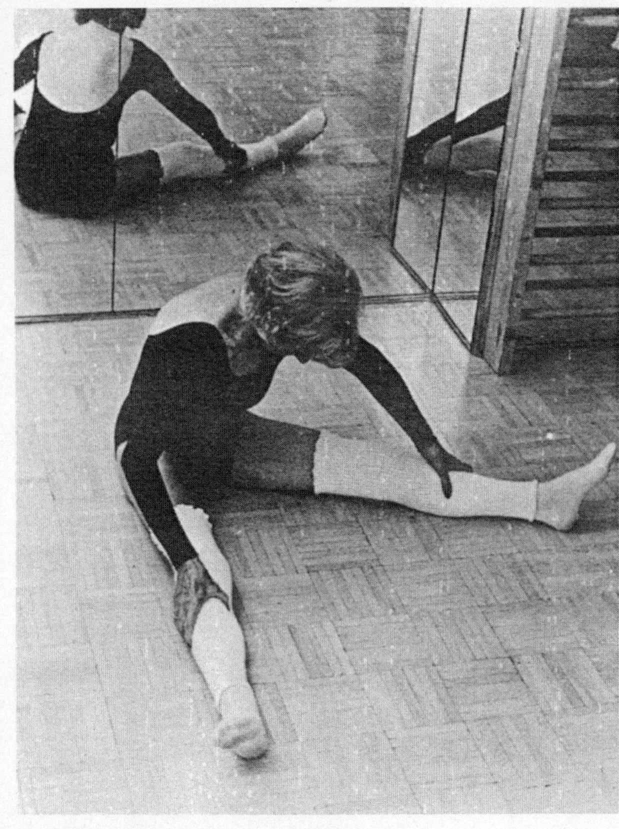

To stretch the inner thigh, sit on the floor and spread your legs as far as you can without forcing or losing balance. Relax your body and legs. Bend your torso forward and place your hands on your legs as close to your feet as is comfortable. Bend your elbows and hold this position for a count of 30. Then move gently up and down a quarter of an inch. Do 30. If your legs don't straighten, bend your knees. ▲

Give your spine and hamstrings a thorough stretch. Lie on your back, resting your head on a small pillow to support your neck. Margaret must use a pillow to protect her neck because of her fusion. Bend your legs at the knee and bring up to your chest. Clasp your hands in back of your knees, calves, or ankles—whichever is more comfortable, and ease your knees toward your chest. This should not be a pulling or jerking motion. Either hold or gently move toward your chest a quarter of an inch and then go back to your original position. Do 20. Gently bend your knees and return your legs to the floor. Take a breather before continuing with the next exercise. ▼

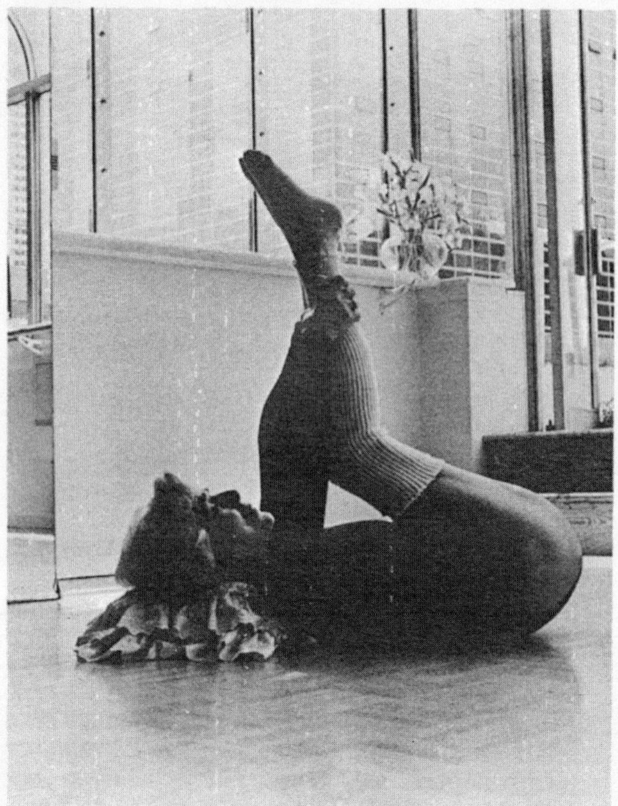

To further stretch the spine, as well as the thighs and stomach muscles, lie on your back with your hands at your sides. Rest your head on a pillow to protect your head and neck. Tighten your behind and push your pelvis off the floor. Gently push the pelvis up a quarter of an inch higher, then lower. Do 20. Keep your arms, neck, and feet relaxed. ▶

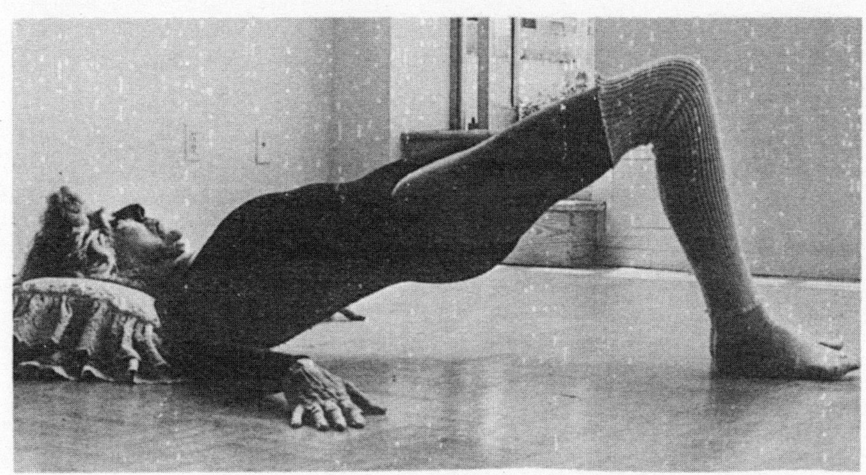

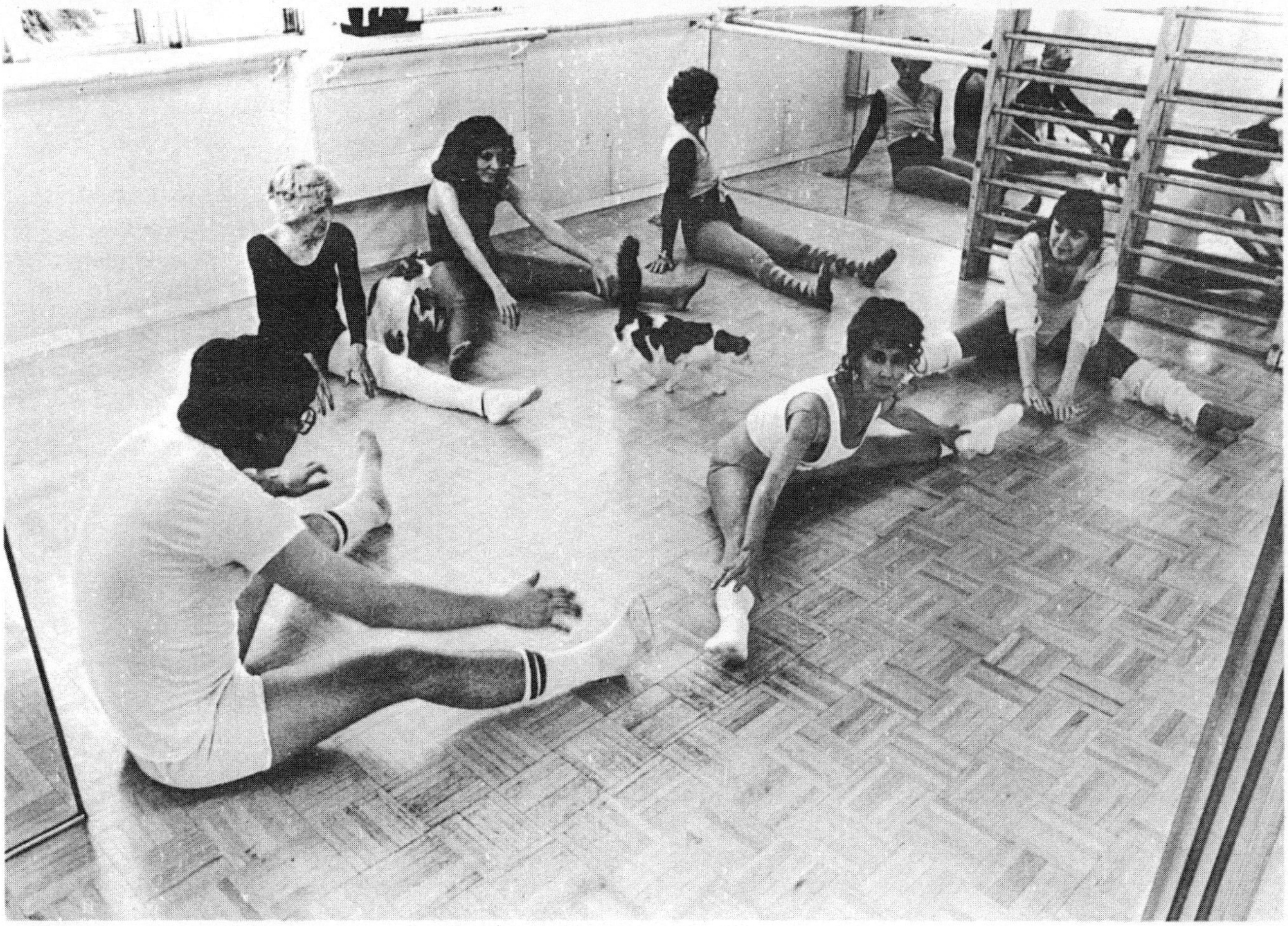

All I ask of my students is that they do as much as they can when exercising. Unlike programs where you are expected to keep up or drop out, I encourage students to rest when they feel tired, then continue when they are rested.

Until your body is ready, you may look a little awkward doing some of the exercises. That doesn't bother me a bit, as I would rather look a little awkward now and have a fabulous figure later on. ▲

CHAPTER TWENTY

Overcoming Problems

An Arabian proverb says:

> *He who has health has hope;*
> *and he who has hope has everything.*

While health can be a relative matter, I certainly agree that hope is the fuel that keeps us going. Hope is the heart of survival.

My personal hope kept me alive throughout my travels. It propelled me as I learned to exercise through pain to strengthen my own body.

One beautiful young woman who had polio as a child proved to me again that even someone with apparent physical disabilities can exercise and become fit. A bride of only a few months, she came to my studio with her handsome husband. As is typical of people who are confined to wheelchairs or who must walk with crutches, her upper body was muscular, though lean. Her lower limbs and buttocks shook as she dragged her feet and legs along the floor, moving across the room on aluminum crutches.

I had told them when they contacted me about classes that I had no previous experience with the physically disabled. My technique comes strictly from common sense and practical personal experience. Knowing this, they still came in for private lessons. As the husband told me, they wanted the lower part of her body to become strong and firm. They heard of my program from students and had seen the incredibly fast results.

I must admit that I was nervous. I honestly did not know the extent of her paralysis or what, if anything, I would be able to do for her. And I didn't know what they expected of me. Surely this woman had been given physical therapy through the years. I had to hold back tears when her husband took her crutches and she sank to the floor, gripping the *barre* with both hands.

I positioned her body for the behind exercises—the same as in the One-Hour Program. Then I showed her how to do them.

I don't know how, but she struggled until she was able to move just a little. When she protested, she looked to her husband for support.

Imagine my shock when he told her to quit being a crybaby and to get on with the exercises! "I love you too much to let you be a complete cripple," he said. She continued. Slowly. Deliberately. She did only what she could.

I was a wreck!

This gorgeous creature took two private lessons with me before she and her husband moved out West. They taped a class so that she would be able to continue working with her body. Even after these two sessions, I learned later, she began to experience muscle tone she never thought possible.

A few months after they left New York, the husband called me to say that she was *still* exercising and that she looked and felt magnificent! He also told me that she did not drag her feet as much as before. Of course, she will always need crutches to get about, but he told me her behind was already getting very tight.

To this day, I cannot understand how she did the exercises. I don't know where this daring couple is today, but I thank them for reminding me in two short hours what determination and willpower can accomplish.

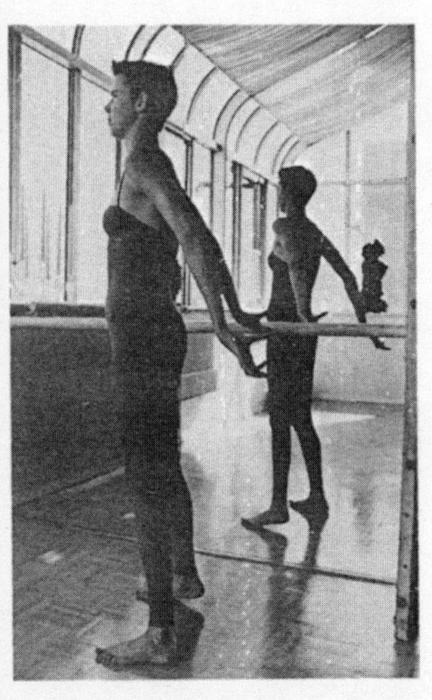

Scoliosis and lupus have limited Tara's flexibility, but have not stifled her determination. She cannot raise her arms in back to do this warming-up stretch for the underarms and pectoral areas, but she does them as well as she can. Her thumbs are pointed upward and her arms rolled over for maximum stretch. As with all of my exercises, each movement is slow and gentle. Notice how one leg is shorter than the other—the result of her back condition. ▲

Another student who is an inspiration to me and to my other students is Tara. Her physical problems are mammoth, but her attitude and emotional strength are empowering to all of us.

In her mid-thirties, Tara has scoliosis so severely that one leg is noticeably shorter than the other. She has a congenital calcium deficiency and milk allergy, which, as a child, affected bone development.

For twelve years, Tara has been treated with cortisone for systemic lupus erythematosus (lupus), a chronic inflammatory and connective tissue disease that involves the vital organs and autoimmune system. It is manifest by extremely swollen joints that become red, hot, and stiff during periods of inflammation.

Despite medical conditions that most of us would consider to be debilitating, Tara has incredible spunk. She has found that if she does not exercise, she loses mobility. Consequently, she makes a concerted effort to improve her body potential. For a while she worked with a chiropractor who helped her to see the wisdom in giving up high heels.

"I was in more pain because I insisted on being in style," Tara laughs. "He helped me see how silly that was and made me stop wearing heels altogether."

Initially, Tara came to me because she had heard that this program was good for people with weak or damaged knees. She *labored* with the exercises, doing the most her body would allow. For her first six classes she could not raise her legs off the floor to do the Open & Close. In very little time she found benefits she never expected from this, or any program. Her lower back is stronger; she has improved flexibility, and now has physical strength that far surpasses the norm for people with her problems.

All this because she does what she can—her best.

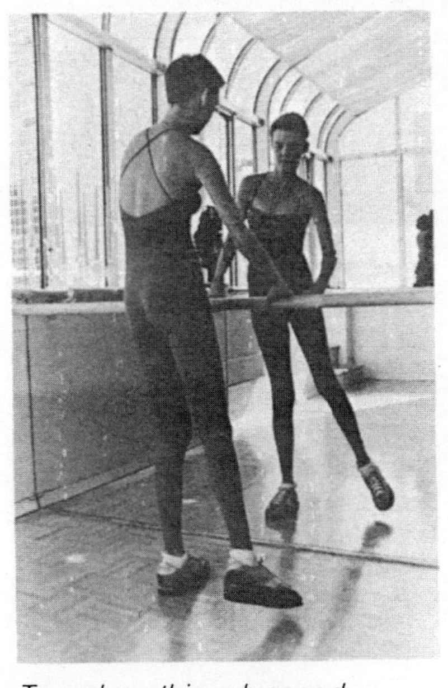

Tara does this advanced exercise for her hips and behind because she can't kneel. I don't teach this to most students because it takes so much control. Tara is very conscious of what her body can and cannot do. It may seem that she is doing this and other exercises incorrectly. Not true. She is doing what is correct for her. She wears specially-fitted running shoes even while exercising for balance. ▲

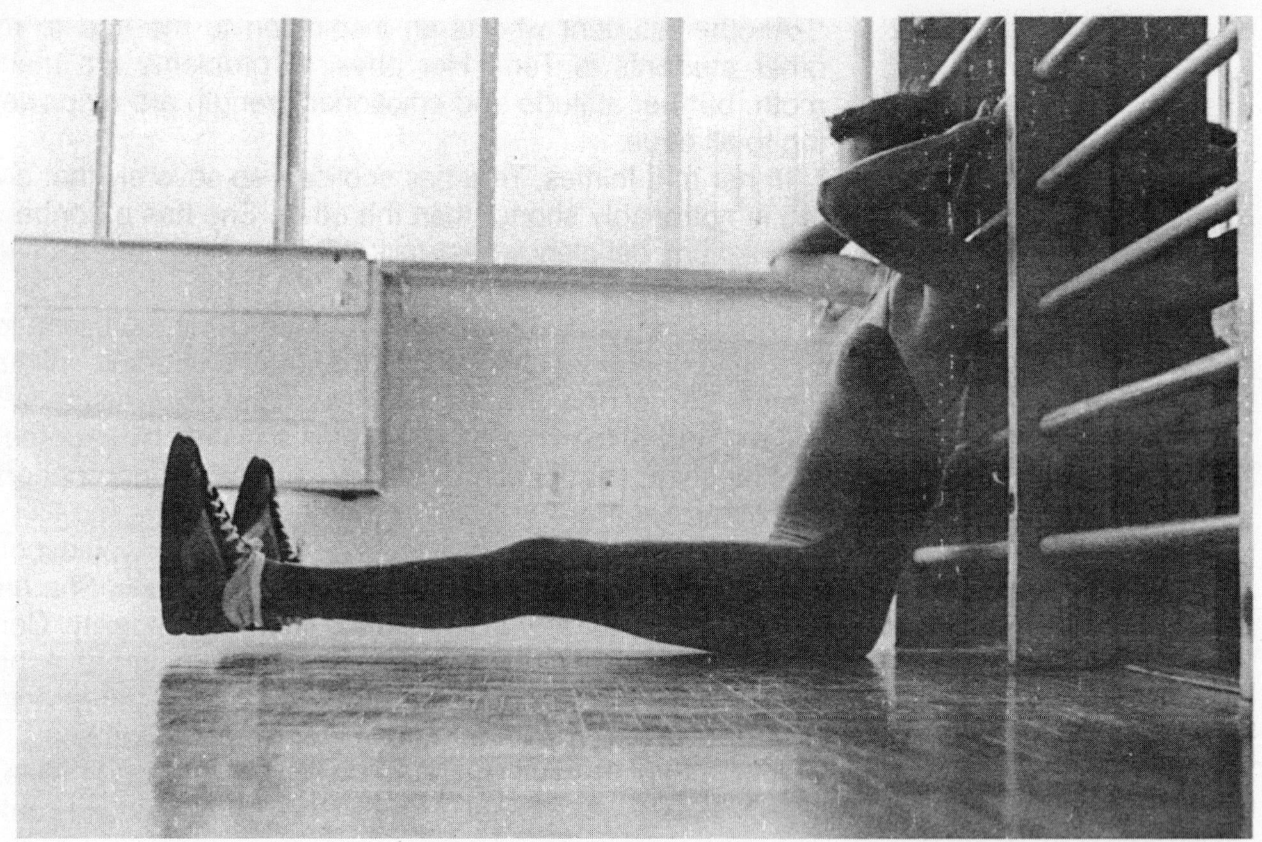

This is possibly the most difficult exercise I teach, yet, because she has such strength in her abdominal muscles, Tara is able to do it with relative ease. She sits with her behind 5 inches from the wall and rests her upper back and shoulders against it. Tara's lack of mobility limits her reach, so she works against the ladder, clasping the rung just above her head with both hands. Because she cannot bend her knees from the starting position to achieve a higher leg lift, Tara merely raises both legs off the floor as high as she can and opens and closes them about an inch off the floor. She can do as many as my advanced students without problems. ▲

CHAPTER TWENTY-ONE

The Advanced Program

Most of my students are not even aware that I have introduced them to a program of advanced exercises until they are well into it. When I see that someone has acquired enough strength and stamina—which is usually after the fourth or fifth class—I give her some new movements to integrate into her program. It may be a new way to tip the pelvis or turn the leg, something subtle that transforms the basic exercises into more powerful, advanced exercises.

The progression from the One-Hour Program to the Advanced Program is a gradual, very individual move. Unless a student demonstrates the physical ability to do more, I keep her at the basic level. I do not compare one student with another, nor do I have a timetable that says that by the fifth class everyone should be doing the advanced behind exercises, or that by the seventh everyone *must* do the advanced stretches. I do not permit my students to begin an exercise unless I have evidence that their bodies are prepared for it.

Do not start these exercises until you have completely mastered the One-Hour Program. You are looking at some very potent movements and your body *must* be ready for them. One advanced stomach or behind movement, for example, is equivalent to twenty of the comparable beginners' movement. These exercises may *look* the same as those in the One-Hour Program. Don't be fooled: They are the same, but with some very precise, subtle changes. If you follow the directions correctly, you will immediately feel the differences.

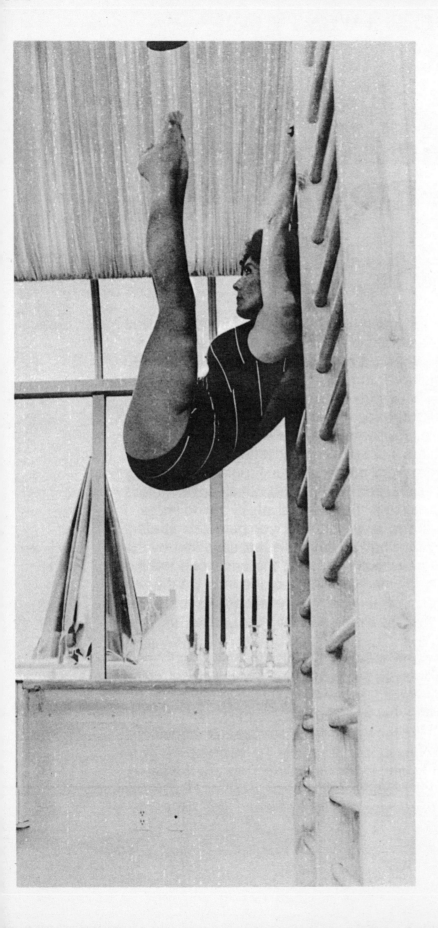

This hanging leg lift is a test in body strength. Do not attempt this unless you have access to a studio ladder, such as I have, a chinning bar, or a gymnasium with proper equipment that can support your weight. You also must have tremendous strength in your wrists, shoulders, and arms to do it safely. It takes incredible abdominal strength and, once mastered, this exercise can be expanded to include opening and closing your legs as you hang. Even now I can only do 20 sequences at this height. ◄

All of the students you saw in the One-Hour Program are beginners, with fewer than three classes at the time their pictures were taken. They demonstrate how to do the exercises quite properly, but they are not ready to go to the maximum level with them. By the time they have mastered the One-Hour Program, they will have the strength and flexibility to execute every exercise I do in this Advanced Program.

The challenge of this upper level plan is another reason to move on. It is a magnificent feeling to master one set of body moves and then reach out even further toward the mastery of even more difficult movements. Ultimately, you will have integrated the two levels of challenge into one totally personal program that takes the same amount of time.

Yet another obvious reason to advance to a more difficult program is boredom. Exercise, I am the first to admit, can be monotonous and boring. If you can introduce some variety into your body work, you will find the time passing like a breeze.

Because of the high level of control needed to do these advanced movements, you will feel and see results every time you do them. I show you how to alter the basic program into advanced movements, explaining in detail how to do the new, more difficult, advanced level. When you are certain you are ready for them, move ahead.

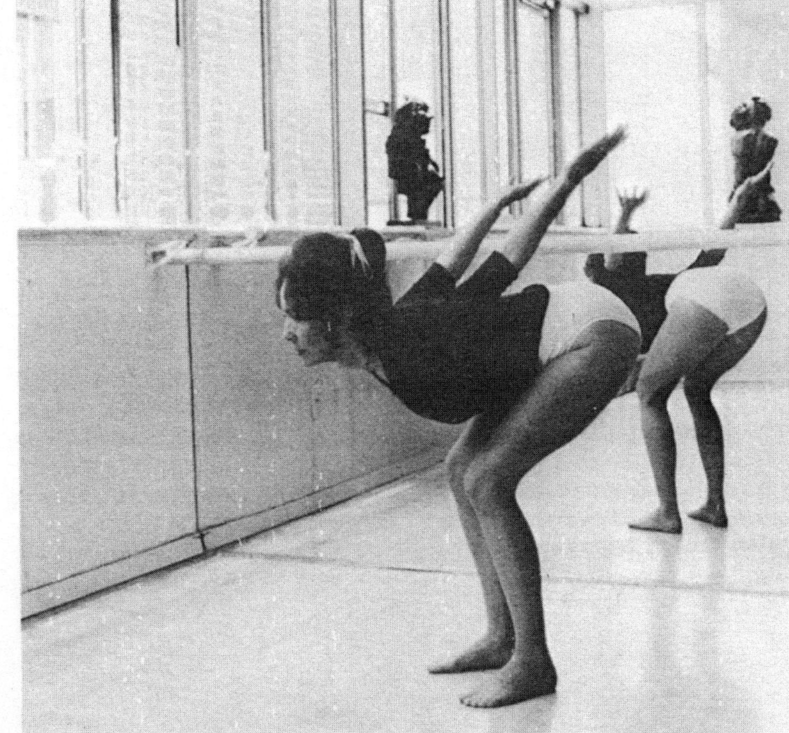

WARMING UP *Stand erect with your feet 12 to 15 inches apart and stretch arms and body upward. Tip your pelvis up, tightening your behind. Bend your upper body forward, arms out in front of you, as though reaching for something just out of reach in front of you. Knees are bent. Continue bending the knees and leaning forward; bring arms up behind you. Return to starting position. Repeat 15 times, keeping your knees relaxed.* ▶

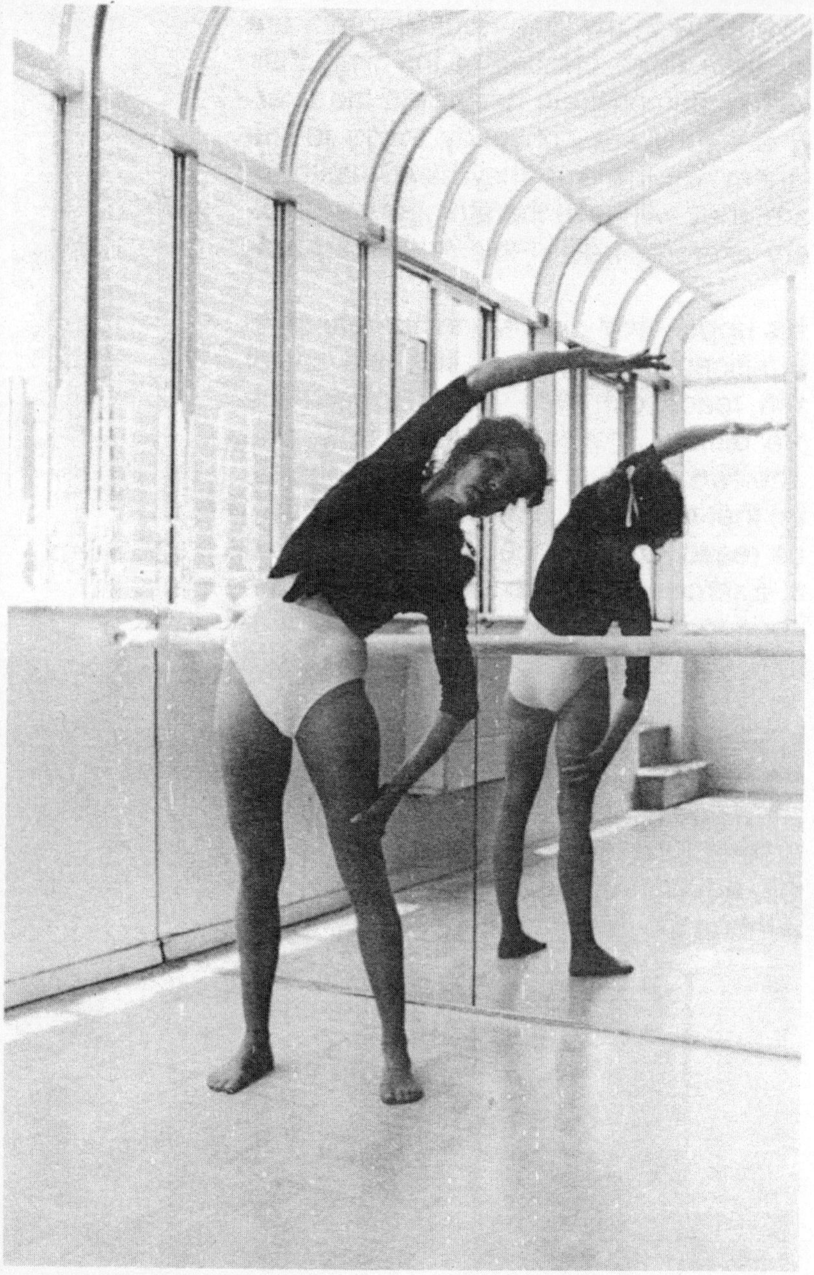

WAIST STRETCH *Reach one arm up and over your head and stretch as far to the opposite side as you can. Rest the other hand on your thigh. Remember to keep this arm out and bent to support your lower back. Notice how straight and even my hips are and how I keep my pelvis tipped upward. Most of my students can stretch over much further than I can because of my back problems. Even so, I am 4 inches smaller in the waist than when I was a teenager. Keep raised elbows straight. Do 100 in each direction.* ▲

FOR TIGHT UNDERARMS
Again, drawing from the One-Hour Program, the underarm tightener begins by standing erect, feet slightly apart, pelvis tipped forward. Stretch your arms out to the sides at shoulder level. Roll arms over and, keeping your arms straight and high, reach behind you as if you were trying to make your hands and shoulder blades meet. Hold head and shoulders up and back. Move arms only a half inch at a time, back and forth behind you. Keep arms as high as you can. Do 100. To learn better balance, do it while standing on one foot. When you reach 50, change feet. ▼

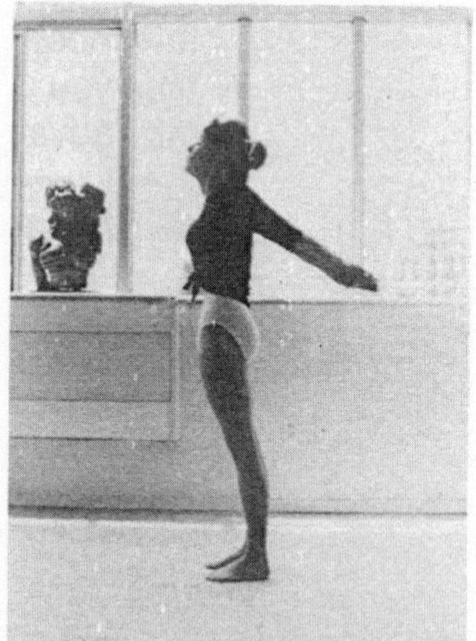

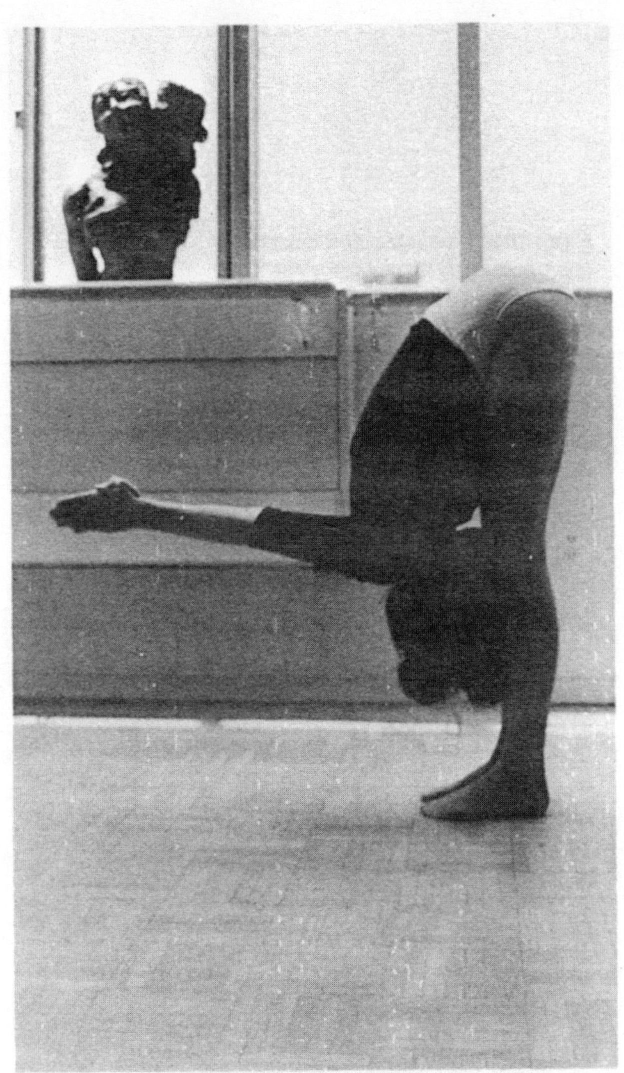

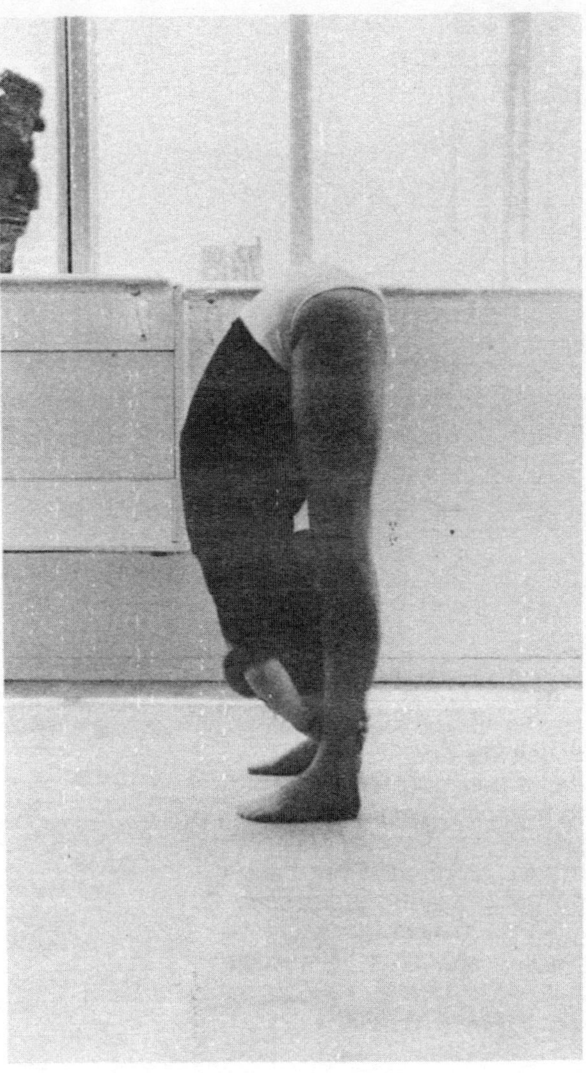

THE ADVANCED STRETCH

From that position, clasp hands, fingers straight, and bend straight over. Keep your arms behind your back. Do not tighten your knees. Slowly put your nose to your knees and move your arms as close to the floor as possible. Hold for a count of 20. This is to be done in triple slow *motion. Do not lock knees. Keep legs relaxed.* ▲

Without straightening up, move your arms down your leg and clasp your ankles from the inside. You probably will have to slip your feet apart a few inches to do this. If you are not ready to grasp your legs from the inside, hold on from the outside for a slow count of 20. ▲

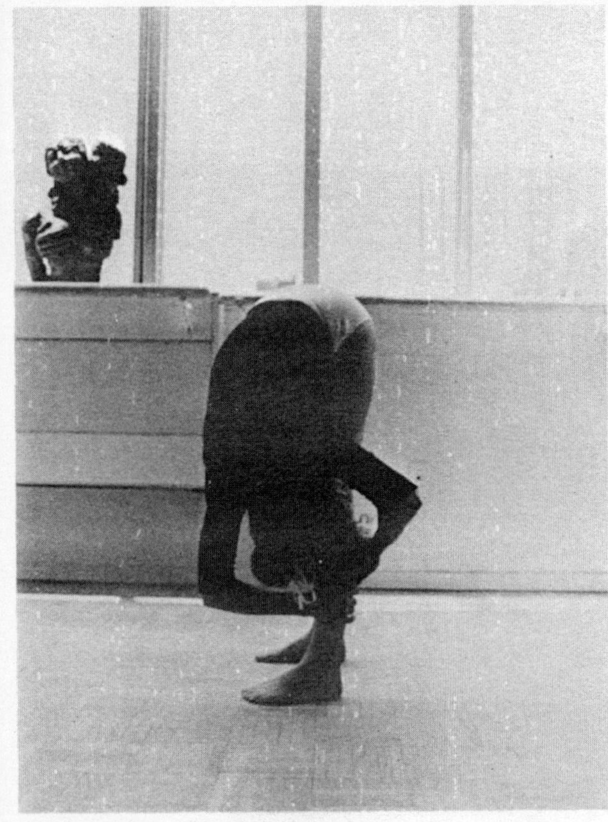

Turn torso to one side as low as you can. Grasp your leg from the outside, keeping your elbows bent out. You can do this with your feet together or apart. Try to move your head past your knee, between it and your outside elbow. Keep both hips even. Do not lock your knees. Do 20. Do not straighten up. Instead, gently move to other side and repeat. ▲

From that position, still keeping legs relaxed, move your hands to the floor, fingers facing each other. Bend your elbows. Gently move your torso a half inch lower and move up and down 20 times from there. If you are unable to move, hold for a slow count of 20. Return to a standing position by curling your shoulders upward as you straighten your spine. This powerful combination stretches your hamstrings, calves, shoulder blades, and lower back. It works wonders on your balance. ▼

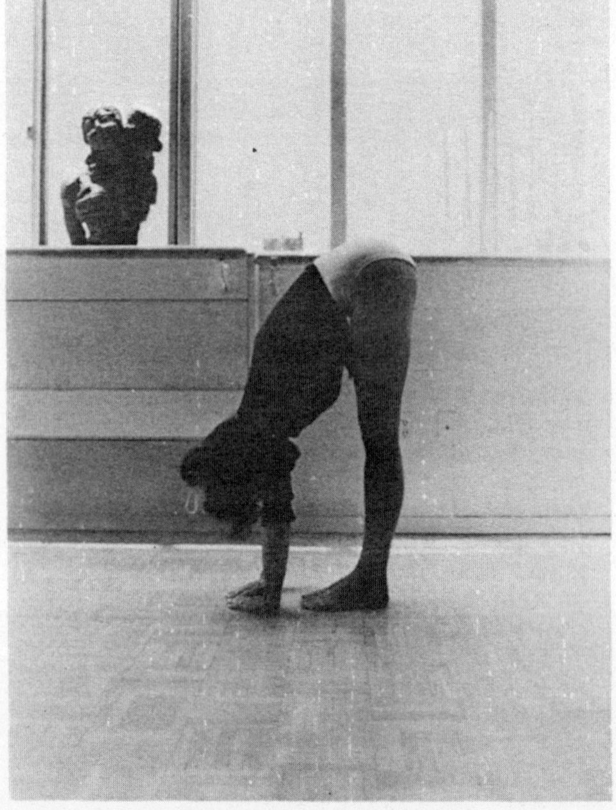

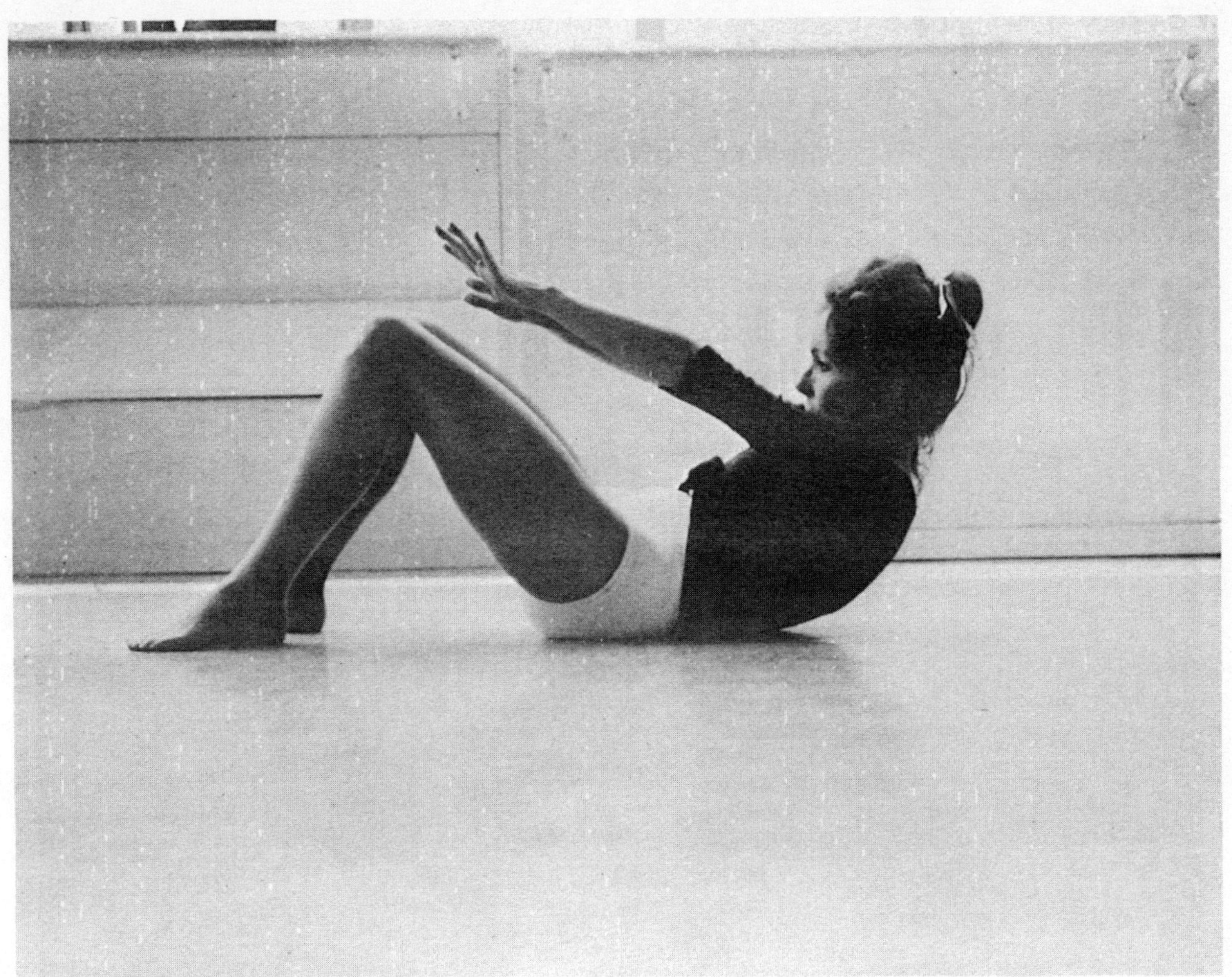

FOR THE STOMACH #1
Begin as you would to do the first stomach exercise in the One-Hour Program. Pull your upper torso upward, keeping your shoulders rounded and your elbows bent outward. Your body and legs should be relaxed. Let go of your legs and gently move up and down from that point. Notice how high my shoulders are. An inch higher and I would be using my back muscles. The object is to work on the stomach and abdominal muscles. Do 100. ▲

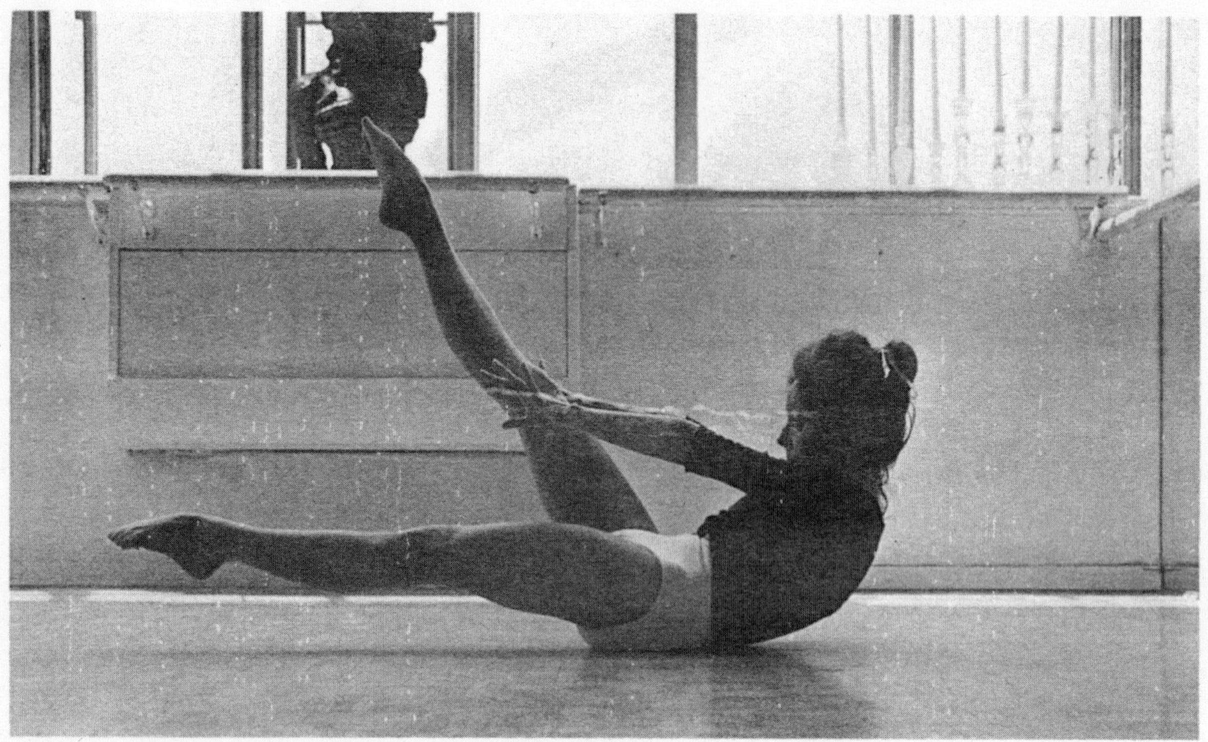

FOR THE STOMACH #2 *Lie flat on the floor. Lift your left leg 6 inches off the floor and raise your right leg perpendicular to your body. Clasp your hands behind your raised knee. Pull your upper torso off the floor, rounding your shoulders and keeping your head pushed forward. Let go of your knee and, without letting your shoulders fall back, move up and down a half inch in both directions. Do 100 with each leg.* ▲

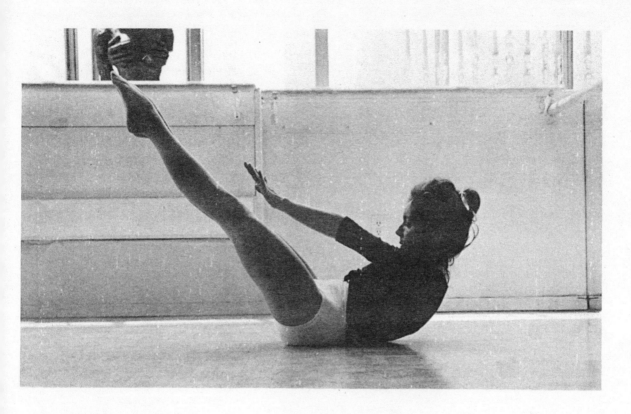

FOR THE STOMACH #3
Rounding out the stomach series is this precise move, done with both legs up. You can move legs lower than this, but be sure that you do not let the small of your back come off the floor. The lower the legs, the more the back will try to take over for your stomach muscles. Be sure your stomach muscles are strong enough to hold this lower position of your legs. As explained in the One-Hour Program, grab your outer thighs to pull your upper body off the floor. Push the small of your back into the floor. Let go of your legs and extend arms out straight. Start to lower your legs without letting your back muscles take over. If you feel pressure, that is your signal that your stomach muscles are not strong enough to lower your legs further. You must raise them to a position comfortable for your back. Do 100. ▲

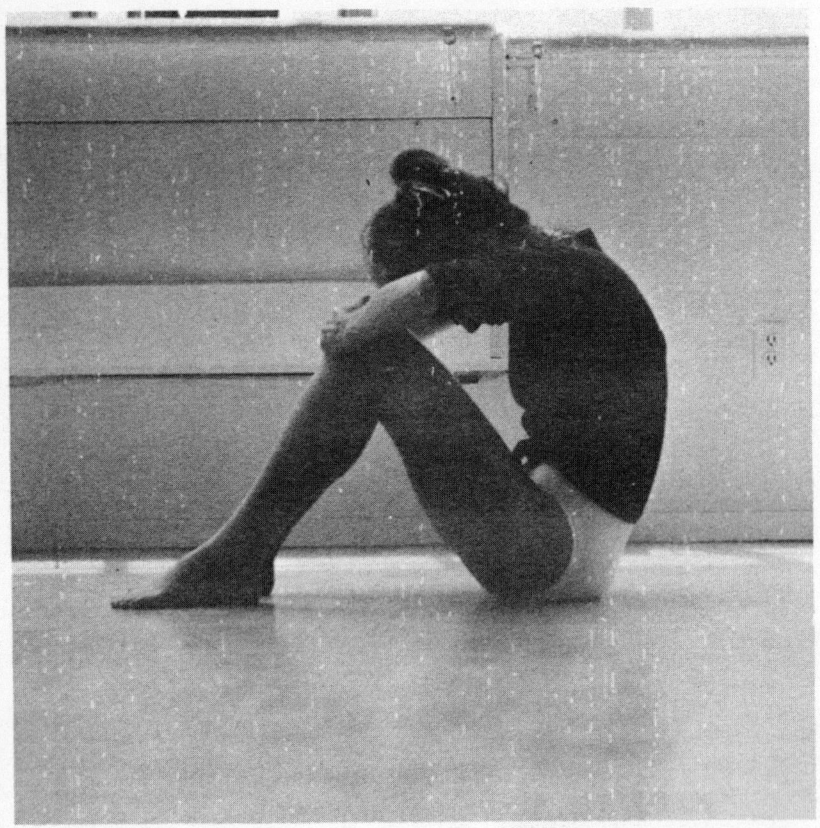

THE ADVANCED STOMACH EXERCISE #1 *Sit up with both knees bent, feet flat on the floor, head and shoulders rounded forward, and pelvis tipped upward. Scoot forward with your bottom so that you are not sitting on your tailbone. Your palms will be on your knees and your elbows out as far as possible. Tuck your head between your arms, resting your forehead on your knees.* ◂

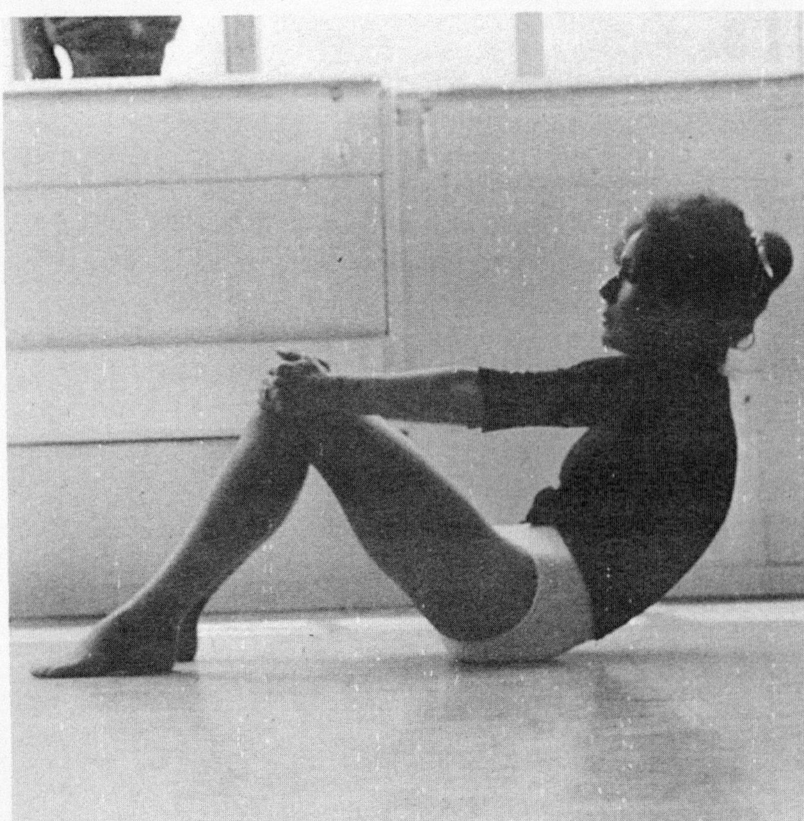

Tighten your behind and, without straightening your back, continue to tip your pelvis upward like a scoop. Your back will automatically stay rounded as long as you just roll your pelvis toward your waist while holding your knees until your arms are straight. ◂

Let go of your knees. Do not let your torso move. Keep your pelvis curled up and your shoulders rounded. Gracefully raise your arms upward, even with your ears. If you feel your feet coming off the floor, straighten your legs a little in front of you. ▶

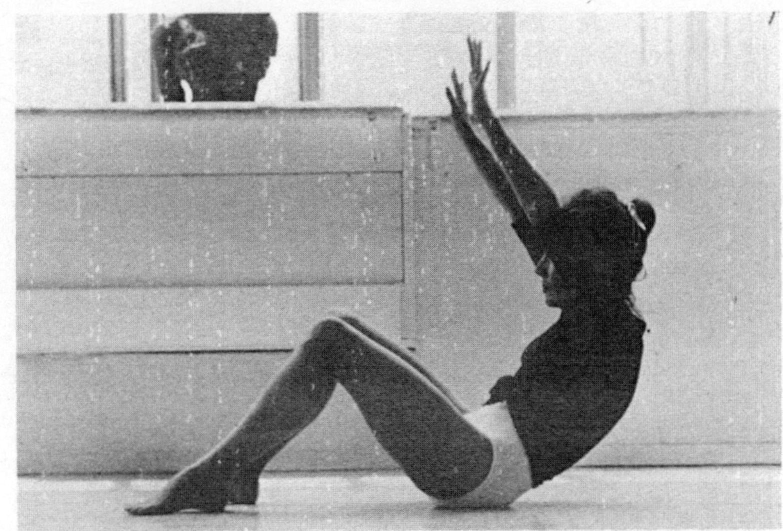

Hold that position without letting your upper body roll backward. Slowly lower your arms until your fingertips touch the floor. Gracefully raise and lower your arms 10 times without letting your body roll back. Breathe easily, normally. This is excellent for learning balance. ▶

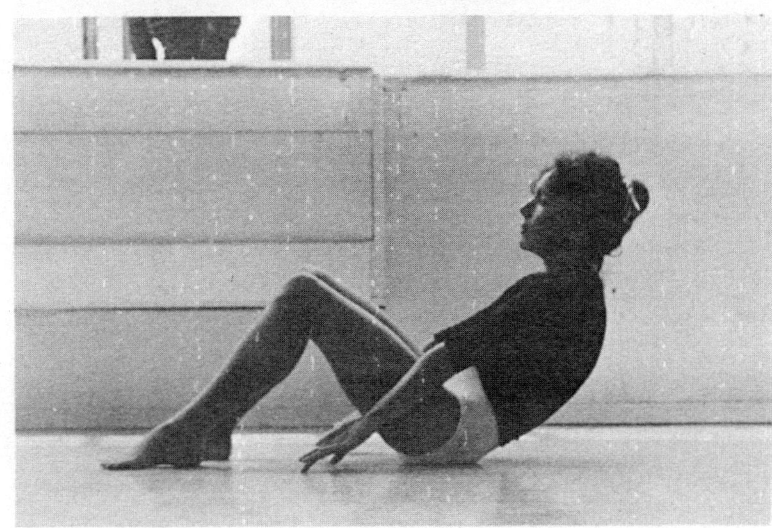

Without moving your body, return your hands to your knees. Arms should be straight and back rounded. Your pelvis should be tipped upward. Without altering your position, take a breather. Curl pelvis up still more, lower your body a little further, and repeat, moving your arms up and down 10 times. To complete exercise, slowly lower your shoulders to the floor vertebra by vertebra. You will feel the strength and power of the abdominal muscles doing all the work. ▶

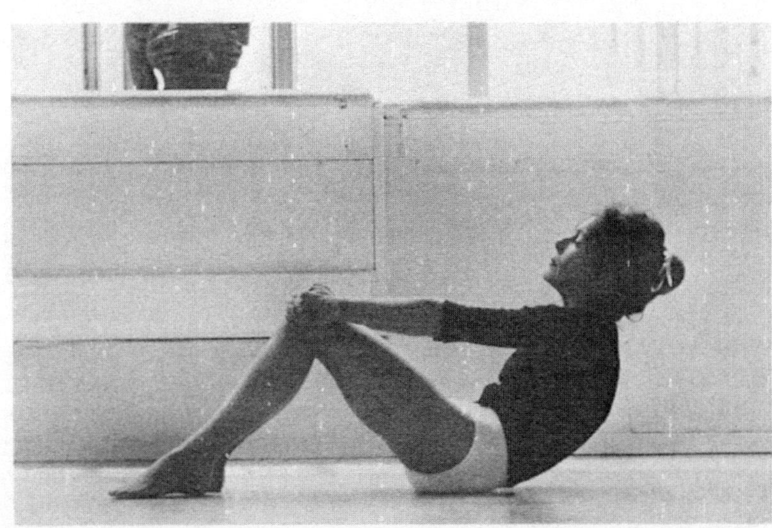

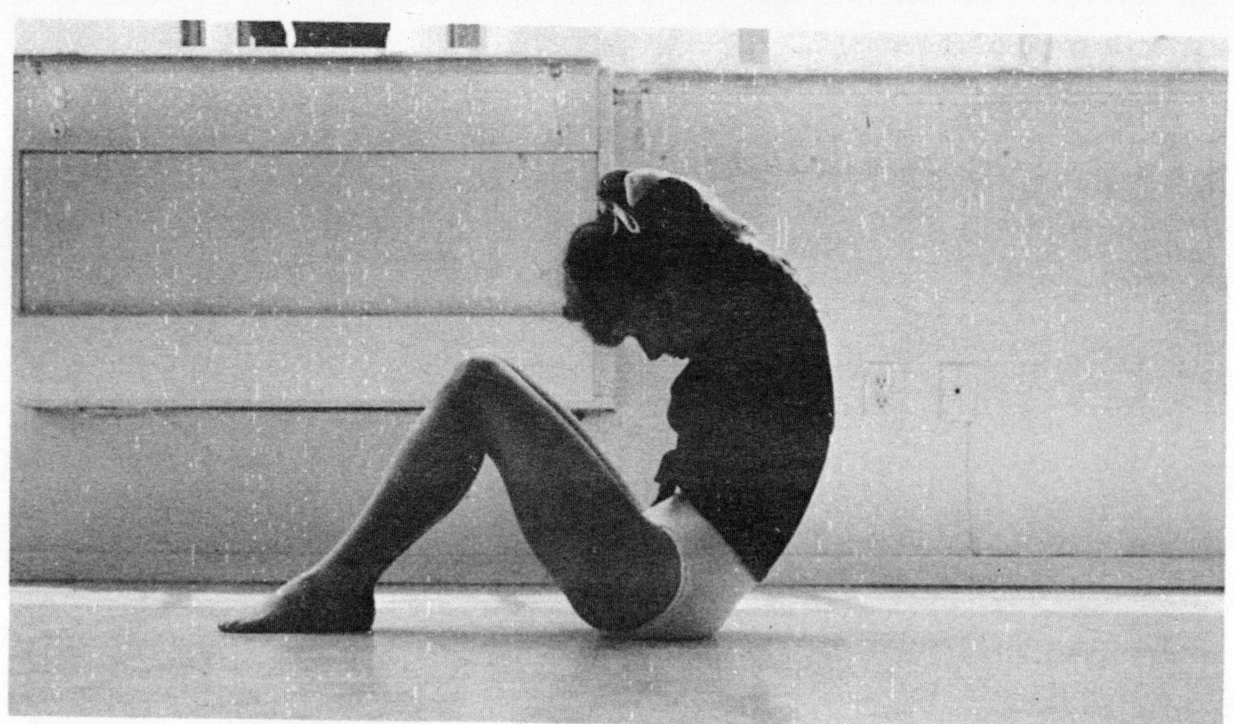

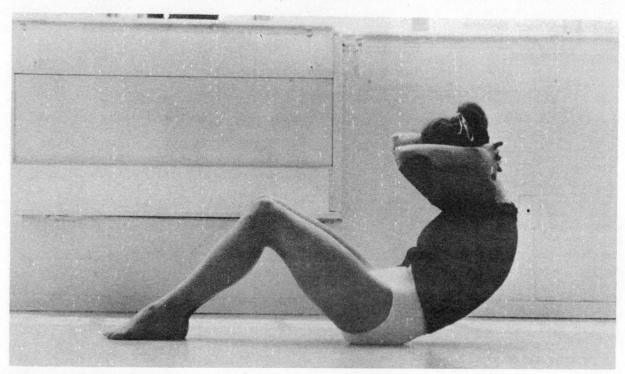

THE ADVANCED STOMACH EXERCISE #2 *From the same starting position as the previous exercise, clasp your hands behind your head and lean your head forward, your chin on your chest, and your forehead on your knees. Lower your body to the floor by curling your pelvis up even further, using your stomach muscles to ease yourself back, one vertebra at a time. The closer your feet are to your behind, the more your stomach will work and you will have to tip your pelvis higher to roll back. Do this extremely slowly with control. Once is enough, if you do this correctly.* ▲

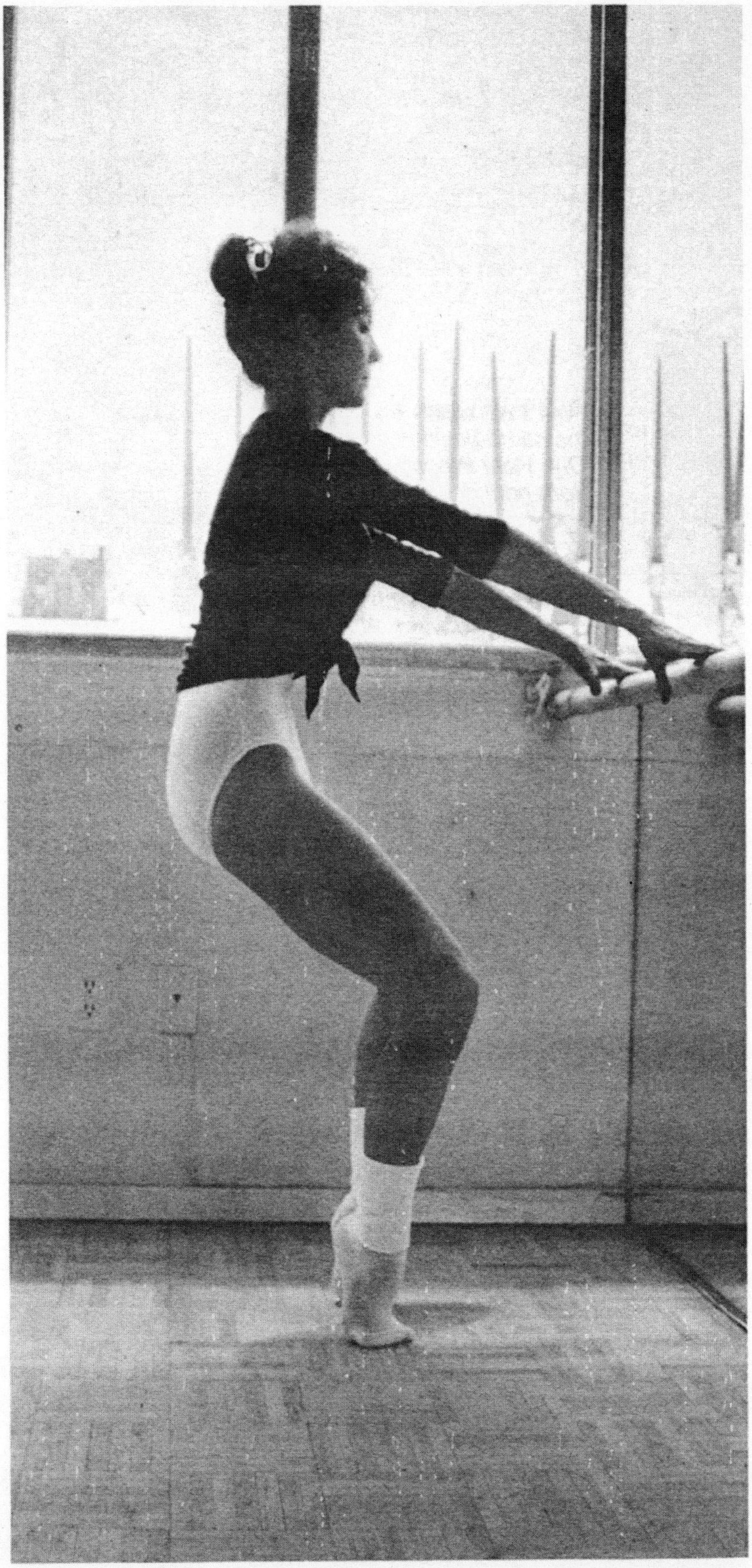

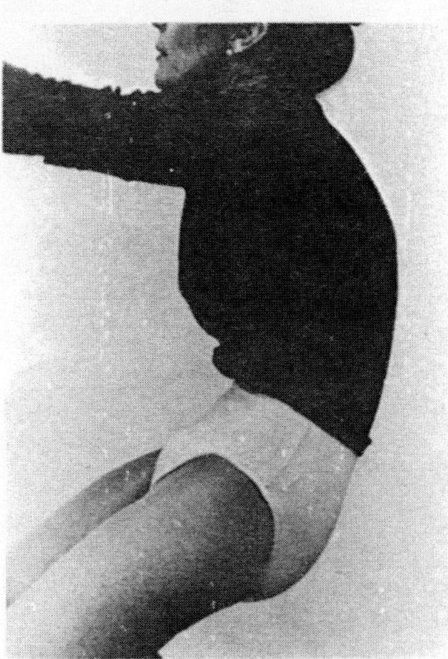

FOR THE LEGS #1 *Face the barre and hold it with both hands. Keep shoulders straight. Go up on your toes (not the balls of your feet), heels together. Move your pelvis upward a half inch farther than you think you can and then back. Go down 2 inches lower. Repeat this process 3 times and then reverse directions until you are back at your starting position. Do not stick out behind.* ◄

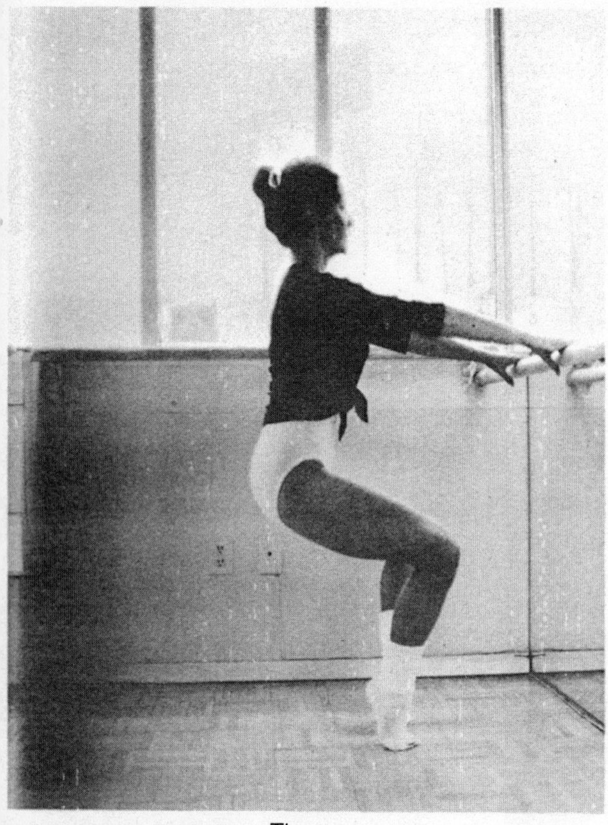

FOR THE LEGS #2 *The second exercise for the legs begins like the first: on your toes, heels together, holding the* barre *with both hands. Lower your body 10 to 12 inches, slowly and gently, then return to the top position. Repeat 20 times. Rest as needed.* ▲

FOR THE LEGS #3 *Start in the same position as in the One-Hour Program. Rest your right heel on the* barre. *Fold your hands across your ankle. Keep your hips even. Do not lock the knee of the leg you're standing on. Stretch your head and body forward. When you can't go any further, hold, letting your head go down further, either resting it on your foot or letting it go to the left. Stretch and relax. Count to 50.* ▼

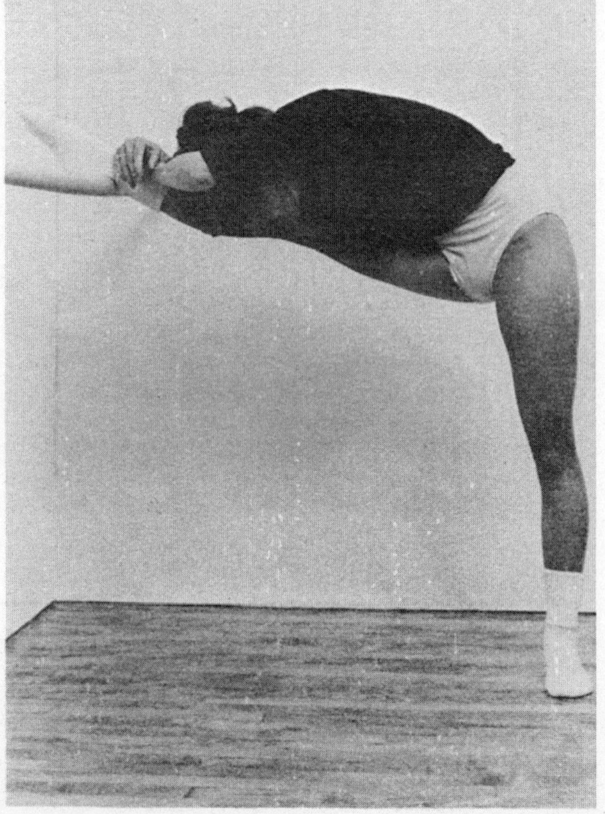

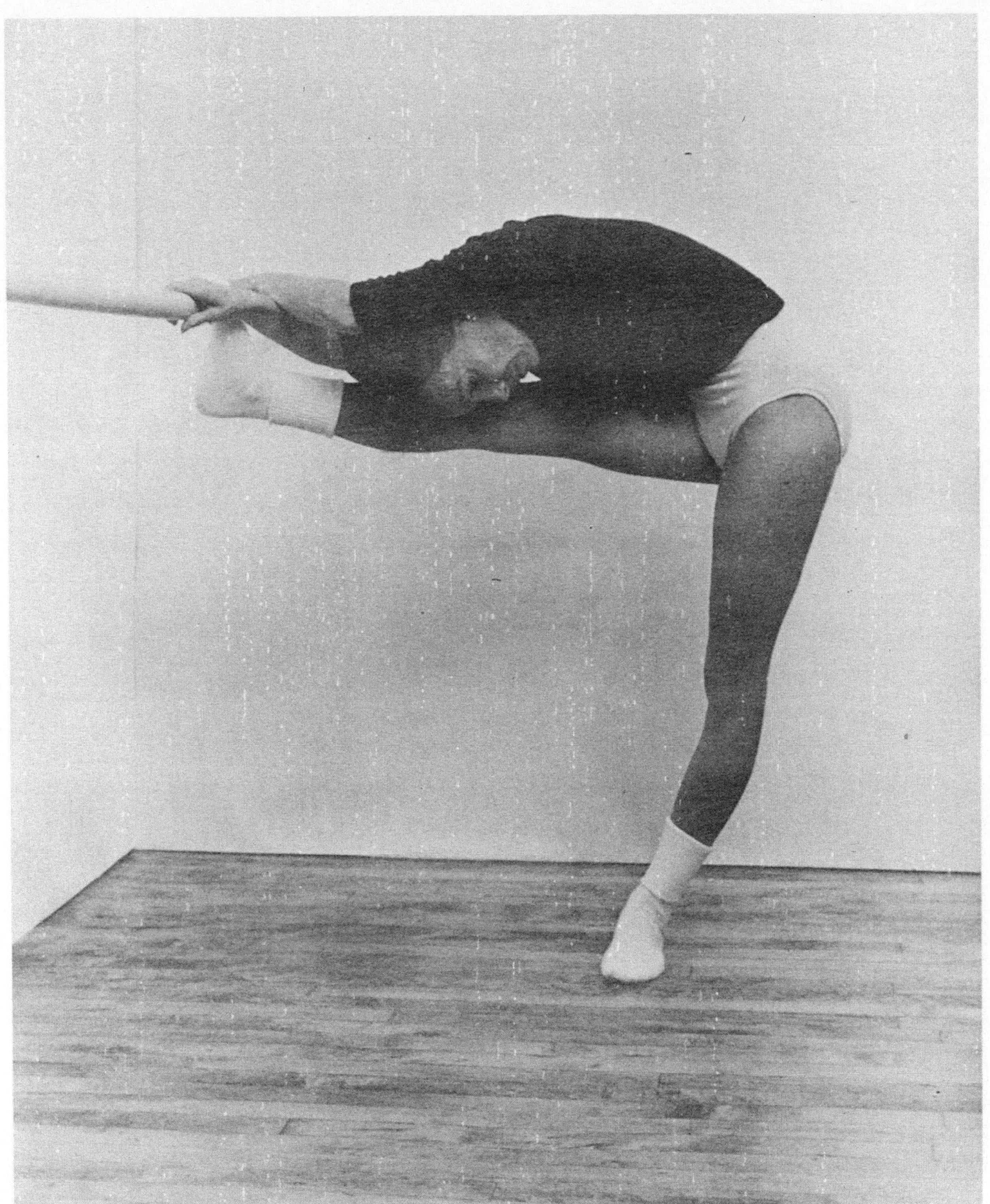

FOR THE LEGS #4 *Place the arch of your foot on the* barre, *holding your hands on each side of your foot. Gently scoot your standing foot toward the* barre *and cross your hands (as in the drawing) over your foot. Gently straighten the bent leg. Bend elbows and put your head between your leg and arm. Straighten your leg to increase the stretch. Gently move your body back and forth—very slowly, please—50 times.* ***IMPORTANT:*** *If you have a tendency toward sciatica, do not do this exercise.* ▲

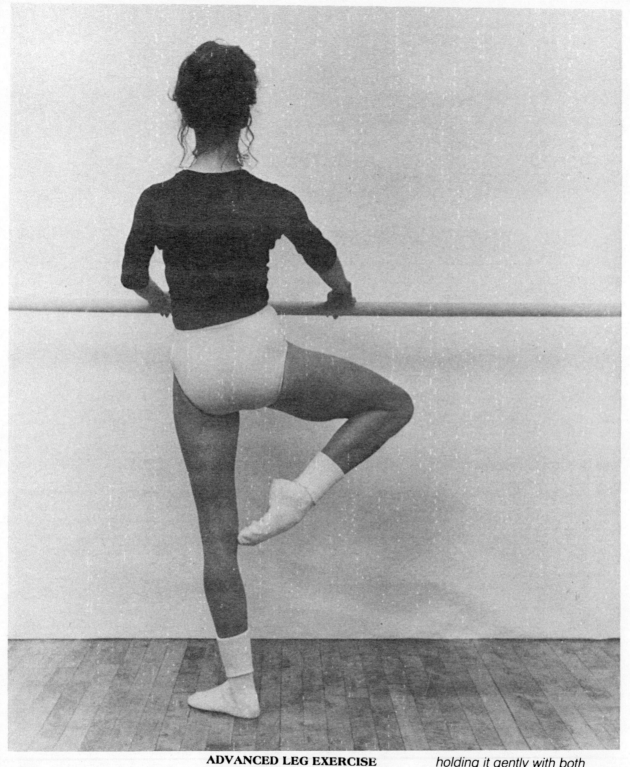

ADVANCED LEG EXERCISE
This graceful leg movement is fantastic for toning and shaping your legs while working on your balance. It is rooted in my ballet training, as you may have guessed. Face the barre, *holding it gently with both hands. Bend your right leg up and out to one side, pointing your toe toward the knee of your upright leg. (Don't lock your knees.)* ▲

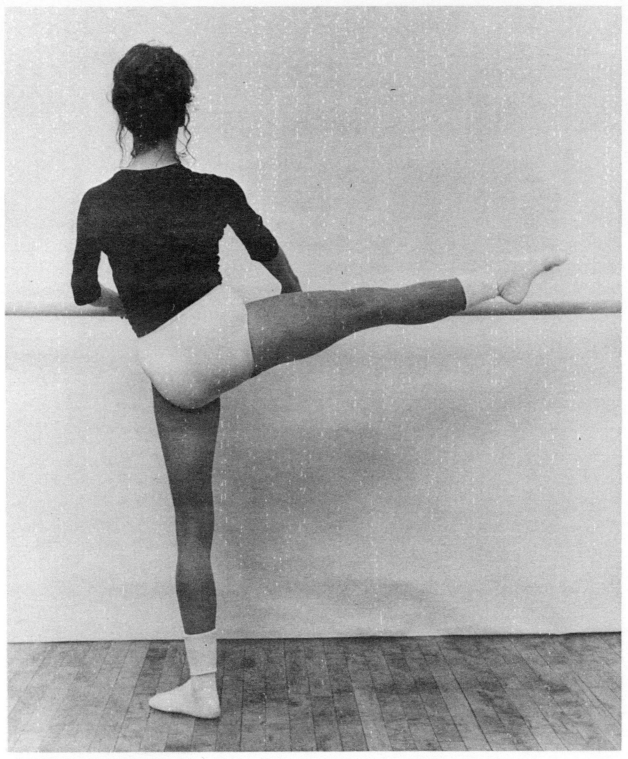

Straighten your leg out to the side without dropping it to the floor. Relax your shoulders. Keep your body erect, head up. ▲

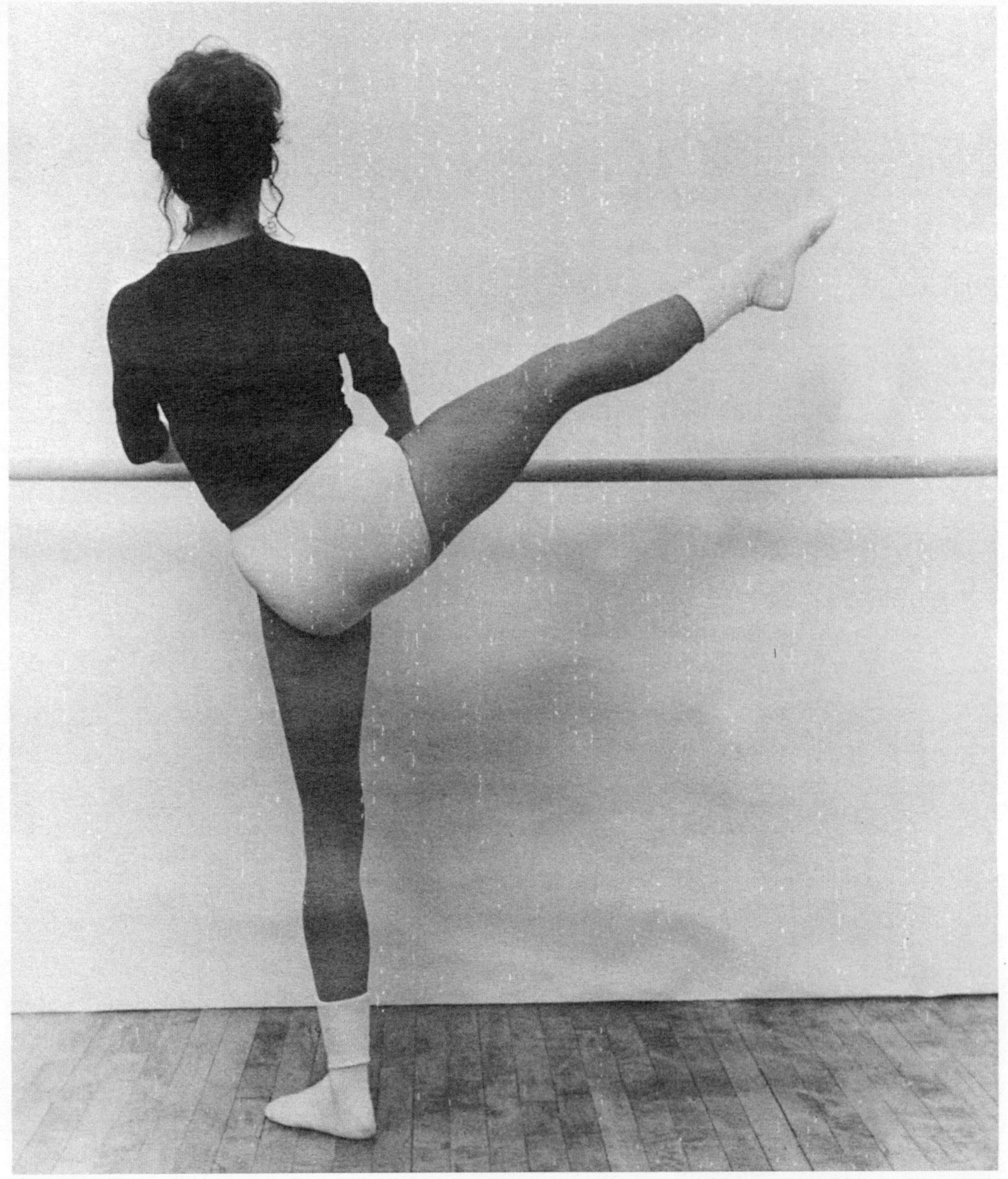

Bend your knee again and raise your leg at least 1 inch higher. Straighten your leg at the higher level. Bend and raise leg still higher, until you can reach this height. Then slowly lower leg to the floor. Do 10 times with each leg. ▲

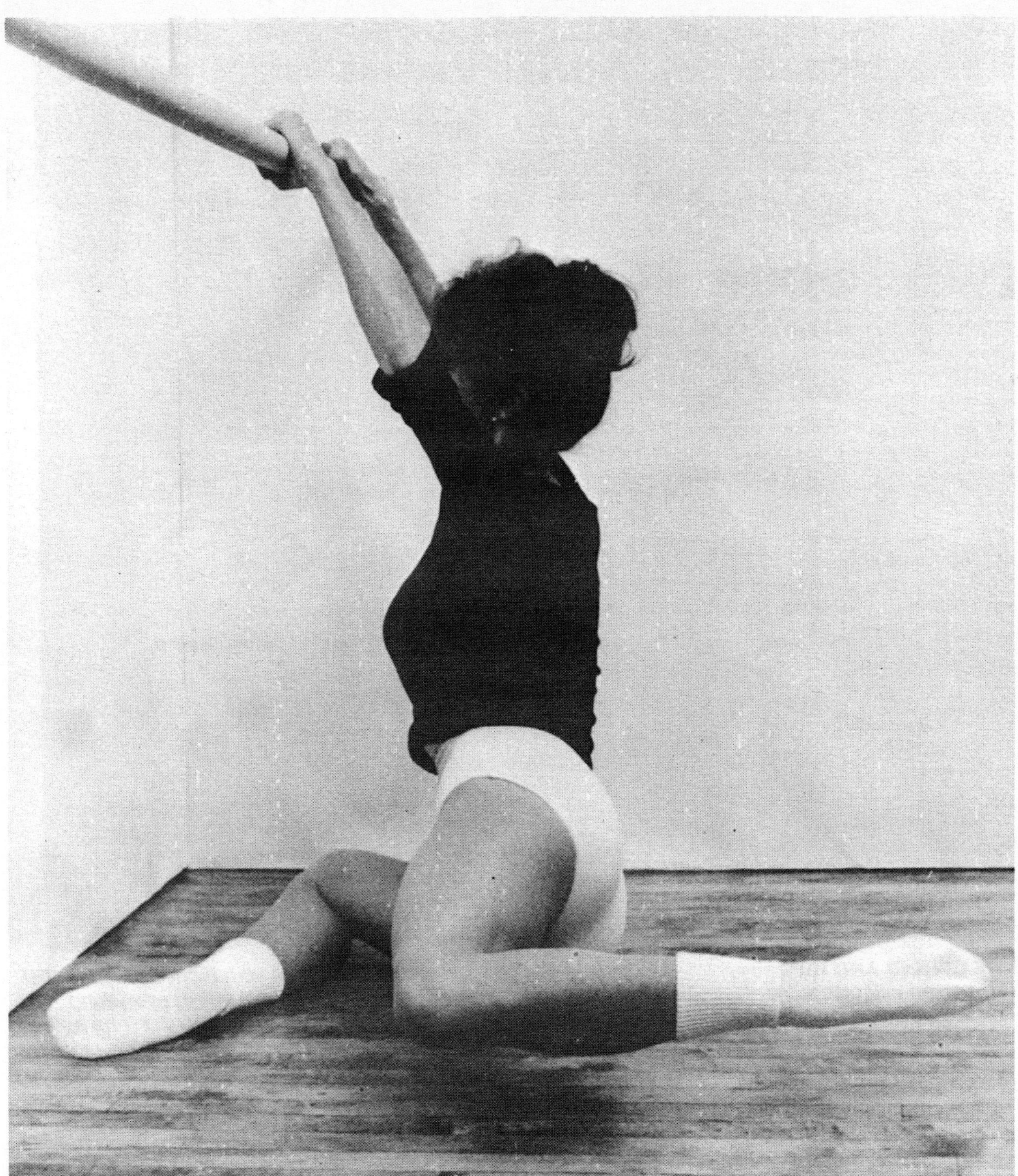

FOR THE BEHIND AND HIPS
#1 *The first of the exercises for the behind and hips is straight from the One-Hour Program. Notice how the left hip is rolled as far forward as possible, much more than in the basic program, and is even with the right hip. You should be able to keep your back straight. Don't lean over. The left knee is even with the left hip, but about 4 inches from the floor. Knee and foot are level. Move knee ever so gently a half inch to an inch back, then return to the side, even with the hip. Do 100 with each leg. Keep behind tight and pelvis tipped up.* ▲

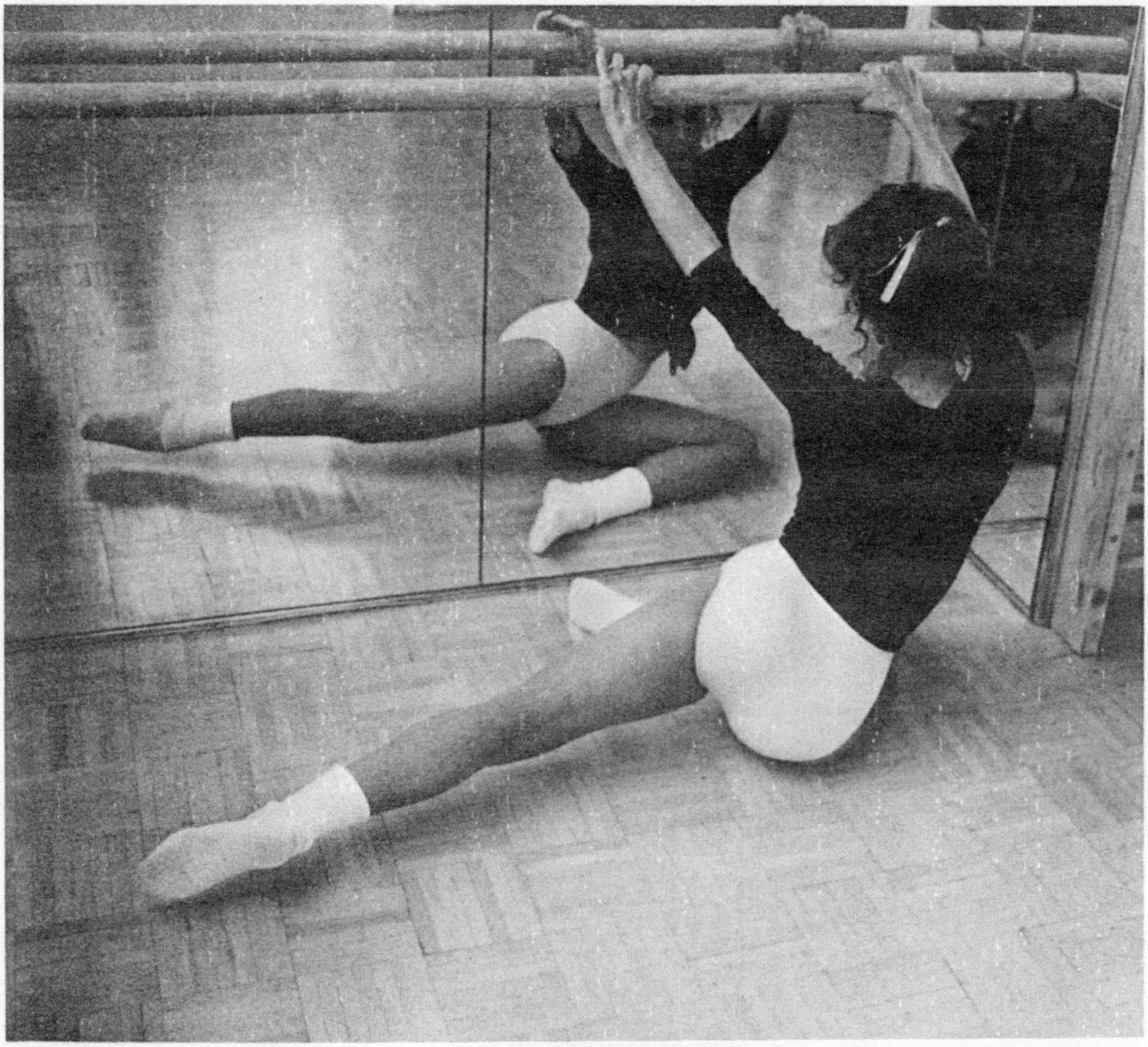

FOR THE BEHIND AND HIPS

#2 *This behind exercise starts in the same way as #1, but with the left leg straight out to the side. Roll the hip forward. Keep behind tight, pelvis tipped up, and foot turned into the floor.*

Try to get your leg as high off the floor as possible. Sit erect with your hip rolled forward. If you are doing everything correctly, you won't be able to lift your extended leg more than 3 inches off the floor. Move leg up and down, a half inch in each direction, slowly and gently. Do 100 with each leg. ◄

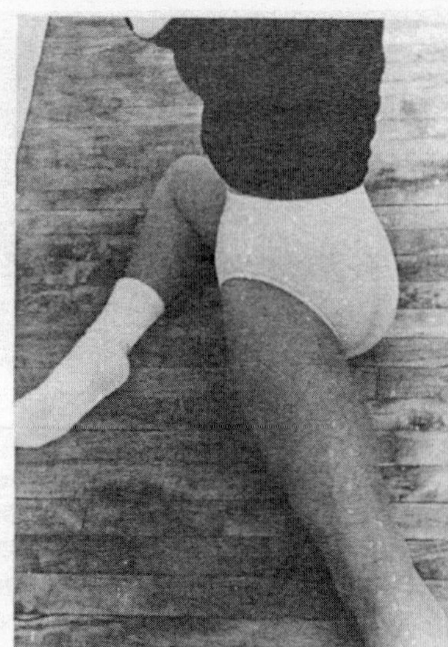

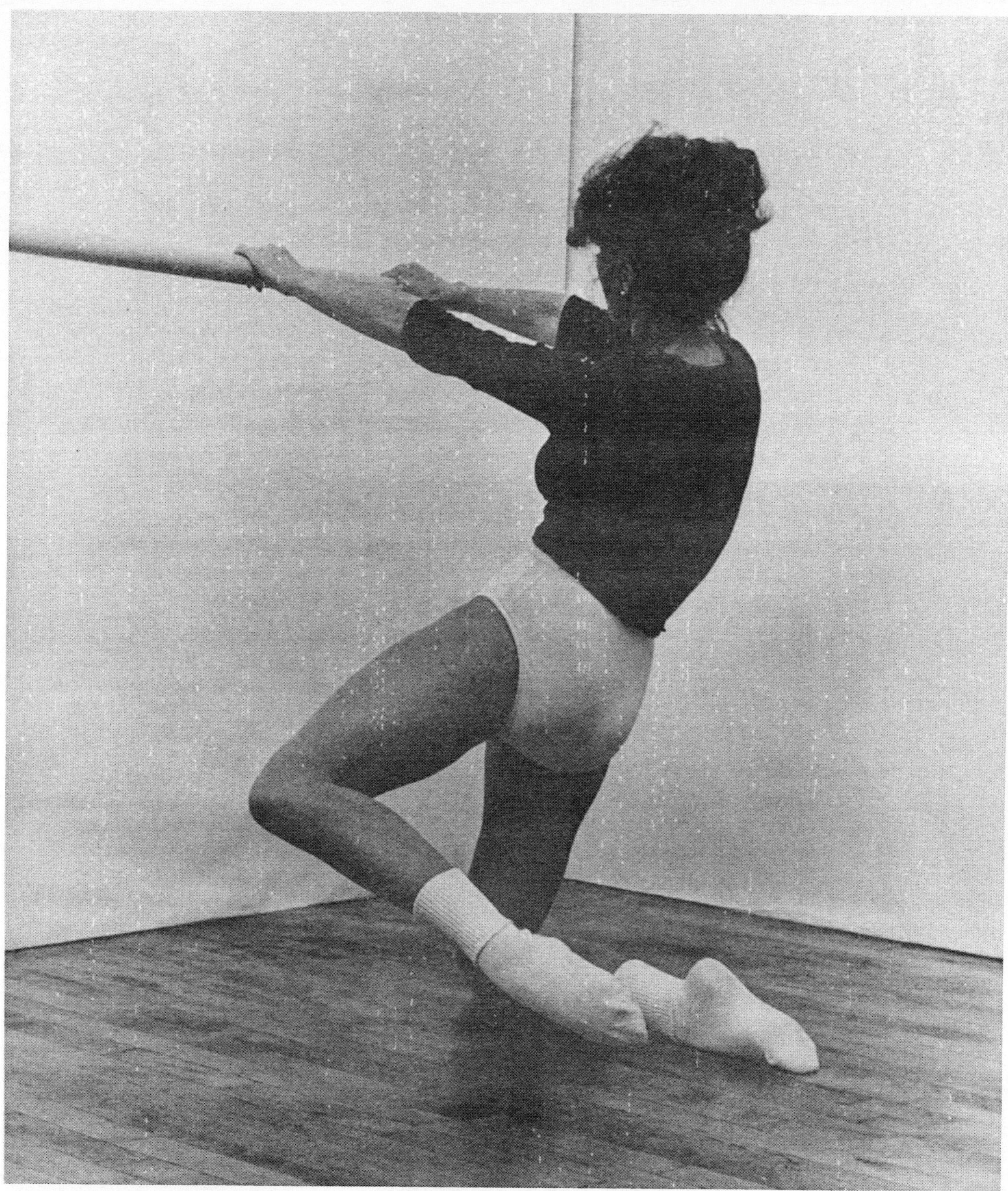

FOR THE BEHIND AND HIPS
#3 *If you do this kneeling exercise for the behind and hips correctly, this is as high as you will be able to lift your foot off the floor. Keeping both hips even, tightening your behind, and tipping the pelvis up, round your shoulders. Lean to the right to take weight off kneecaps. Raise your left knee out to the side, concentrating on keeping your hips even. Turn your knee to the ceiling. Notice how it is higher than my foot. Also notice how straight my lower back is and how rounded my shoulders. Move back and forth in tiny, precise movements, a half inch to an inch in each direction, but not in front of your hips. Only bring knee even with hip. Do 100 with each leg.* ▲

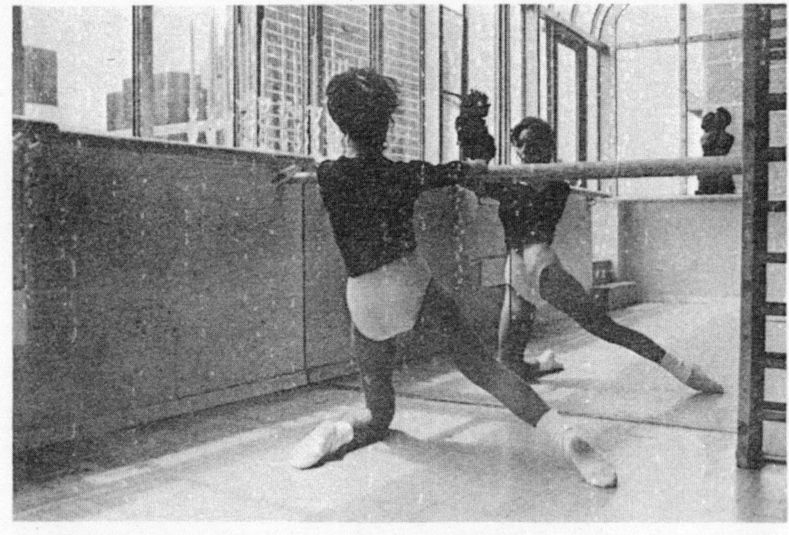

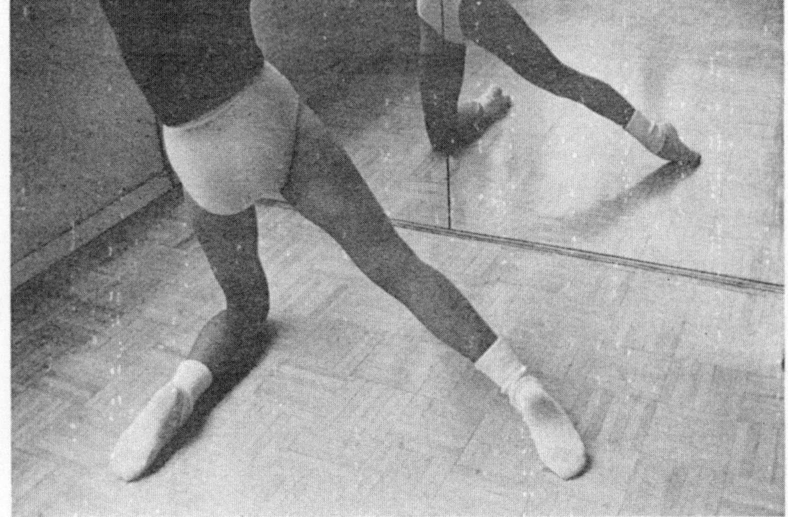

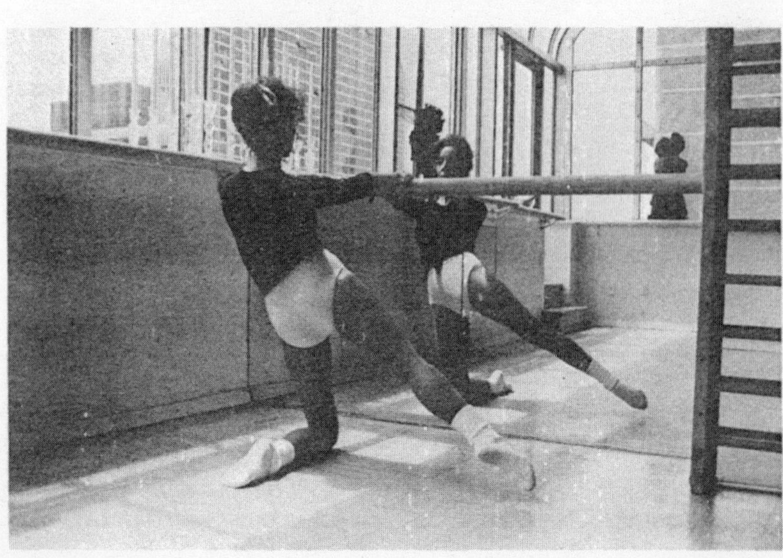

FOR THE BEHIND AND HIPS
#4 *Kneel facing the* barre, *holding it with hands at shoulder width. If possible, stretch right leg straight out to the right. Keep lower back straight and shoulders rounded, hips even. Lean your body to the left, pulling your leg to your body without bending knee. You can see how far by noting the tape mark on the floor. This takes your weight off your left kneecap. Keep foot turned to the floor. Tighten behind. Tip your pelvis up. Then lift your right leg off the floor 2 inches—or as high as you can—and move up and down. Do 100 with each leg. Keep your leg relaxed without locking your knee.* ◂

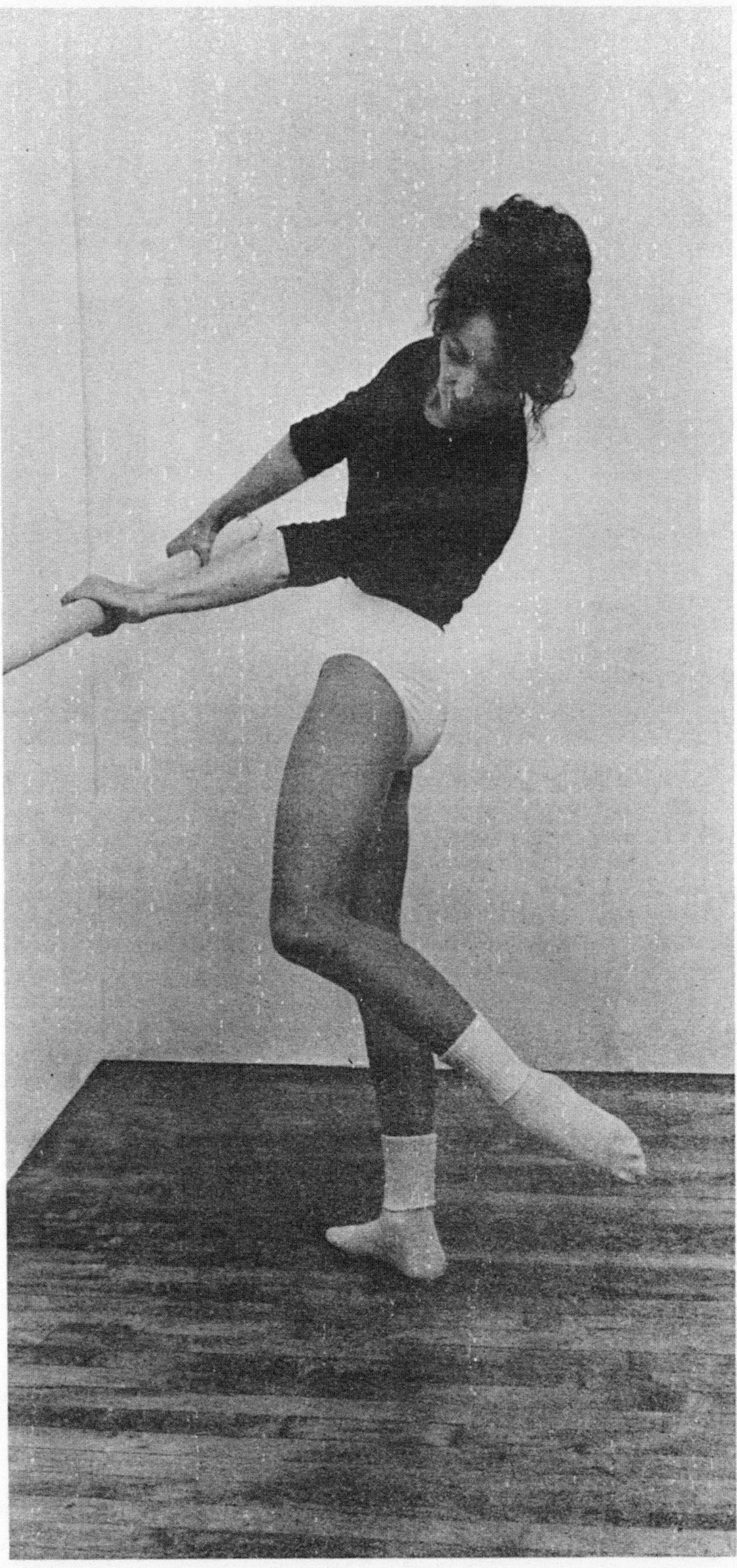

ADVANCED BEHIND AND HIP EXERCISE #1 *This advanced exercise is never taught until a student has had 4 or 5 hours in class and their bodies are strong enough to be in control. It only* looks *simple! Stand with your feet together, facing the* barre. *Raise your left knee to the side, turning it upward and pointing your foot behind you. Tighten your behind and curl your pelvis up. Lean your shoulders toward your raised leg. This keeps pressure off your back and helps you to keep your pelvis up. Keep hips even. Move your leg to the back in tiny, precise movements, keeping your knees up. Do 100 on each side. Do not lock right knee. This and #2 are substitutes for the kneeling exercises in the One-Hour Program if you have bad knees or bruise easily.* ▶

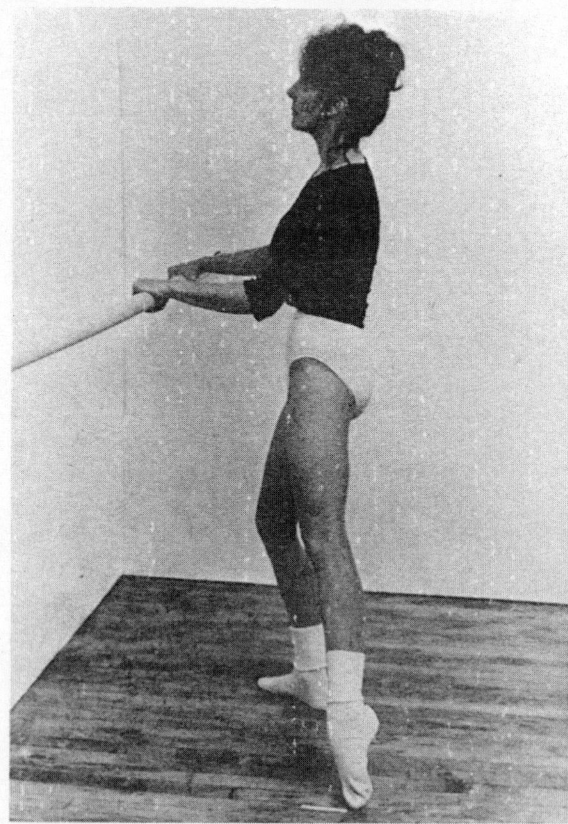

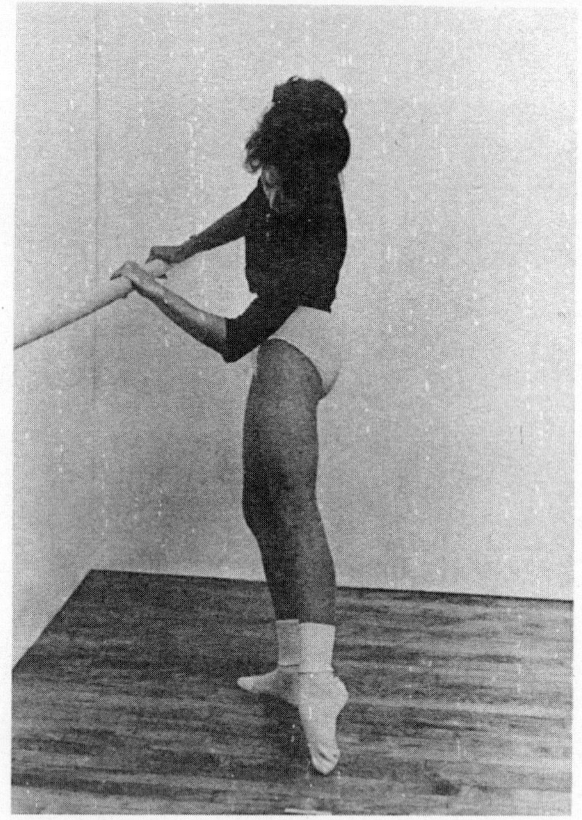

ADVANCED BEHIND AND HIP EXERCISE #2 *As you stand facing the* barre, *keep your hips even and your right knee bent just a little. Take your left leg straight out to the left side, still keeping your hips even and your back straight. Head is up, shoulders relaxed.* ▲

Bring your left leg toward your right foot. Lean your body to the right, keeping your behind tight and your pelvis tipped upward. Notice how far I have brought my leg from the marker. Lean your shoulders over to the left, relax.

Then lift your leg up and down. If you are standing properly, you won't be able to get your foot more than 5 inches off the floor. This is especially true if your hips are even and pelvis is curled up. Do 100 on each side. ▲

OPEN & CLOSE *Sit against the wall with your behind 3 to 6 inches from the baseboard and your shoulders against the wall. Grasp the* barre*—or whatever you are using—with both hands. If you feel you want to stretch your spine further, lean your chin forward. With your legs together, bend your knees and raise your legs up in a jackknife in front of your body. Straighten your legs, keeping them high, and slowly open and close. Do not lock knees. The higher you raise them and the wider you open them, the more your thigh muscles will tighten. Do 100—4 sets of 25, if necessary.* ▶

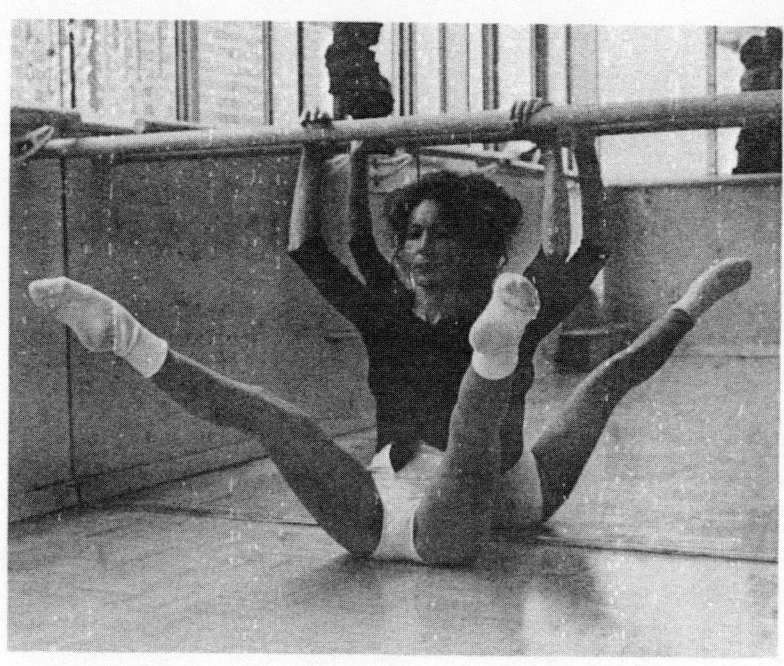

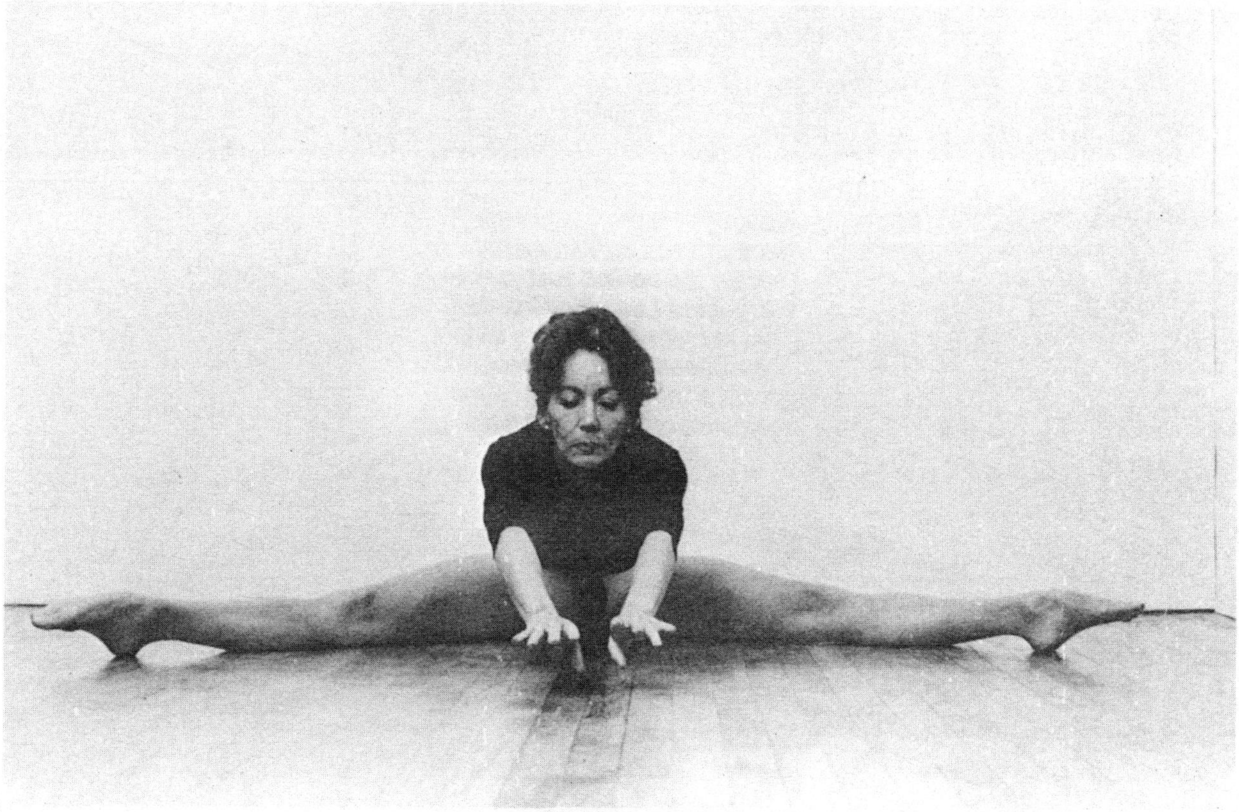

STRETCH #1 *Spread your legs as far as you can. Point your toes but keep them relaxed. Stretch your arms forward and lean your upper body forward as far as you can. Move forward from there gently until your chest is on the floor. Then stretch to each side, resting head and arms on leg. Do 50 in each direction.* ▲

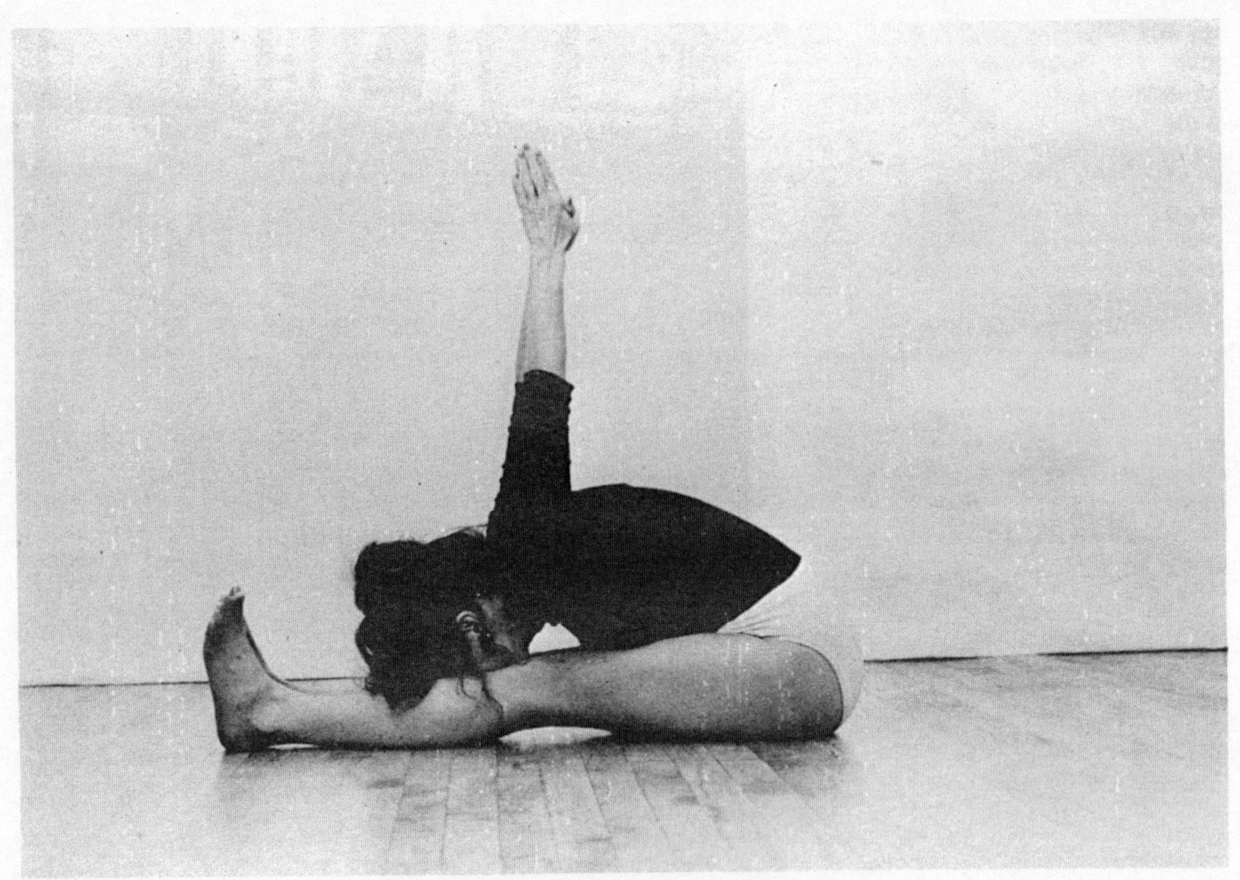

STRETCH #2 *With legs together sit erect. Reach your arms out behind you, palms together. Lean forward, feet flexed, stretching over to rest your head on your knees with your arms up in back. Hold for a count of 25. Do not force.* ▲

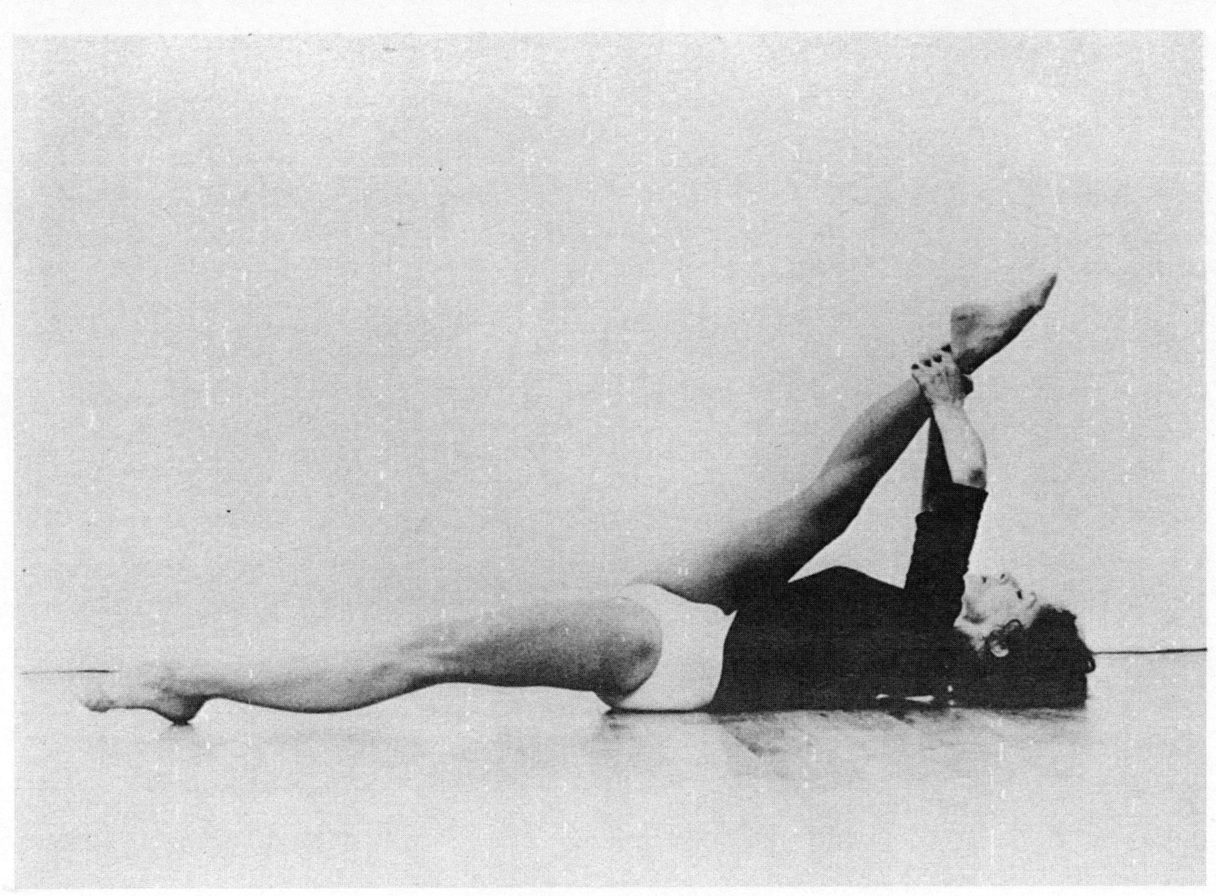

STRETCH #3 *This is a beautiful hamstring stretch. Lie flat on the floor, back and shoulders relaxed. Bend your right knee to your chest then straighten leg upward. Clasp your right leg gently with both hands at the ankle and ease it softly toward your chest. Keep your arms relaxed, elbows bent outward. Gently bring leg toward chest. Relax. Do 50 times with each leg.* ▲

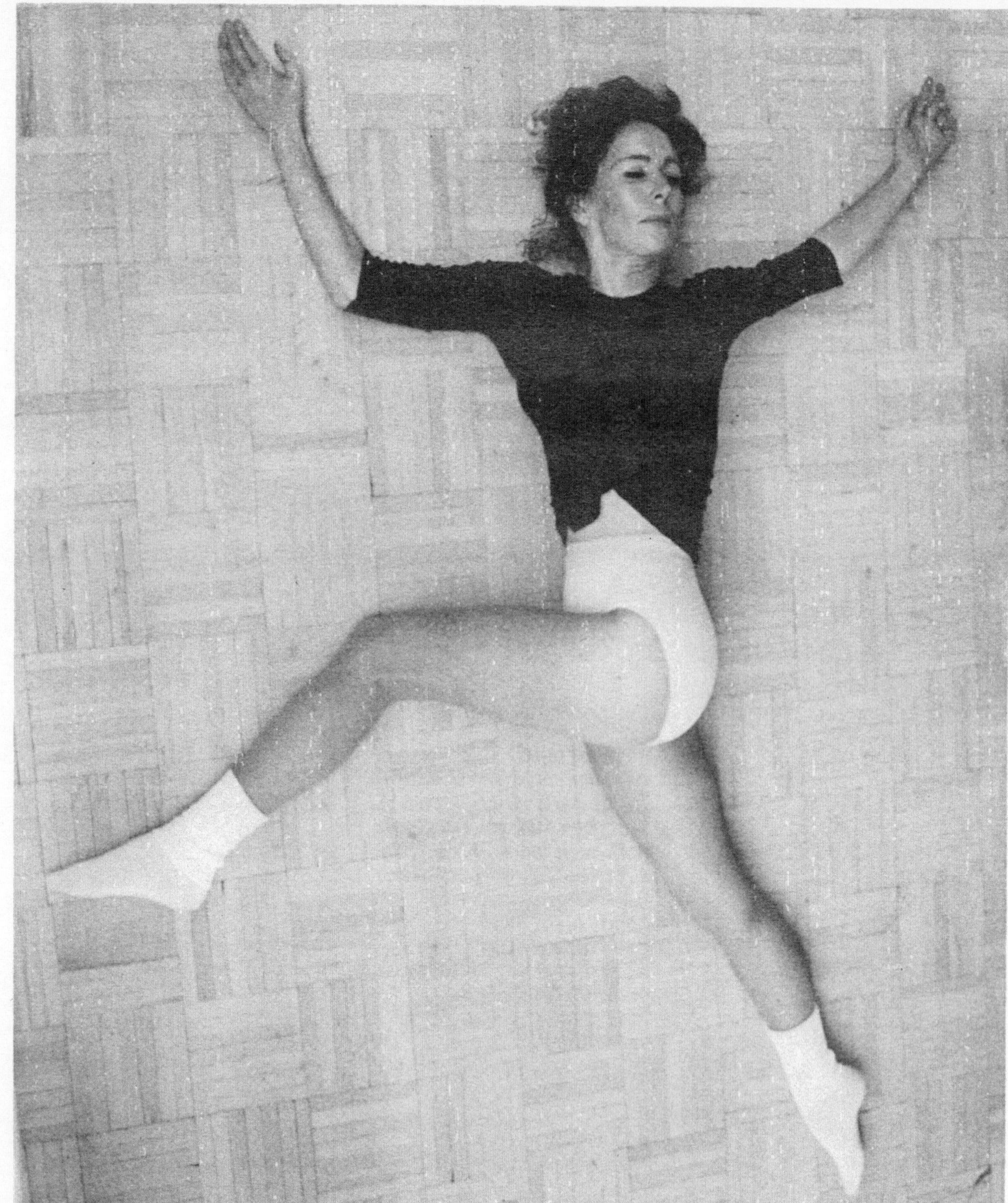

STRETCH #4 *For someone with the least hint of back pain, this could be called the best stretch. Lie flat on the floor, arms bent at shoulder level. Keep elbows on the floor. Raise your left leg up and cross over to the right side, as though you are trying to touch your right elbow with your left knee. Keep your right leg on the floor. The higher you can take your knee to your arms and the straighter you can keep your right leg, the more stretch you will feel through your pectorals, your spine, between your shoulder blades, even your sacrum, hamstrings, and thighs. Hold for a count of 40 on each side.* ▲

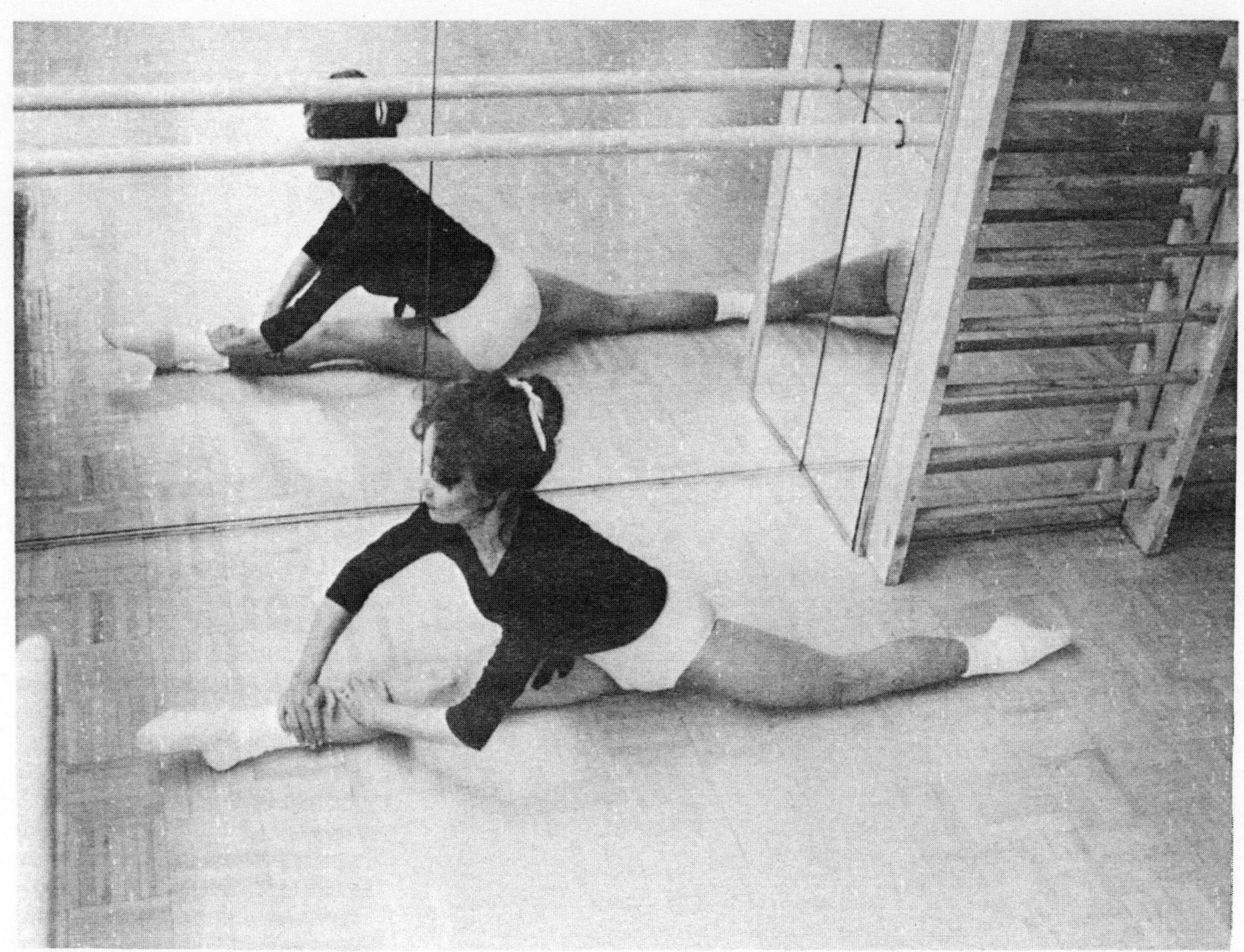

STRETCH #5 *This is a grown-up version of the split everybody learned in phys. ed. or dancing school. I give it to some of my advanced students and do it myself for flexibility, letting hand rest on leg for balance. My students like to do it because they feel like gymnasts! It's a superb stretch for your thighs. Do not force. Hold for a count of 30.* ▲

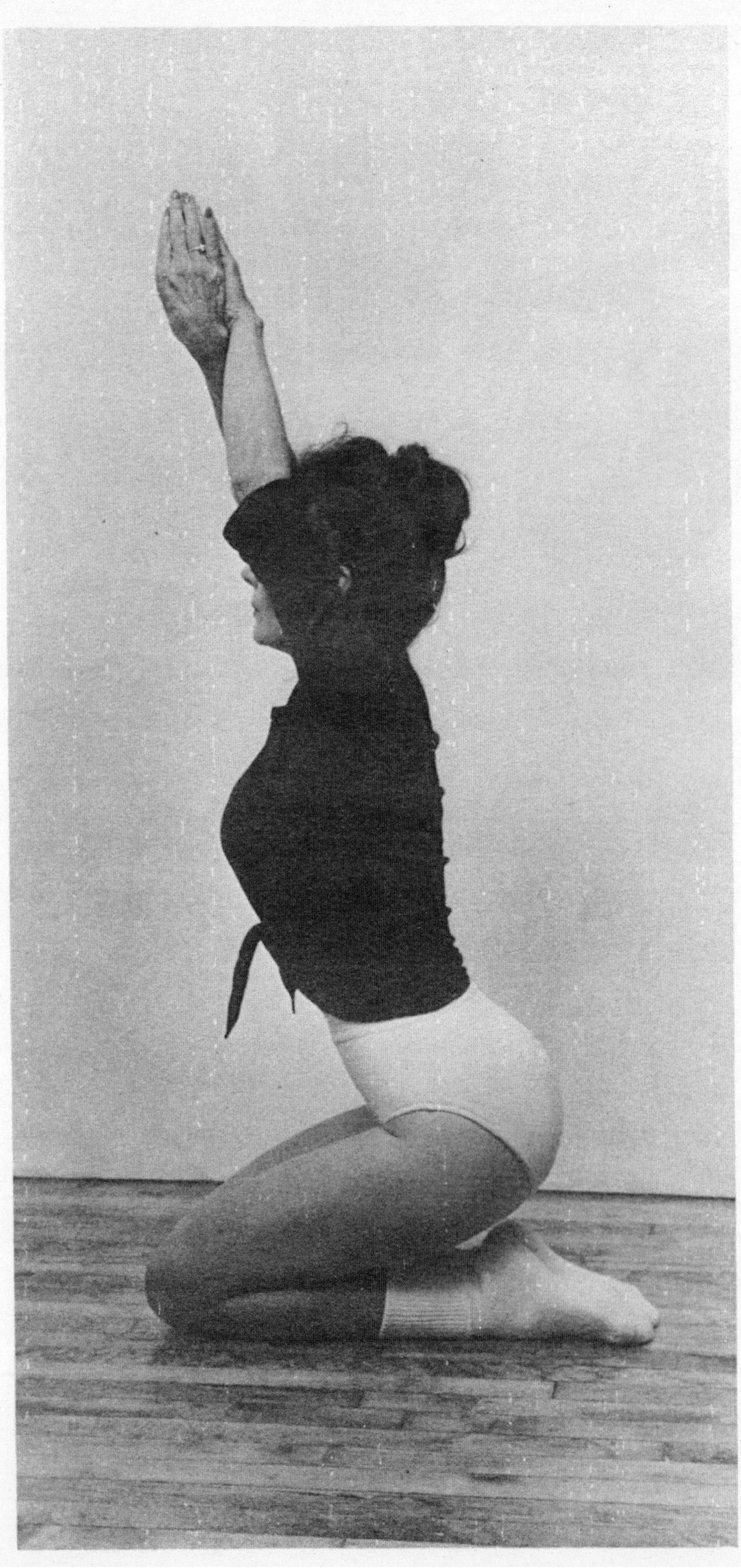

PELVIC ROTATIONS *As with the Scoop, Pelvic Rotations are wonderful for the pelvis and lower back and they give your thighs a wonderful stretch. Sit on your heels, hands clasped and arms stretched high over your head. Raise your body 3 inches from your heels and move your hip to the right. Now curl pelvis up in front, then over to the left, and finally back to complete the circle. Move only your pelvis (like a belly dancer) without dropping your behind to your heels. Make large, smooth circles. Do 20 clockwise and 20 counterclockwise. For variety, you can move your hips and pelvis in a Figure 8.* ◂

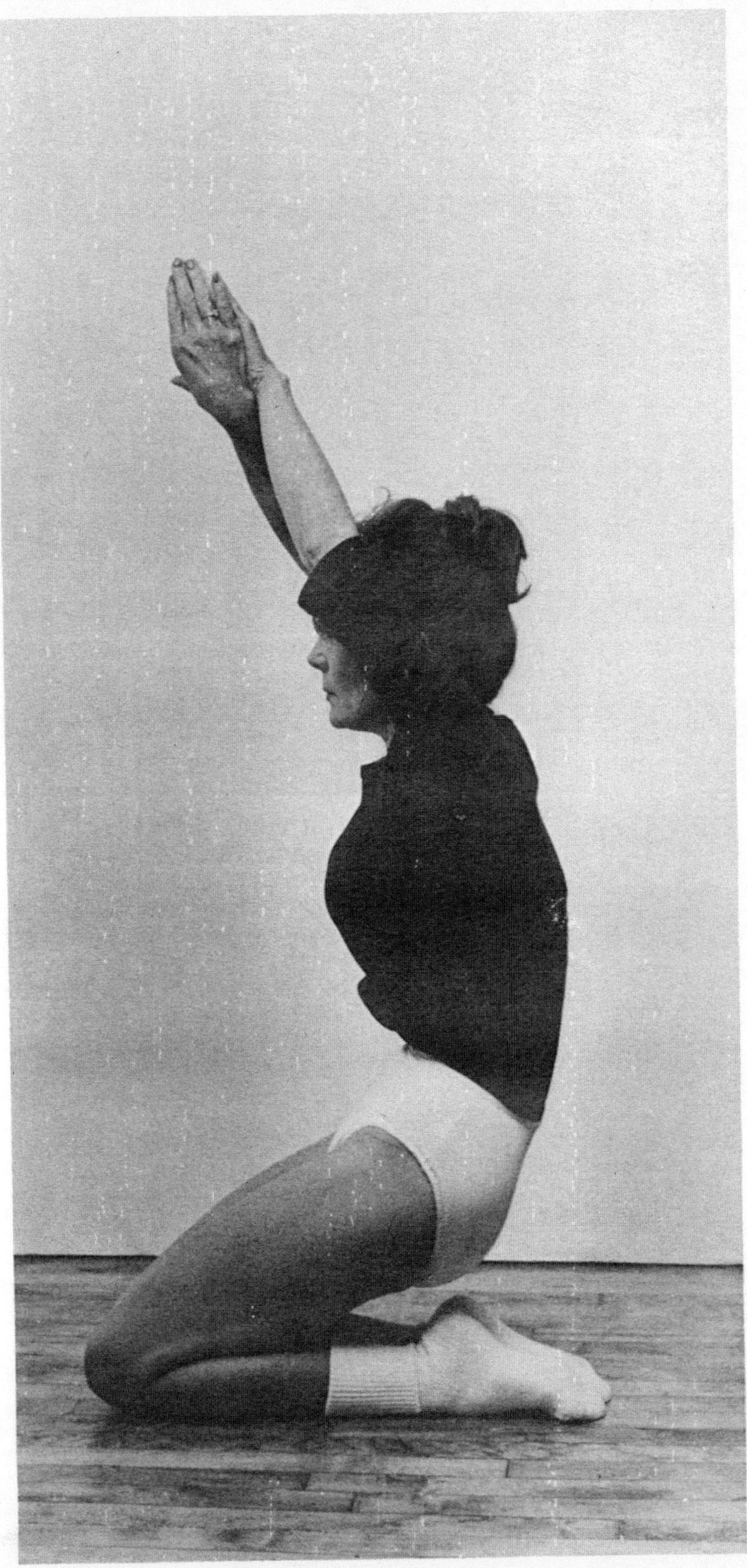

THE PELVIC SCOOP *The Pelvic Scoop increases flexibility in the pelvic area and tightens the inner thighs and the abdominal muscles. Kneel with your arms over your head. Stretch your body and arms high. Then aim your behind down to your heels. Curl your pelvis upward like a scoop and tighten your behind muscles. Keep your knees together. Continue tipping your pelvis upward, lifting your body up to the starting position. Do 20.* ▸

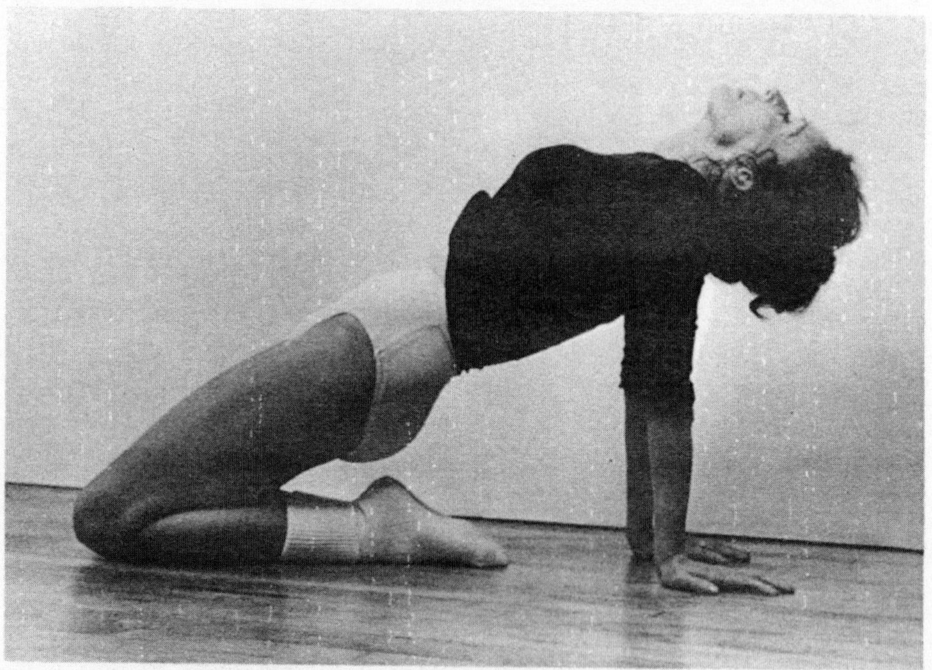

THE THIGH STRETCH *This powerful stretch gently stretches your pectorals, thighs, neck, stomach muscles, as well as your spine. Kneel, sitting on your heels. Put your hands behind you on the floor behind your feet. Relax your neck and let your head fall back toward the floor. Tighten your behind and curl your pelvis upward, raising your behind off your heels. Push pelvis up as high as you think you can and then push up even higher.* Relax. *Do 20 times.* ▲

THE INNER THIGH SQUEEZE *Do the Inner Thigh Squeeze, as taught in the One-Hour Program, as you have already learned. Hold for a count of 300. See the photos in the One-Hour Program to refresh your memory on how to do this.*

MY DEEPEST APPRECIATION TO MY STUDENTS WHO ARE PICTURED ON THESE PAGES

Faye Beckerman
Shira Boardman
Ellen M. Godowitz
Audrey Hagemailer
Tobi Himmel
Susan Kent
Kelle Kerr
Harvey Koeppel
Lisa McElroy
Lynne Meena
Jane Pinckney Middleton
Lane Middleton
Page Middleton
Janet Milazzo
IdaMay Otto
Hernando Perez
Margaret Pfeiffer Pinckney
Karl S. Sabo
Melanie Schor
Ellen Sthika
Harry Sloofman
Carolyn Smith
Katie Studley
Tara Terrell
Neal Thompson
Anna Tipton
Mary Tipton
Janet Valente Ben-Ami
Susan Wallace

SUPER CALLANETICS

THE ADVANCED EXERCISE PROGRAMME FOR THE BODY YOU'VE ALWAYS WANTED IN MINUTES A DAY

CALLAN PINCKNEY

With the assistance of Karen Moline
Photographs by Stuart M. Gross

Dedication

To Edwina Sandys.
How I have enjoyed tremendously all the wonderful laughs we have had throughout the years.
Thank you.

Acknowledgments

I love every minute of preparing books and videos that will help people get stronger and shapelier. It is a complicated process that always requires a strong support group.

I would like to extend very special thanks to Gail Rebuck and Amelia Thorpe of the Random Century Group, who have published my books with such verve and enthusiasm for the past several years; to my attorney, Marc Bailin, and my agent, Mitch Douglas—and finally, to all of the wonderful people around the world who do Callanetics and Super Callanetics; and especially to those who have written to me about how my programs have improved their bodies and given them self-confidence.

A Note of Warning

Do not *ever* attempt to do any of the Super Callanetics exercises until you are completely familiar and comfortable with the Callanetics philosophy, movements, exercises, and terminology.

You *must* have completed and mastered at least ten hours of the one-hour Callanetics program before attempting *any* of these exercises.

There are risks inherent in any exercise program. The advice of a physician should be obtained prior to embarking upon a rigorous exercise program like Super Callanetics. This program is intended for people in good health who have already mastered the one-hour Callanetics program.

If you are pregnant, these advanced Super Callanetics exercises are *not* suitable.

A Note About the Neck

By this time, after having completed at least ten hours of the one-hour Callanetics program, you should feel nothing in your neck except for a lovely, wonderful stretch.

But because most people are not trained (or able!) to relax, your neck and/or upper back may ache the first time you do the stomach exercises. If so, you can support your neck by clasping your hands lightly around it, with your elbows pointed out to the side. Always keep your neck relaxed during these exercises.

If you still feel pain at the back of your neck after you have completed at least ten hours of the one-hour program, consult your physician.

A Note About Knee Problems

Callanetics has helped many people strengthen their knees and relieve chronic pain. If you have severe knee problems, do these exercises only with the consent of your physician.

A Note About Back Problems

Callanetics has also helped thousands of people relieve their back problems. However, it is advisable to use discretion when doing Super Callanetics if you have any back problems. If you have any history of backaches or other physical complaints, you should consult a physician before attempting these, or any other, exercises.

Sciatica Syndrome and Other Chronic Problems

You will notice that some of the exercises have notes about what to do if you have sciatica. Please follow these instructions carefully.

If, however, your sciatica or any other condition continues to give you discomfort and seems to have been aggravated by any of these exercises, discontinue doing them.

Three Professionals' Reactions to Doing Callan's Program

Now, I consider myself to be in excellent shape, but she put me through a workout that had me very surprised about my own athletic strength . . . it was an incredible experience.

ALBERT BIANCHINE
A Professional Ski Instructor

I felt a lot more confident about my body. It got much stronger, and this helped free up my breathing. I feel like the notes are just flowing right out . . . .

ANN WHITNEY
Singer

The (Program) not only shaped my buttocks, but it helped the muscles a ballet dancer uses to "turn out" into position, and because my legs became so much stronger, I found I could leap higher.

CINDY BENNETT
Dancer

CONTENTS

Buttocks – Outer Thighs – Hips

The Entire Body

Stretches

Pelvis-Front and Inner Thighs

The Twenty-Minute Super Callanetics Routine

Why Super Callanetics?

One day, back when I began teaching Callanetics in the early seventies, a student of mine was working hard during a class. Suddenly, she turned to me—and I remember that when she first started doing Callanetics, she'd had really soft, gooshy buttocks, and her body was very weak—and she said, 'Callan, this is getting too easy. I don't feel anything!'

I realized I felt exactly the same way.

I wanted to feel more, that wonderful sensation of the muscles working deep that is the basis for all the Callanetics and Super Callanetics exercises. Not only that, but my students wanted more of a challenge; they were getting so tight and so strong, so quickly, that I needed to take them further. (And most of these students were people like you and me—who despise exercising, and who will sometimes look for excuses not to spend an hour shaping their bodies. Sometimes I think that exercising is worse than washing your hair. And sometimes I'd rather plow a field . . . but I don't live near a field and where do you get a mule and, besides, I don't know how to plow . . . so I end up scrubbing between the kitchen tiles with a toothbrush!)

That's when I began to develop what has become Super Callanetics.

It's human nature, of course, to get lazy about whatever it is you're doing—work, play, sports, even relationships—once you become really good at it. And when I found myself getting very nonchalant because the one-hour Callanetics program had become too easy, I slowly began to develop a new and more intense version of the familiar Callanetics exercises—Super Callanetics. I wanted to get the same fast results in an even shorter amount of time. At first, I wasn't even certain that I would succeed, but I did already know that after your body becomes stronger from doing the one-hour Callanetics program, you'll have found that you can do the same amount of exercises in a shorter amount of time. Would the same principle apply to Super Callanetics? The answer, of course, is yes. Some of the movements may look the same as the basic ones—but when it comes to Super Callanetics, looks can be very deceiving.

What Super Callanetics Can Do for You

Several years ago, I was invited to West Berlin to teach Callanetics to some of the American Green Beret and Special Forces soldiers stationed there. Before I began their training, I was more than happy to teach some of the other soldiers on the base—particularly those from other countries who were competing in different sports—who were interested in Callanetics. There was one in particular, an expert in martial arts from Britain's Royal Air Force, who really was a lovely chap. He watched me demonstrate Callanetics with intense interest. 'God, this is *incredible*,' he said in his lovely clipped accent. 'It doesn't seem like you're doing *anything*. You're not even *moving*!'

I laughed. 'That's the whole point! Less *is* sometimes better,' I said. 'If you talk to most of the chaps stationed here, you'll find that many of them are suffering from back problems, and the reason is that they've never been taught to isolate their muscles, or how to relax. And when people can't relax and their bodies are tense all the time from using muscles they don't need to use, they wind up wasting all their energy, and wearing themselves out.'

His eyes grew wider. 'I can't *believe* you said that,' he exclaimed. 'You are so right! I've always believed that was true, but no one would listen to me. And I know it's got to be correct, because I've taught myself how to relax, and where the results really show are in competition. One of the reasons I'm so good is that I can outlast my competitors, because now I know how to save my energy by *relaxing,* and only concentrating on the muscles that are working.'

His enthusiasm was infectious. Because, frankly, he was the only person I've *ever* run into who totally understood what I was saying without having experienced Super Callanetics or even the one-hour Callanetics program. The one-hour program was so revolutionary when it was first developed that even the doctors I talked to looked at me as if I were some kind of female Tarzan, still living in the deepest jungle. Now, of course, many of the same doctors who pooh-poohed Callanetics not only recommend it to their patients but recommend Super Callanetics as well. The original Callanetics program was designed to alleviate my personal medical problems. At the time, some of what I was saying seemed positively revolutionary. But the various Callanetics routines have always been based on nothing more complicated than common sense. I first began developing Callanetics, as you may know by now, because my bad back and knees were getting worse—and they certainly weren't helped by what they experienced when I took exercise classes. Some of the movements I was allegedly 'taught' in these classes were so violent that they became the final straw of abuse my body could take. I feared I would be spending the rest of my life in a wheelchair. Thankfully, I have been able to put those fears to rest.

And I would also just like to tell you one more little thing about those Green Berets and Special Forces soldiers in Berlin. Growing up with Hollywood movies as I did, I always rather expected these soldiers to be brawny and indefatigable, the most physically fit people in the world. They were so funny at first—they wanted to know why the general had sent someone like me, who barely came up to most of their chests, to teach them these Tinkerbell exercises. And then they found they couldn't even do twenty Open and Closes, which is an exercise some seventy-five-year-old men and women can do in a breeze once they've built up their muscle strength. (I must confess that this made me a teeny bit nervous, because these are supposed to be the men whose job it is to protect people like me against our enemies!) Those soldiers certainly ate their words after a few Callanetics sessions . . . especially when their backaches went away.

You don't have to be a soldier or a fitness fanatic to do Super Callanetics. It can work for you, because it's you working your own muscles at your own pace. There are no weights involved, no use of any pressure on your body other than what your own muscles can do. Super Callanetics allows people of any age and ability to feel and look so much better, without fear of exhaustion or injury. It does not take years, as it does with ballet or yoga, to become proficient in Super Callanetics. And it only takes an hour or two a week or a few minutes a day for you to see some truly amazing results.

I am also certain that by now you have noticed not only a transformation of your body, but a lovely feeling of self-confidence that comes with learning how to be in control. That is because Callanetics and Super Callanetics are like meditation in motion.

Think of how delightful it is to take a vacation in Ibiza or Greece or a Caribbean island, to lie in the relaxing heat, listening to the soothing waves of the ocean—not from a headset!—or watching a glorious sunset, and then sitting blissfully underneath the spectacle of millions of stars glowing in a clear night sky (if you're fortunate enough to be somewhere with no pollution). That lovely feeling of relaxation, of flowing, of being soothed by the sound of the ocean . . . combined with the wonderful knowledge that you *can* be in control of your body, is what I want Super Callanetics to be for you. (To say nothing of how marvelous you will wind up looking in your bathing costume.)

But you don't have to spend thousands of dollars on a vacation at the beach (although a trip there, if you forget about the indignities of the airports and the flights, can certainly be a fabulous—and definitely relaxing—experience) in order to be able to take it easy and detox yourself from everyday stress. One of the first things I teach my students is that it's perfectly all right and safe to relax. That's the biggie. Our entire lives are now nothing but stress. We go to sleep with stress and wake up with stress. And the more hectic the city or place where you live, inevitably the more stressful your life will be.

Super Callanetics can counteract all of that. Every time you do Super Callanetics, you're actually teaching yourself how to relax. It's why you'll hear me saying, *Relax your body*, over and over, during the different exercises. I can never say it enough, and you can never be too relaxed while doing Super Callanetics. As many of my students have told me, Super Callanetics really is a fabulous substitute for a tranquilizer. And so much healthier! Thousands of people have been able to stop taking diuretics and laxatives, tranquilizers and other drugs, because Super Callanetics has improved the overall state of their bodies so much that they've no longer needed any synthetic help for problems they thought would never go away. And if you're exhausted, or worn-out, or angry, or just plain frazzled, Super Callanetics is better than any drug—because it's your body working for you.

Not only that, but as you learn to control your muscles, it's impossible not to begin to truly appreciate just how wonderful a creation your body is. Every muscle in your body is meant to be used. Your muscles are there for a *reason.* And when those muscles are used, they strengthen all the other parts of your body, including your bones. I recently had a physical, and I thought the doctor would tell me I was shrinking. Instead, I was completely shocked when I was told that I, at fifty-one years of age, measured a half inch taller than I had ever been! I thought there had to be a silly blunder, and I made him measure me again and again. It was no mistake. I was actually half an inch taller, and this is at an age (and with my history of back and bone problems) when I thought I'd be shrinking! Doing Super Callanetics is like getting a healthy shot of preventive medicine. I attribute my 'growth' to all the wonderful stretching of my spine, as well as the strengthening of the muscles that support my skeleton. I no longer slump over. It's almost like having a guarantee that you'll be standing, erect and firm, when you're eighty years old.

The Difference Between the One-Hour Callanetics Program and Super Callanetics

Do you remember how you felt after your very first hour of Callanetics? You felt an incredible internal sensation—and a wonderful awareness that your muscles had been working. Many people have remarked to me that they didn't know exactly *what* that feeling was—only that it felt *amazing.* That's how you feel when your muscles are getting stronger. With Callanetics, you can build up an *incredible* amount of muscle strength after only one hour, and as you continue stretching your spine and strengthening your muscles, you keep getting stronger and more flexible. Your body is becoming tighter and more beautiful, and that means you're doing Callanetics the right way.

Super Callanetics will allow you to feel this even more. Learning to do these intense exercises is a revitalizing experience. It's also an excellent challenge.

The basic difference between the one-hour program and Super Callanetics is simple. Each motion of Super Callanetics is basically the equivalent of *twenty* of the one-hour movements. So the results are *twenty* times as effective and noticeable.

The minute you do Super Callanetics, you will feel just how much deeper these exercises work, for faster results.

If you have already seen the Super Callanetics video, you'll know that I often say, Curl your pelvis up more than you think you can. Staying curled up helps deepen the contractions of the specific muscles you're working, and helps your body perform quite efficiently.

I also realized when I began teaching Super Callanetics that if you are curled up more, the little motion you need to do when you are curled up becomes even smaller. Being able to control your muscles in such a short range of motion requires a great deal of strength, and helps explain why Super Callanetics is so effective at tightening up your body faster—and keeping it tight. The better and more advanced your position, the less you will be able to move. That is how it should be.

By now, you will have noticed that some of the movement in the exercises seems almost imperceptible. Well, you're not wrong in thinking that. Many of the Super Callanetics exercises use only one-sixteenth to one-quarter of an inch of motion. Take out a ruler and see just how tiny one-sixteenth of an inch really is. It's *minuscule*!

You may also remember, if you have seen the video, that I often tell you to move one-half inch, not one-sixteenth to one-quarter inch. This is because so many people have written to say that after they have become stronger, they find that they are easily able to move *less* than one-half inch. So you can start off by gently moving one-half inch for all of the exercises. When you feel that you have comfortably mastered them, gradually work up to one-quarter inch. Your ultimate goal is to move no more than one-sixteenth inch. Look at your ruler again. It certainly *is* a challenging goal.

Remember, in Super Callanetics, *Less is more.*

And don't be deceived by these little movements. They are incredibly powerful!

When You Are Ready to Begin Super Callanetics

Please: You must read the section A Few Tips Before You Begin on pp. 33 before you start doing any Super Callanetics exercises.

Before *ever* attempting any of the Super Callanetics exercises, you must be completely familiar with all the movements, terms, and exercises from the one-hour program, and have built up strength from doing them regularly. I cannot stress this enough. Even Mike Tyson couldn't begin to attempt Super Callanetics without having mastered the entire one-hour program, even though we all know how 'strong' he is. You need *at least* ten to fifteen hours, depending on the individual, of solid experience with the one-hour program before ever attempting Super Callanetics.

Many of my students are very surprised when I tell them that I have already taken them—unknowingly—into some of the Super Callanetics movements *if* I have seen that they have the proper muscle strength for them. It all depends on the individual. Some people find the Buttocks exercises very difficult during their first few hours in Callanetics, and the Stomach exercises very easy (or vice versa). If you find that's true for you, you might want to gradually incorporate some of the Super Callanetics exercises in your regular Callanetics exercise program, while still remaining in the one-hour program for all the other exercises. When you have comfortably improved in other areas, then move on to Super Callanetics.

Other people are never able to stretch as much as they like, because flexibility is really based on genetics (and their genes pooped out in the stretching arena!). You can either do splits and try out for the cheerleading squad, or wonder just how those girls can extend their legs so easily when you can barely lift yours off the floor! (To say nothing of those glorious chaps on the gymnastics teams.) There are also other factors involved—how flexible you were when you were younger, and how quickly you might be able to regain some of the flexibility; how stiff you might be after a hard day sitting at your desk at work; and how tired you might be that morning, for example. Of course, some other people possess a terrific stretching ability and don't even know it . . . because they've never attempted it! But most body types do have the ability to improve their flexibility to a greater extent.

What *you* can do is make the most of *your own potential.*

It doesn't matter what shape you're in—stretching is as important as brushing your teeth. What you should *never* do is torture yourself if you find stretching to be difficult. You cannot expect miracles when you first start. If you aren't very flexible, you must keep at it at *your* level, or chances are you could have problems and injuries later in life. Be patient. Never force yourself into a position that might feel uncomfortable. Do not compare yourself to anyone else who may be stretching in the room with you—what is a tremendous and successful stretch for that person might not be the same for you. (For this reason, you should never stretch with another person. He or she will not know your stretching abilities on that specific day, and can pull you just a tad too much—and this can create an injury.) Even some ballet dancers, who have been training their bodies since they were children, do not have and will *never* have the ability to fully stretch and extend themselves as much as they would like to. That knowledge does not keep them from stretching every day. They know—and *you* should know by now—that one should only do as much as one can, gently, and listen to one's body. If you start to feel any strain, ease up on either the stretch or the exercise. Cut back on your repetitions. Modify your Super Callanetics program for the particular day. And if ever your body says stop, *Stop!*

How Often Should I Do Super Callanetics?

You certainly don't have to do Super Callanetics every day! Since Super Callanetics is so much more powerful and effective than the one-hour program, some of you—if you do all these exercises correctly, with your heart and soul—will find that you may only have to do it once a week. One hour of Super Callanetics per week is much more than the equivalent of two one-hour Callanetics sessions.

Or you may wish to alternate between one one-hour Callanetics and one Super session each week. And because there are more exercises in Super Callanetics, you can pick and choose from the exercises you like and do the best and create your own individualized Callanetics exercise program.

Others will find that two sessions of Super Callanetics are necessary to maintain that lovely tight body. However many sessions of Callanetics you are accustomed to doing, Super Callanetics should halve that number.

Once you become even stronger, you can gradually increase the reps of some of the exercises, for more of a challenge. Doing so will not take any longer than a few extra minutes.

Don't forget that if, for instance, you find yourself with an unusually heavy workload one week and unable to do a full session of Super Callanetics, you have other choices. You can try the Twenty-Minute Program on page 155, or it's quite simple to incorporate some of the exercises into your daily routine. Stuck in line at the supermarket or waiting for the lift? Try some of the standing Buttocks—Outer Thighs—Hips exercises, such as Out to the Side. Or perhaps you need a pick-me-up in the office and the doughnut-and-tea cart is rolling by. Stand up and do a few Underarm Tighteners or Neck Relaxers—or even an Up and Down if you have the room—and see how your vitality returns in an instant. Super Callanetics is certainly a lot better for your figure than a jelly doughnut!

And what is most important . . . is to have fun with Super Callanetics. Be creative. You are doing Super Callanetics for you. It's your body, and you know how well it can work, at its own speed. Every time you make that little motion, moving only one-sixteenth to one-quarter inch, you are gently tightening and shaping your body even more.

How Super Callanetics Can Help You

Using Super Callanetics as a Warm-up

Athletes are often surprised when they find out that Super Callanetics is one of the best warm-ups there is before their intense workouts. Anything you do that raises your body temperature is, really, a warm-up. Your body needs to be warmed up before strenuous sports activity or it is very likely that injuries will result to muscles, tendons, and ligaments. They need a chance to warm up and become more pliable before being vigorously stretched. And your body also needs to be stretched *after* exercising to counteract all the work your muscles have been doing. Stretching itself is not a warm-up! If you try to stretch when your muscles are 'cold,' you can really hurt yourself.

With Super Callanetics, your muscles will be working extremely deeply without your worrying about how warm they are. Super Callanetics *is* a warm-up! You don't need to do the entire Super Callanetics program as your warm-up. Choose which section works best for your particular sport or art.

And people who do Super Callanetics properly don't get injuries. Why? Because your muscles will work *only* when they are ready—not when you command them.

How Super Callanetics Can Improve Your Performances

SKIERS

Professional skier Albert Bianchine lives and teaches skiing in Vail, Colorado, and he discovered Callanetics when he was browsing in a bookstore two years ago. 'When I was going through the Callanetics book, I quickly saw that these were very good exercises, and as soon as I started skiing, I noticed a tremendous difference in my abilities—my mobility, endurance, and flexibility all improved a great deal. And my inner thighs would never get as tired.

'There's a tremendous problem with skiers in the West,' he continues, 'which is that people arrive here from all different elevations, which is quite taxing on the body. Not only is skiing incredibly demanding physically, especially when armchair athletes are not in particularly good shape when the season starts, but they suffer the additional altitude stress here when they hit the slopes. This leads to all sorts of injuries, especially if people aren't properly warmed up.

'This is why Callanetics has helped me, and other skiers, so much. I knew that some skiers were skeptical about how Callanetics works, since it's not aerobic exercising, but when I looked at the program, I was basically more curious than skeptical. I also knew Callanetics was soundly designed. I was also lucky that Callan herself came to Colorado for workshops, and I learned from her. Now, I consider myself to be in excellent shape, but she put me through a workout that had me very surprised about my own athletic strength. Boy, was I fooled! Doing Callanetics is an incredible experience.

'What I'd also like to say is how much Callanetics has helped my lower back. Skiing, especially when you hit the moguls, always stresses your lower back. I suddenly realized that I could ski all week with no pain—Callanetics has helped relieve much of the stress and tension on my lower back.

'I only wish that Callan would move out here! Hopefully a Callanetics franchise will open here soon, so that other skiers can benefit from all the exercises that have helped me so much.

'I am ready for Super Callanetics.'

SINGERS

Ann Whitney is a professional opera and musical-comedy singer, and when she began doing Callanetics, she found some surprising results. 'When you sing, you especially use your diaphragm, stomach and back muscles,' she explains. 'I found that Callanetics had strengthened these muscles so much that I could expand my rib cage much more to take bigger breaths, and I could hold my tones and phrases much longer as well.

'I also felt a lot more confident about my body', she adds. 'It got much stronger, and this helped free up my breathing. I feel like the notes are just flowing right out, instead of sounding tight and constricted.'

Another benefit of Super Callanetics is how it helps your posture, which is especially important for performers who might be onstage for hours. 'When you sing you need to be "grounded,"' Ann explains. 'If you start slouching, your whole chest can cave in. You not only have no room to breathe properly, but you sound terrible! Callanetics and Super Callanetics have taught me how to open myself up and stand comfortably. I now know that all the muscle strength I need is there, to expand and work for *me.* I also know that I control my body, rather than its controlling me. Now I never have to worry about how I'm standing or what I'm doing when I'm singing. All I have to do is sing!'

BALLET (AND OTHER) DANCERS

Cindy Bennett is a professional ballerina, and she also found some very interesting results when she began doing Callanetics. 'I used to think I knew everything and was really strong,' she says, laughing at herself. 'Doing Callanetics was really quite the humbling experience.

'You see,' she continues, 'I didn't think the exercises would be difficult at all for me to do because I have been trained to be in perfect control of my body. And dancers have to be especially aware of everything going on with their bodies, because that's our *life*!

'But when I started doing Callanetics, I actually could not do the Hip and Buttocks exercises. You'd think they would be the easiest ones of all for a trained dancer. I was *so* embarrassed!'

She stuck with it, however, and soon found—much to her surprise—that her buttocks, which had been as tight as they could be from years of dancing and stretching, actually became even tighter. Their entire shape changed . . . for the better, of course!

'Callanetics not only shaped my buttocks, but it helped the muscles a ballet dancer uses to "turn out" into position,' Cindy adds. 'And because my legs became so much stronger, I found I could leap higher. My work *en pointe*—in toe shoes—became better and more precise. And all the stretching at the end improved my leg extensions—how high my legs can go.'

Other dancers have had similar results. But as you already know, you don't have to be a professional *anything* to use and enjoy the benefits of Callanetics.

Cindy is ready for Super Callanetics.

How Super Callanetics Can Help Your Posture

When I first left home to conquer the world (don't you love the arrogance of youth?), I ended up traveling for over a decade. Because I lived in so many foreign countries, I intentionally learned the manners and customs of each country where I stayed in order not to offend any of the local inhabitants. These usually were countries where the male was 'the god' and the female was 'the mule' (and often 'the plow' as well). Continuing on my innocent merry way from country to country, I didn't realize how instinctively I had changed my posture to take on the submissive appearance of the female and remain unobtrusive.

Japan was the straw that broke the camel's back. There, I was always bending over in order not to draw attention to myself (which only served to aggravate my bad back condition even more), placing my hand in front of my mouth before and after speaking, and holding my head down when I would be talking to men which is the custom for women there. But when I arrived back in the United States, I found that the appearance I gave to Westerners was that of a pathetic wimp, and that I had become the unwitting yet perfect target for bullies.

One of the things that changed my wimpiness through the eyes of the Westerner was, obviously, my posture. The more I did the program, the more erect I stood and walked . . . the more self-confidence I had, the more people accepted me as their equal. As I moved on to Super Callanetics, my posture became even more erect, and my confidence became so much stronger that whenever I entered a room filled with people, almost everyone would stare at me, wondering who I was. Again, through their eyes, I had become more than their equal. It wasn't so much that it was me—it was their perception of who I was because of my *posture*.

The way you hold yourself is sending messages to the world, whether positive or negative. Imagine walking into a room with the CEO and all the board members of an excruciatingly important company waiting to interview you for the job of your lifetime, representing their firm. First impressions are always the most important. You will never get this coveted job—or any other of consequence—if you walk in slumped over, your stomach protruding, your buttocks sticking out, and your head hanging.

And posture can give away so many of your inner feelings. Why do you think the muggers in the street know whom to mug? They judge their victims by their energy and posture. As horrible as that is—it's their profession.

Super Callanetics has freed me from worries about my posture. What is so amazing for me is that I remembered how I had been taught as a child to walk with a book on my head. I had forgotten these silly but all-important childhood lessons, and paid a very high price for becoming unaware of how my body looked to the rest of the world. Thanks to Super Callanetics, I can now enter any room, head high, body erect yet relaxed, and know that no one will ever think I am a subservient female again!

How to Do Super Callanetics

I've heard every excuse in the book not to begin Callanetics and Super Callanetics! People say they're too old . . . it's too late . . . they're fat because it's 'hereditary' . . . they know Super Callanetics can't work for them. My favorite is the 'thyroid problem.' These people are convinced that all their weight and body problems stem from underactive thyroids. For a very very small percentage of people, that may be true—but if you do think your inability to lose weight is caused by a medical problem, you *must* see a doctor immediately.

Others try one session and never return. They want to look good, but aren't willing to commit themselves and do what they have to do for a beautiful body. Instead, they spend all their time complaining about how dreadful their bodies look and make them feel.

They don't know what they're missing!

You don't need any special clothing, special props, or special preparation to do Super Callanetics. You can do Super Callanetics whenever and wherever you want . . . in the morning, afternoon, or evening. In a special exercise room with a barre, or on a mat in your bedroom, even watching your favorite television program, using a piece of living-room furniture for balance. In the backyard, or even in the dark, if that's what you prefer! All you need is an hour of uninterrupted time (although, I must confess, sometimes I do talk on the phone when I'm doing Super Callanetics—as long as it's a *cordless* phone!).

About the Barre

You will notice that many of the exercises in Super Callanetics are done at the barre. As you know from *Callanetics*, *Callanetics for Your Back*, or *Callanetics Countdown*, sturdy furniture can always be substituted for any of the barre exercises.

Do, however, use a padded exercise mat or folded towel for any floor exercises that involve kneeling, so that you can protect your knees from accidental bruising. You may also want to keep a suction-cup type of bath mat handy, to place under your feet in case you feel like you are about to slip during any of the standing exercises.

And don't forget that you should *never* use a towel rack to support your weight during the Open and Close exercise. They aren't designed for anything other than towels!

About Hanging

If you have already browsed through this book or have seen the Super Callanetics video, you may have noticed that one of my favorite warm-ups and spine stretches—the Hang—is nowhere to be found. There is a very good reason for this. I have found that too many people were 'hanging themselves' irresponsibly. One woman wrote to tell me she was hanging from a sapling branch—and it broke! Well, what did she expect?

I absolutely adore hanging. It stretches the spine so beautifully. But most people do not have access to the type of high ladder barre I have in my exercise studio, and they find it uncomfortable to hang from a door (as I suggested in the *Callanetics* book).

If you are determined to hang, please make a small investment in a durable chinning bar, and install it properly. Then you can hang from it to your heart's content. Start with a hang that lasts no longer than a count of three. As you build up the strength in your wrists, gradually work up to about a count of sixty. Never, as you know by now, hang longer than is comfortable. Your body should always remain perfectly relaxed.

What Not to Wear

SHOES

As you will have noticed from my other books and videos, I never wear anything on my feet other than ballet slippers. (Actually, I prefer to go barefoot, but my feet get a wee bit too dirty during a photo session for me to show them to you. Eagle-eyed viewers will notice, however, that I am barefoot in several of the photographs in this book!) Feel free to wear ballet slippers, socks, or just be barefoot—whatever you prefer. (If you are exercising on a slippery floor, be sure to keep a suction-cup–type bath mat nearby to place under your feet should you find yourself losing your balance.)

Shoes are simply too heavy to wear during any Super Callanetics exercises. If you tried wearing aerobics shoes during the Buttocks exercises, they'd end up feeling like five hundred-pound weights after only a few reps! They can also throw you off balance.

If, however, your physician has prescribed orthotics for you, and you are accustomed to wearing them in your workout shoes, please feel free to continue wearing them, but only for the standing exercises.

TIGHTS

The only thing I insist upon when I am teaching is that my students *do not* wear tights that act as a girdle, unless your doctor recommends them. They can affect your circulation. The only girdle you should be wearing is that of your own muscles! That's the best and the most natural.

And then there is the problem of pulling these 'tight' tights on and pulling these 'tight' tights off—this can aggravate preexisting back problems (as well as ruin a perfectly good manicure!).

And frankly, my experience has been that using clothes to disguise your true shape is not good for you during a Super Callanetics session. Then you will always think that your body looks better than it actually does. If you can't see your body or feel what your muscles are doing, you won't work as hard.

Mirrors

Before you get carried away admiring your new Super Callanetics–shaped body, however, I do need to say something about all those mirrors you might find yourself staring in. Although mirrors are extremely useful for you to be able to see your positions during many of the Super Callanetics exercises, it is very important that you not become *obsessed* with them. You should be able to *feel* your body working for you. Your muscles respond to what you tell them to do. You *don't* need a mirror if you *feel* the exercises properly. Remember what happened to Narcissus!

About Music

You may recall that I also have fairly strong feelings about music. When you first began the one-hour program, I advised that no music be played. For one thing, it's almost impossible not to try and keep up with the beat when you hear it; moving to rhythm is instinctive. (That's great if you're out dancing, but not when you're doing Callanetics and Super Callanetics!)

For another, many people who have done aerobic dance–type exercise have become accustomed to hard, pushy music. Even when I tried exercising to loud music, I felt great immediately afterward, but not long after that I would suddenly find myself completely wiped out, instead of having energy that would last for days.

Well, since you already know that my philosophy is the total opposite of almost everything that's out there in the universe, I must confess that all the screaming and hollering and thrusting that goes on in some exercise classes is enough to have most people carried off to the loony bin (if only for a rest).

So I've found that exercising to either no music, or very soothing sounds such as those you'll hear on the Super Callanetics video, is much more conducive to a relaxing session. It's like going to a house of worship or spending time alone with your Creator: many people like to go even though they're not particularly religious, because it's so peaceful and calm. It gives them a little chance to get away from all the noise out there. And noise bombards you, practically every second of the day. It hits your nervous system and has a definite, negative effect. And I've found that the older you get, the more you need to find a haven of calm in which you can surround yourself. Loud music is great if you're eighteen, but most people as they grow older find that they prefer something that will soothe their souls and ease their spirits (and not make their ears ring for hours).

Instead, use the time you spend doing Super Callanetics to cleanse your mind of all negativity. Feel that your body is so light you could soar and glide in the air like a bird—but not a hummingbird. You can get exhausted watching those precious little darlings flap their wings in triple fast motion!

I must add, however, that if you do prefer to do your Super Callanetics to punk rock or heavy metal or house music (or whatever else there is blaring on the radios all day long), don't despair (but do be careful not to damage your hearing). Once you've mastered Super Callanetics, you will possess such tremendous control of your muscles that you will be able to exercise to any kind of music you want—for you will have trained your mind and body to respond only to the delicate, tiny, controlled motions. Music will have no effect on how you perform Super Callanetics—other than to please your ears.

About Breathing

When I first started teaching, some of my students were so used to 'heavy breathing' that it often got out of hand in class! People were so deeply involved in their breathing technique that they would forget how to do the exercises! It would also become very disturbing to the other students, who were relaxed and calm—all of a sudden they would hear this great big *whooosh!* of an inhale, and then this great big *whooosh!* of an exhale, usually followed by some rather revolting slobber! I'd even see people sitting and taking their pulse during class. How conditioned we humans can become.

And so I kept thinking . . . something is not quite right. Here are all these people whose hearts, supposedly, are in top-notch condition—but their bodies: yuck! Just *unbelievably* unpleasant to look at, especially the gooshy hanging skin.

When you're doing Super Callanetics, just remember to breathe *naturally,* and you won't have any problems.

The Key Words

There are certain words and phrases I love, and by now you should know them all by heart. Yet these are the keys to what makes Super Callanetics so effective for you. So here they are—again!

- ❑ *Always work at your own pace*
- ❑ *Listen to your body*
- ❑ *Never, ever force*
- ❑ *Gentle, delicate little motions*
- ❑ *Light as a feather*
- ❑ *Flowing like a feather*
- ❑ *Relax your entire body*
- ❑ *Your body is like a rag doll*
- ❑ *Let yourself drip into the floor*
- ❑ *Never compare yourself with anybody else*
- ❑ *Triple slow motion*

Using the Key Words to Do Super Callanetics at Your Own Speed

All of us are different. Thank goodness for that! And all of our bodies are shaped and sized very differently as well. Which is why I have always stressed that you should *never compare yourself with anybody else.* Super Callanetics is not a race. The clock is not ticking. No one is timing you, or expecting you to reach the finish line with everyone else. It doesn't matter how many reps anybody else has counted. You can only compare yourself with what you are capable of doing. So, always remember to *work at your own pace.*

Most important, *listen to your body.*

And *never, ever force.*

One of my favorite words is *gentle.* It's a kind, kind word, and it even sounds sweet. When you are gentle with your body, you are showing it the respect it deserves. If you don't, it's like putting fine bone china in the dishwasher (and that's asking for trouble!). All of your movements in Super Callanetics must be gentle. Flowing, and delicate. *As light and flowing as a feather.*

Relax your entire body.

Listen to your body.

Always work at your own pace.

A Few Tips Before You Begin

Some of the terms I have been using ever since I developed the first Callanetics program can easily be misinterpreted by those of you who are unfamiliar with my exercise vocabulary. Please read this section before you begin any Super Callanetics session.

REPS

A 'rep' is simply an abbreviation for 'repetition.' This means how many times you should repeat an exercise.

REPEAT TO OTHER SIDE

Super Callanetics exercises always begin on the right side. If, for example, you are doing your exercises for the buttocks, you will be sitting on your left side, but you will be *working* your *right* side. Nearly every exercise is repeated on the other side.

COME OUT OF POSITION

After you have finished doing your exercise, relax, and, in triple slow motion (see page 35), come out of whatever position you were working in. Instructions on how to come out of each position are provided at the end of each exercise.

TAKE A BREATHER

People have written me, saying that they thought 'taking a breather' meant they could get up, go to the kitchen, have a cup of tea, talk on the phone with a friend, and then resume Super Callanetics whenever they felt like it. *It doesn't* (although I must say I like the idea)! At that pace, it would take you three days to do a one-hour program if you 'took a breather' every time this book says 'take a breather'!

What 'take a breather' really means is a little bit different. If you find that the exercise you are doing is becoming difficult, *take a breather.* Take yourself out of whatever position you are in, breathe deeply for a few seconds, just relax, and then resume the correct position.

And remember to keep breathing naturally throughout all of the exercises.

Never hold your breath!

WORK AT YOUR OWN PACE

Each and every day is a different one, and your body responds differently to exercise as well, for many reasons. On some days, you will be loose and limber, and exercising will seem a breeze. You'll be able to do one hundred reps without a second thought. But the next day, you might only be able to do twenty, and start to panic. It may be simply that the weather is lousy or your car might have broken down or you ate something that is just lying there in your stomach or work is incredibly taxing and you're so stressed-out that you don't know which way to turn. Or your muscles may simply be tired. *Don't worry!*

Relax. Respect your body. Take it easy. Do a lighter session than usual, with fewer reps of exercises that might seem particularly difficult. If you are really having a tough time, perhaps you might want to stop for that day. Or you can go back to the one-hour program, and return to Super Callanetics for your next session.

Always listen to your body.

One of my favorite letters came from an eighty-year-old man in Arizona. He wrote to tell me that he couldn't wait to go to bed at night, because he knew that when he woke up, he would be doing Super Callanetics. Whenever I'm having a bad day, I think of him, and instantly feel inspired. I am certain that this man always listens to *his* body! If he didn't, he could never do Super Callanetics!

HIP-WIDTH APART

Stand up, and place your hands on your hipbones. Now look down at your feet. They should be lined up with your hips. This gives you better balance. For most people, hip-width is about a foot apart. Try placing a ruler between your feet so you have a perfect idea of what twelve inches looks like!

CURL YOUR PELVIS UP

By now, you should be able to curl your pelvis up in your sleep! This movement, as you know, is so crucial to all Callanetics and Super Callanetics that I am repeating how to do it.

I still find that when I'm teaching, I need a lot of patience working with new students on the pelvis. Many—both men and women—don't even know where it is, much less what to do with it. (No wonder there are so many divorces!) And then when they do find it, learning how to move it flowingly makes them feel incredibly exposed and vulnerable. It can be an excruciatingly self-conscious area for many people. And feeling that way is nothing to be ashamed about. Super Callanetics will help you dislodge your fears and self-consciousness about this area as it shapes and tones your body.

The pelvis, you see, is absolutely crucial for supporting your entire back. The pelvis is the key to your entire body posture. It affects how you sit, stand—how you *move.* The better you can move your joints in a smooth, fluid motion, the more you can stand tall and walk like a peacock. And being able to curl your pelvis up more than you think you can will contract your muscles even more. Curling your pelvis up is a terrific stretch for your lower back.

Remember: Tighten your buttocks. Curl your pelvis up and in toward your navel. Your back will automatically round.

You can always curl your pelvis up more than you think you can!

TRIPLE SLOW MOTION

By now, you should also be very familiar with this phrase! I know I've said it before, but I can never say it enough, and I think this is the best way to say it: All you are doing is watching a slow-motion sequence in a movie . . . slowing it down even more . . . and you are the star. Whatever move you make, you can slow it down even more . . . make it gentle . . . keep it flowing like a feather.

Special Note for All the Standing Exercises

At this advanced level, whenever you are instructed to stand with both feet on the floor, you may keep your legs straight but always have your knees relaxed—never locked.

Warm-Ups

Up and Down

THIS EXERCISE WILL HELP YOU STRETCH YOUR SPINE, AS WELL AS LOOSEN YOUR KNEES.

❑ Stand with your feet a hip-width apart. Stretch both your arms up to the ceiling as high as you can. Tighten your buttocks, and curl your pelvis up. Now stretch even more. Relax your knees—don't lock them—and keep your feet flat on the floor.

❑ In one smooth motion, gently bend your knees as much as you can, and lower your upper body towards the floor, with your arms reaching forward. It's as if you are trying to grasp an object on the floor in front of you. Your torso is stretching out and away.

When you're in this position, do not curl up your pelvis.

❑ Gently swing your arms back, raising them as high as you can behind your body. Your knees will straighten slightly and your buttocks will raise with the motion of your arms going to the back and then up.

REMEMBER: *When you have swung your arms back, this will be one of the few instances where your pelvis will* not *be curled up.*

❑ Just as you're about to reverse the motion to go back up to your starting position, tighten your buttocks and curl your pelvis up even more than you think you can. Keep it curled up until you return, arms once again stretching up towards the ceiling.

5 TO 15 REPS

DOS AND DON'TS

- ❑ **If you have a swayback, tip your pelvis up as much as you can.**
- ❑ **Do not arch your back while stretching your arms up to the ceiling.**
- ❑ **Totally relax your knees.**
- ❑ **Keep your shoulders relaxed.**
- ❑ **Let go of your neck.**
- ❑ **Your entire body is relaxed, including your feet.**

The Swing

❑ This is basically the same gentle swinging stretch as Up and Down, except you will stay in a semicrouching position.

Your entire body is a rag doll.

❑ Just relax your knees. Relax your entire body. You are a rag doll sweeping your arms backward and forward as your knees gently move up and down.

❑ When you have finished, return to your standing position, vertebra by vertebra, remembering to tighten your buttocks and curl your pelvis up.

10 TO 15 REPS

Dos and Don'ts

❑ Totally relax your knees.

❑ Keep your shoulders relaxed.

❑ Let go of your neck.

❑ Your entire body is relaxed, including your feet.

The Waist-Away Stretch

❑ Stand with your feet a hip-width apart. Put your left hand on your left hip, with your elbow out directly to the side. (Or, if it's more comfortable, place your hand on your thigh.) Reach your right arm up as high as you can. Bend your knees slightly.

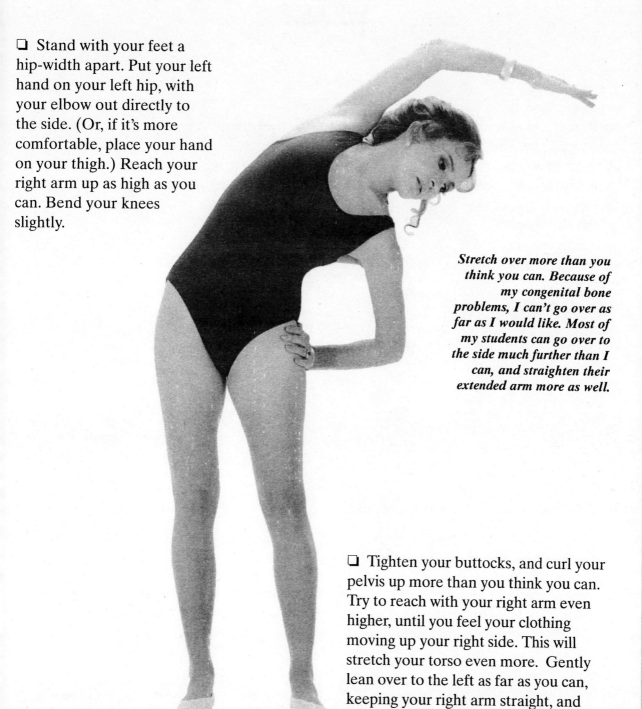

Stretch over more than you think you can. Because of my congenital bone problems, I can't go over as far as I would like. Most of my students can go over to the side much further than I can, and straighten their extended arm more as well.

❑ Tighten your buttocks, and curl your pelvis up more than you think you can. Try to reach with your right arm even higher, until you feel your clothing moving up your right side. This will stretch your torso even more. Gently lean over to the left as far as you can, keeping your right arm straight, and then reach just a wee bit more.

❑ Move your torso up and down, not more than 1/16 to 1/4 inch, while stretching your right arm to the left in a smooth, continuous motion.

100 REPS

❑ To gently come out of this stretch, do not stand up straight. That would put pressure on your lower back. Instead, bend your knees as much as you can and gently stretch your right arm and torso, in front of you and then to your right, in one smooth, continuous motion. Feel your spine stretching.

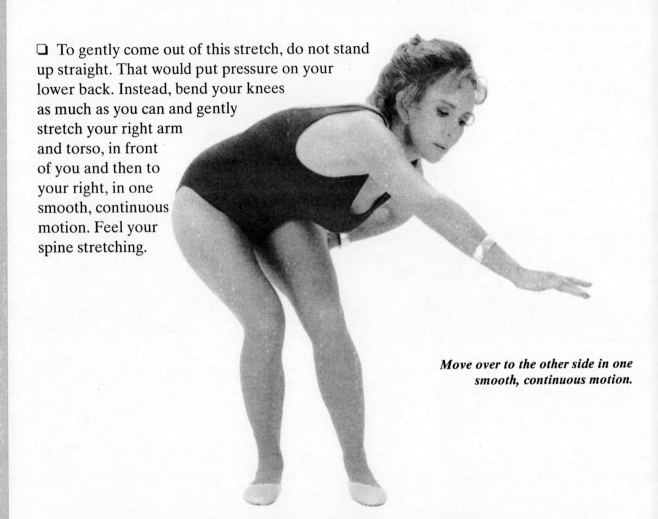

Move over to the other side in one smooth, continuous motion.

❑ When you feel that your back is totally relaxed and that you can't go any further to the right, slowly come up to your original, starting position by tightening your buttocks, curling up your pelvis, and rounding up your torso, vertebra by vertebra.

❑ Repeat this exercise on the opposite side.

100 REPS

Dos and Don'ts

- ❏ You can always stretch over more than you think you can.
- ❏ Relax your shoulders.
- ❏ Keep your outstretched arm as straight as you can, and as close to your head as possible.
- ❏ If you feel crunched on the opposite side you are stretching, you can always stretch that side of your body up even more.
- ❏ Relax your neck.
- ❏ Never bounce up and down; your movement during this stretch is almost imperceptible.
- ❏ Relax your knees.

Underarm Tightener

❑ Stand erect, feet a hip-width apart. Bend your knees a wee bit. Take your arms up and out to the side, keeping them perfectly straight and even with your shoulders. Slowly start rolling your hands forward so that your palms are face-up, thumbs aiming towards the ceiling.

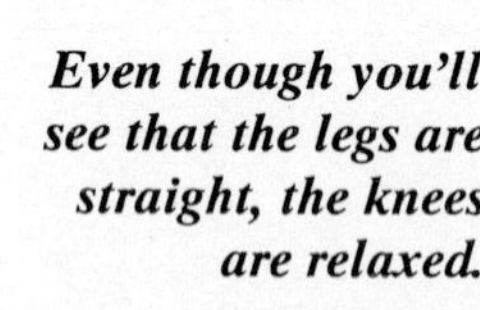

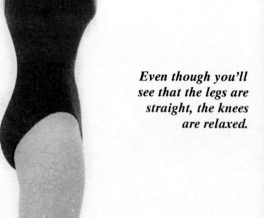

Even though you'll see that the legs are straight, the knees are relaxed.

❑ With your knees still bent a wee bit, tighten your buttocks, and curl your pelvis up more than you think you can. Make sure, too, that your spine is straight, your head is erect, and your shoulders are back and relaxed.

❑ Gently move your arms behind your back, trying to keep your hands even with your shoulders and your arms straight. Without jerking, move your arms 1/16 to 1/4 inch backward and forward.

100 REPS

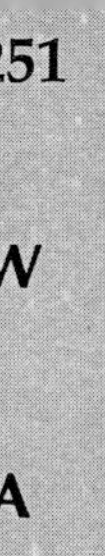

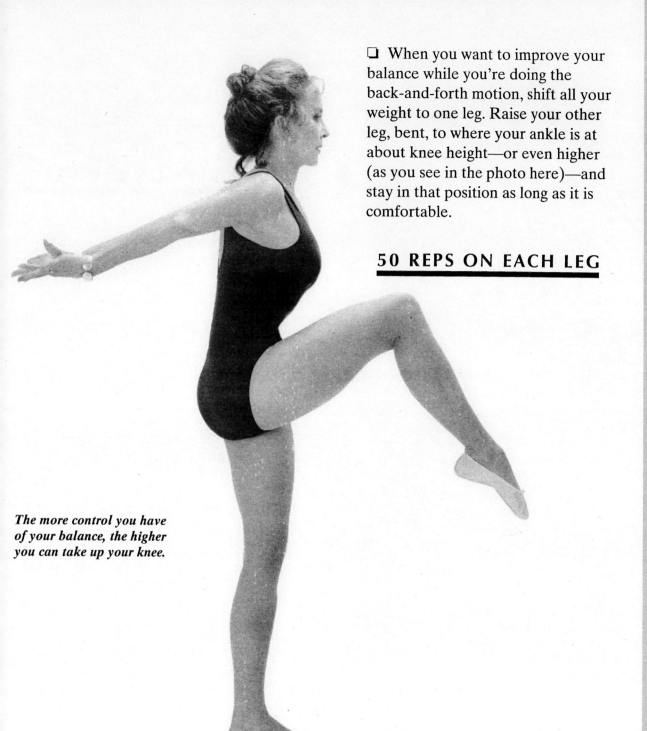

❑ When you want to improve your balance while you're doing the back-and-forth motion, shift all your weight to one leg. Raise your other leg, bent, to where your ankle is at about knee height—or even higher (as you see in the photo here)—and stay in that position as long as it is comfortable.

50 REPS ON EACH LEG

The more control you have of your balance, the higher you can take up your knee.

ONCE YOU'VE MASTERED THAT BALANCE POSITION: *Try straightening your leg out, away from the body, as high as you can. Be sure, however, to keep your shoulders and hands even, your torso erect, and your raised leg relaxed.*

50 REPS ON EACH LEG

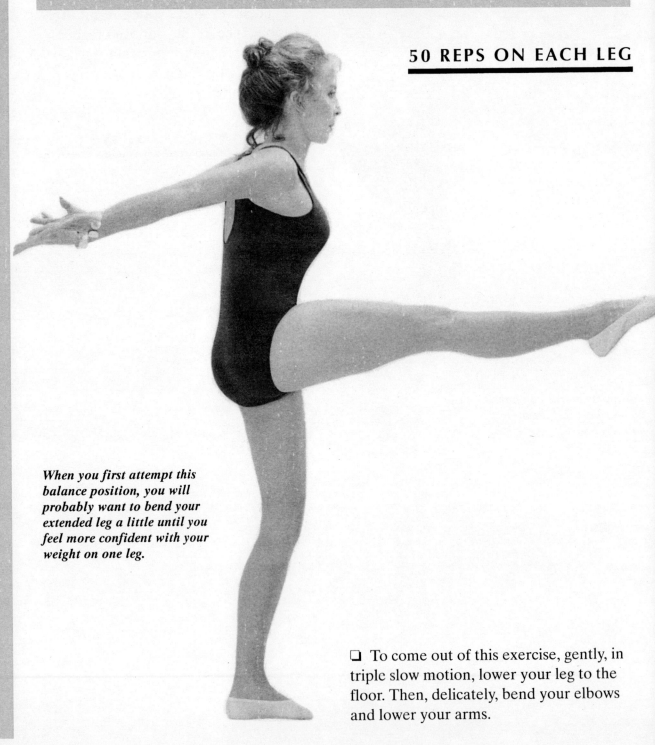

When you first attempt this balance position, you will probably want to bend your extended leg a little until you feel more confident with your weight on one leg.

❑ To come out of this exercise, gently, in triple slow motion, lower your leg to the floor. Then, delicately, bend your elbows and lower your arms.

REMEMBER: *The more erect your torso, the higher your arms are raised behind your body, and the more you can rotate your wrists, the more you will tighten your underarms, loosen the area between your shoulder blades, and stretch your chest muscles. Stretched chest muscles allow your shoulders to go back more. This is essential for correct posture.*

Dos and Don'ts

- ❑ **Keep your pelvis tipped up while both feet are on the floor.**
- ❑ **Gravity is always trying to pull your arms down, so keep them up as high as you possibly can.**
- ❑ **Relax your entire body, especially your neck.**
- ❑ **Don't lock your knees; keep them relaxed.**
- ❑ **When you are working on your balance, try to alternate standing on each leg for a count of 50.**

Standing Hamstring Stretch

This stretch is what I enjoy doing when my lower back has become stiff after sitting for hours in one position.

(If you have mild sciatica, always keep your knees bent during this exercise, to relieve pressure on your sciatic nerve. If you have more than mild sciatica, avoid this stretch.)

❑ Stand erect with your feet a hip-width apart. Clasp your hands behind you, and gently try to raise your arms to the same level as if you were about to do the Underarm Tightener. Make sure your knees are relaxed.

❑ Very slowly, round your torso over, trying to touch your nose to your knees, or as far as you possibly can. Do not arch your back.

❑ If you are able to touch your nose to your knees, slowly continue to take your arms towards the floor as far as you can without forcing. If you are not quite that stretched, gently move your torso in triple slow motion, back and forth, 1/16 to 1/4 inch.

20 REPS, OR HOLD FOR A COUNT OF 20

REMEMBER: *Take advantage of this time to totally relax your neck. It should feel as if it is dripping into the floor.*

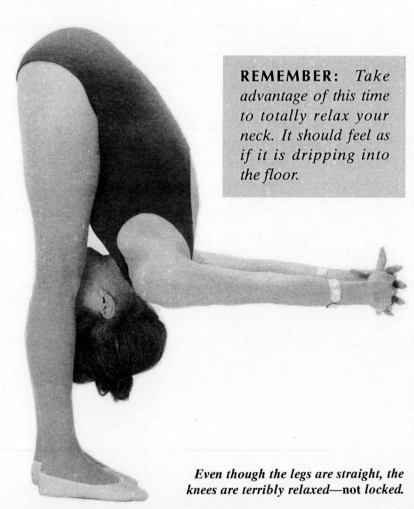

Even though the legs are straight, the knees are terribly relaxed—not locked.

❑ In one slow, smooth, and continuous motion, unclasp your hands and place them on the inside of each ankle. Your elbows are aimed out to the side, and your knees are still relaxed. If you need to move your feet apart another few inches for better balance, please do.

❑ Then slowly ease your head between your legs, as far as it will go, and move your torso back and forth, 1/16 to 1/4 inch.

20 REPS

❑ Gently move your torso over to your right side, clasping the outside of your right ankle with both hands. Bend your elbows out.

❑ Try to place your head in between your leg and your right elbow, and move your torso back and forth, 1/16 to 1/4 inch.

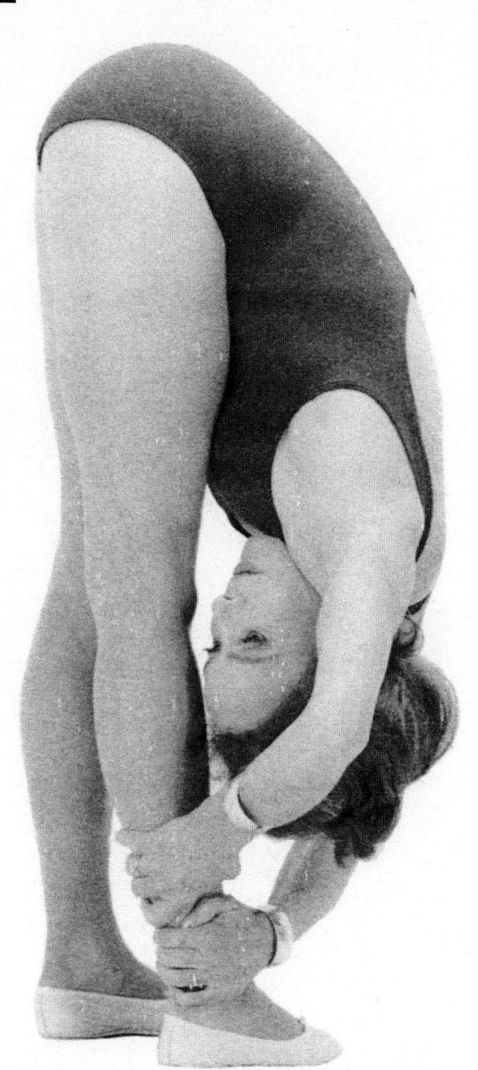

Keep your neck relaxed.

FOR MORE OF A STRETCH: *Bend both knees and move your left hip out to the side; this will shift some of your weight to that side. You should also feel this stretch in your lower back and buttocks muscles.*

FOR EVEN MORE OF A STRETCH: *Move your feet closer together. (You must have good balance for this position.)*

20 REPS

❑ Keeping your knees relaxed, gently move over to your left side, clasping the outside of your left ankle with both hands. Keep your elbows bent and out.

❑ Place your head in between your leg and your left elbow, and move back and forth, 1/16 to 1/4 inch.

FOR MORE OF A STRETCH: *Bend your knees even more, and shift your weight over to your right leg.*

20 REPS

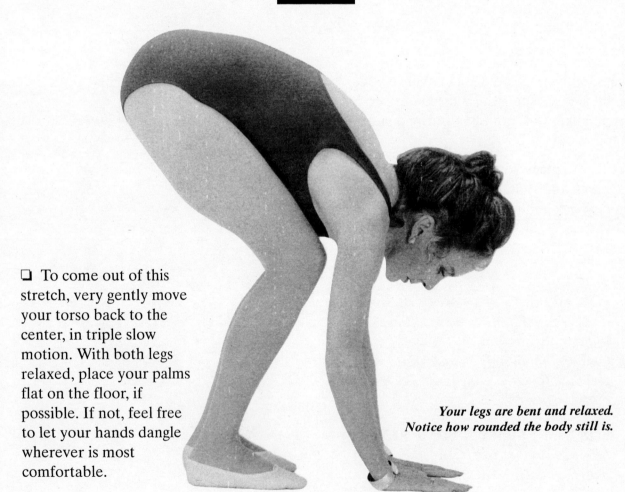

❑ To come out of this stretch, very gently move your torso back to the center, in triple slow motion. With both legs relaxed, place your palms flat on the floor, if possible. If not, feel free to let your hands dangle wherever is most comfortable.

Your legs are bent and relaxed. Notice how rounded the body still is.

❑ Bend your knees as much as you possibly can, bringing your buttocks down so you are in a crouching position, with your hands still flat on the floor, or wherever is most comfortable.

❑ Tighten your buttocks, curl your pelvis up, and slowly round your torso up one vertebra at a time. Your arms should be hanging straight, loose and relaxed.

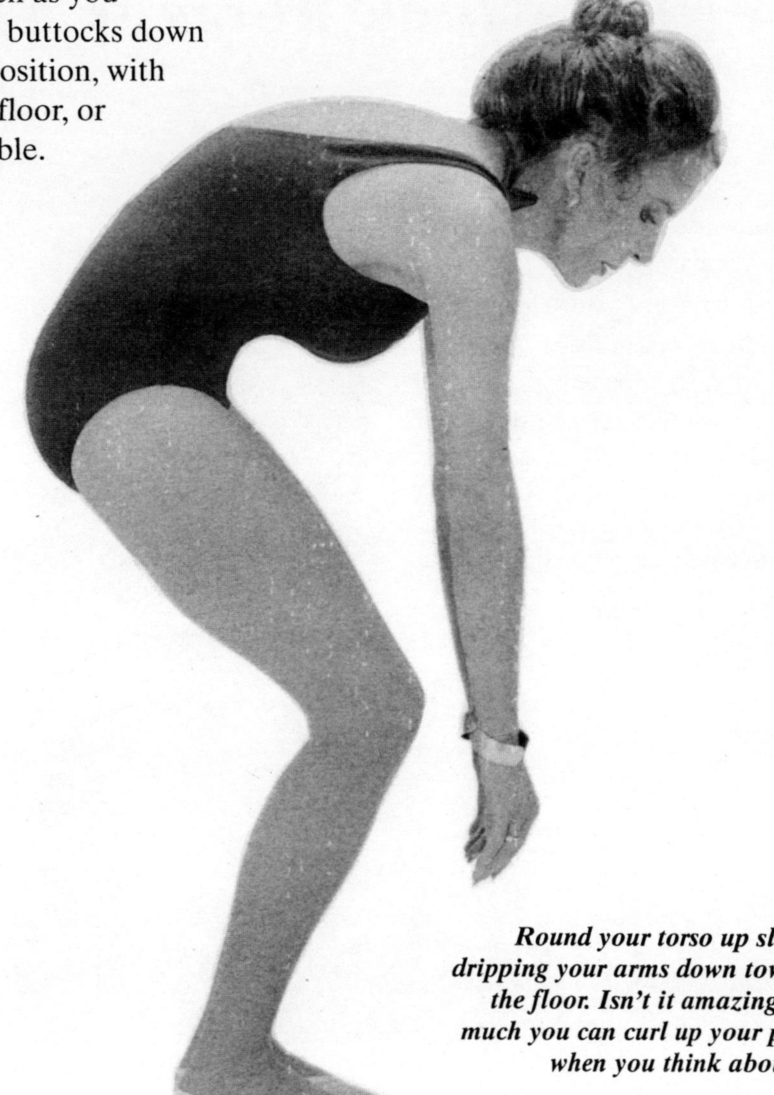

Round your torso up slowly, dripping your arms down towards the floor. Isn't it amazing how much you can curl up your pelvis when you think about it?

Dos and Don'ts

- ❑ **Do not tighten or lock your knees.**
- ❑ **Keep your hips even.**
- ❑ **Keep your entire back relaxed.**
- ❑ **Keep your movements fluid and small. Do not ever make hard, jerky movements.**
- ❑ **Relax your neck.**

Neck Relaxer #1

❑ Stand erect, feet a hip-width apart. Your body is totally relaxed. Pretend your shoulders are melting to the floor. Tighten your buttocks, and curl your pelvis up more than you think you can.

❑ In triple slow motion, roll your head down, resting your chin on your chest.

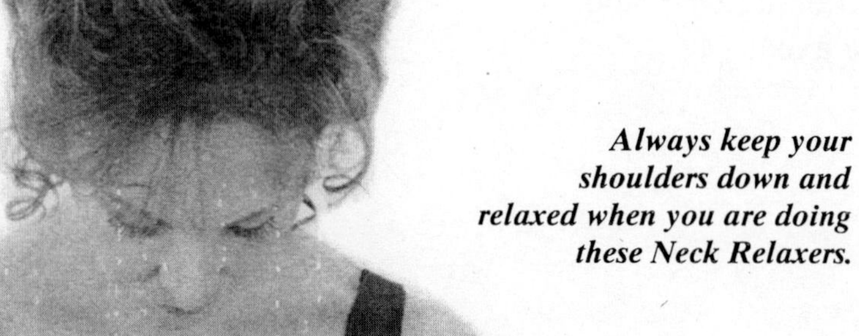

Always keep your shoulders down and relaxed when you are doing these Neck Relaxers.

❑ Still slowly, move your chin over to your right shoulder as far as you can.

❑ Then aim your chin up towards the ceiling, as high as you can, at the same time stretching the back of your neck. You can stretch your neck more than you thought possible.

❑ Next, stretch your neck up even more than you thought possible.

❑ Delicately bring your chin back down to your chest.

❑ Gently move your chin over your left shoulder, and then stretch it up as high as it will go.

❑ Bring it back down to where your chin touches your chest again.

5 COMPLETE HALF-CIRCLES TO EACH SIDE

Neck Relaxer #2

❑ In the same stance, with your body relaxed, shoulders melting into the floor, buttocks tightened, pelvis curled up, and knees relaxed, gently look over to your right side as if you were having a conversation with someone standing in back of you, and hold for a count of 5.

❑ In triple slow motion, turn your head to where you are looking over your left shoulder, and hold for a count of 5.

❑ When you are finished, move your head back to center.

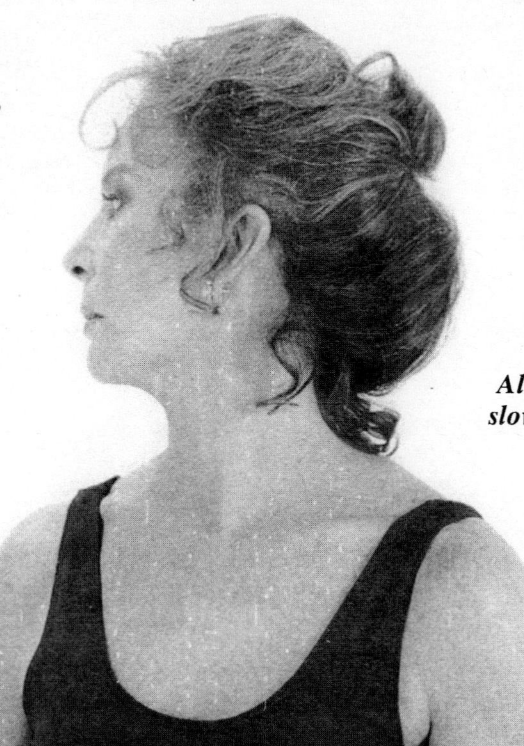

Always move in triple slow motion and think beautiful, soft thoughts.

5 REPS

Dos and Don'ts

- ❑ **Do not tense your shoulders; they must stay relaxed, dropping down to the floor. Don't let them move up—as they tend to do naturally if you're not thinking about it—when you are stretching your neck up.**
- ❑ **Do not move your body or your shoulders.**
- ❑ **Keep your buttocks tight and pelvis curled up.**
- ❑ **Keep your knees relaxed.**
- ❑ **Stretch your neck extremely gently when you move it.**

STOMACH EXERCISES

Since you have already mastered Callanetics, you will be very familiar with the starting position for these exercises.

But please, it is absolutely crucial for you to remember that there are several very important differences between the stomach exercises in the one-hour Callanetics program and in Super Callanetics.

1. Starting Position

Before you even begin any of the stomach exercises, don't forget to have a towel or exercise mat handy, to place under your spine to protect it while you're on the floor.

I have noticed that many of my students become very nonchalant about the correct position for these exercises once they are familiar with how to do them. Yet rounding yourself up properly is so important! Do not get sloppy or lazy, because maintaining the lovely 'round' is what prevents you from putting pressure on your lower back, and too much force on your neck. The results are also much more noticeable!

REMEMBER: *When you are rounding up, your arms, neck, shoulders, and upper back flow as if they are one. Do not ever jerk your arms or neck to help you round up. Think gentle . . . think flowing . . . think* beautiful *round.*

2. How Much You Move

REMEMBER: *I've said that* Less is more? *Well, you will soon be noticing, if you haven't already, that many of the movements in Super Callanetics are actually* smaller *than those of the one-hour program. This is because it is actually* more *of a challenge to use a smaller range of motion—you have to have more control of your body to do this. (And because certain exercises require that you curl your pelvis up* even more *than you think you can, you will find that this actually* prevents *you from making a larger motion with your body.) Take out a ruler and measure 1/16 to 1/4 inch. It's barely even there! Even when you have mastered Super Callanetics, you must remember at all times to keep your movements tiny and almost imperceptible.*

3. Rounding Your Torso

In *Callanetics*, *Callanetics for Your Back*, and *Callanetics Countdown*, you will recall that your upper back was resting below your shoulder blades. Look at the photographs in this section, and you will immediately notice how rounded my shoulders are, and how far off the floor my upper back is. My stomach muscles are strong enough to maintain this position without straining the back.

Also bear in mind that the more you can grasp your legs and take your elbows out and up, the better the stretch of your upper back muscles. This, in turn, rounds your torso even more, allowing your stomach muscles to contract and work efficiently. The result is that you become stronger more quickly.

4. How to Get Up Off the Floor to Protect Your Back

One of the worst things you can do for your back is to jerk yourself up off the floor and just get up. It is very simple to learn how to get up gracefully, in a fluid, easy motion.

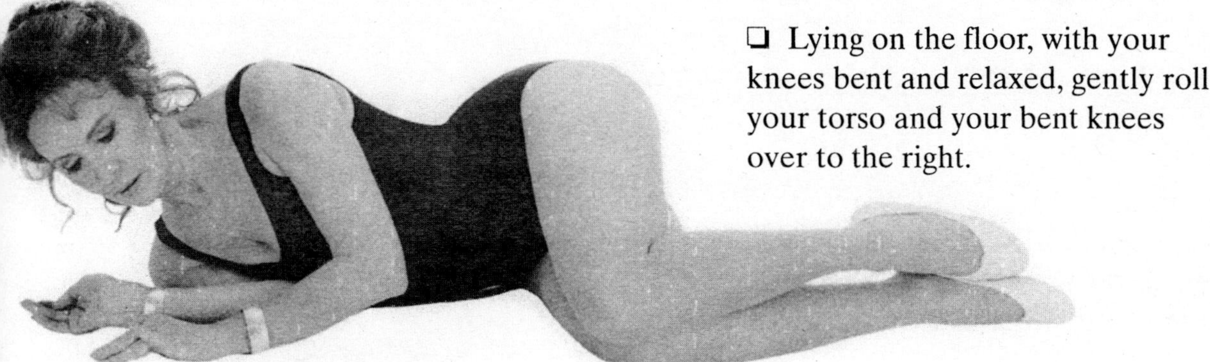

❑ Lying on the floor, with your knees bent and relaxed, gently roll your torso and your bent knees over to the right.

To begin getting up off the floor, roll onto your side.

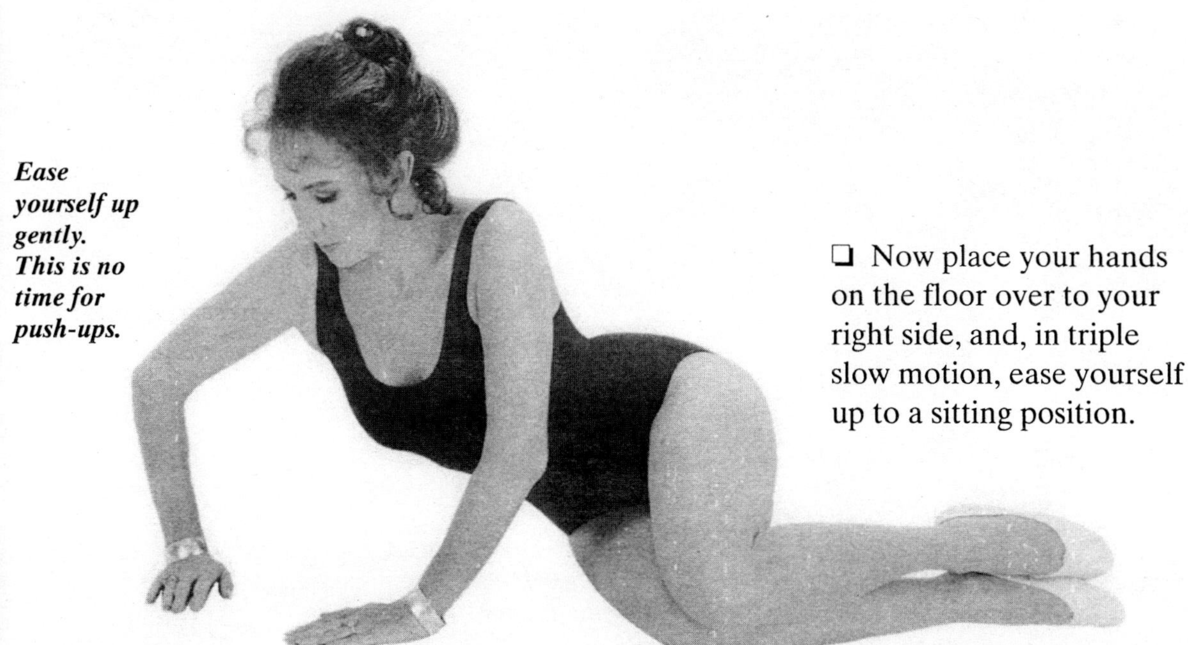

Ease yourself up gently. This is no time for push-ups.

❑ Now place your hands on the floor over to your right side, and, in triple slow motion, ease yourself up to a sitting position.

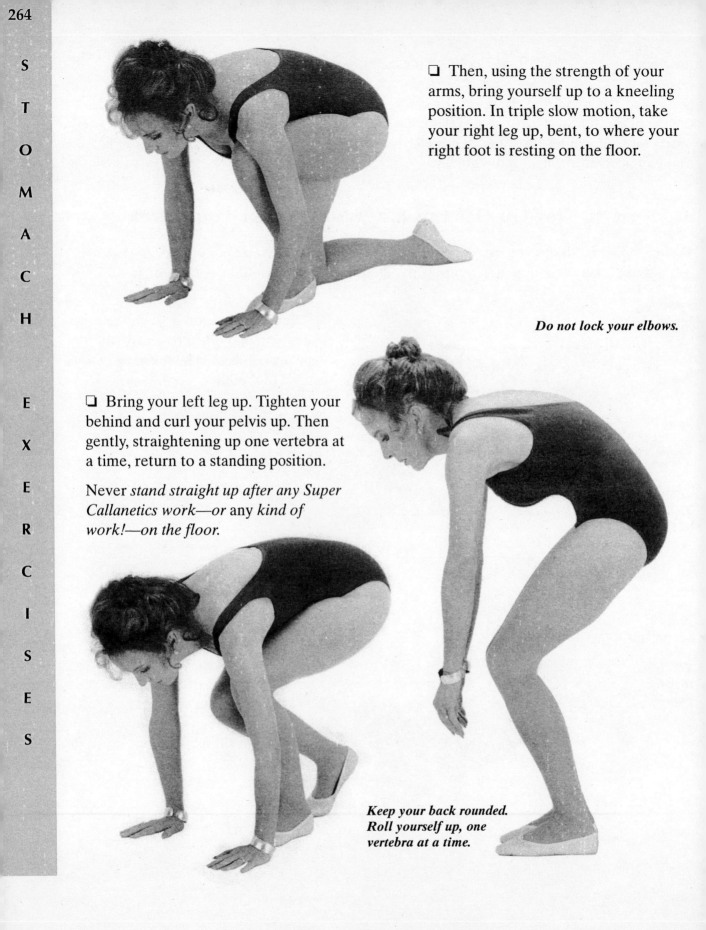

❑ Then, using the strength of your arms, bring yourself up to a kneeling position. In triple slow motion, take your right leg up, bent, to where your right foot is resting on the floor.

Do not lock your elbows.

❑ Bring your left leg up. Tighten your behind and curl your pelvis up. Then gently, straightening up one vertebra at a time, return to a standing position.

Never *stand straight up after any Super Callanetics work—or* any *kind of work!—on the floor.*

Keep your back rounded. Roll yourself up, one vertebra at a time.

5. Don't Forget Your Neck

If your precious neck feels uncomfortable or hurts while doing any of the stomach exercises at the Super Callanetics level, this could be a sign that you may have a medical problem. Do not shrug off neck pain. It could be an indication that there is a long-standing problem, one that comes to your attention only after you begin doing certain kinds of body motions. For most people, this has turned out to be a blessing in disguise—because they went to their doctors and found out what was causing their problems. From there, they were directed to solutions.

Preventive medicine is like using plain old common sense. As I have said many times, *listen to your body*. Many people tend to ignore warning signals of potential problems—and then by the time they have to go to a doctor, it is often too late to correct a condition that could easily have been rectified earlier on.

Your body is the only one you have!

REMEMBER: *For all the stomach exercises where your body is resting on the floor, you can, if you prefer, put your hands behind your head, with your elbows out to the sides. In the advanced exercises, you will feel the stomach muscles working just as deeply.*

Bent-Knee Reach

❑ Lie on the floor, knees bent, feet flat a hip-width apart, and arms at your sides. Grab your inner thighs with all your might. Take your elbows out to the side as much as you can, and then aim them up towards the ceiling.

❑ Letting the small of your back be relaxed and melting into the floor, slowly round your head and shoulders up, off the floor. You will be rounding your nose into your chest. At the same time, bring your elbows out and up toward the ceiling even more. When you have rounded your torso as much as you possibly can, gently take your hands off your inner thighs and, keeping them inside your legs, grab the back of your legs higher to where you can round your torso and bring your elbows out and up even more.

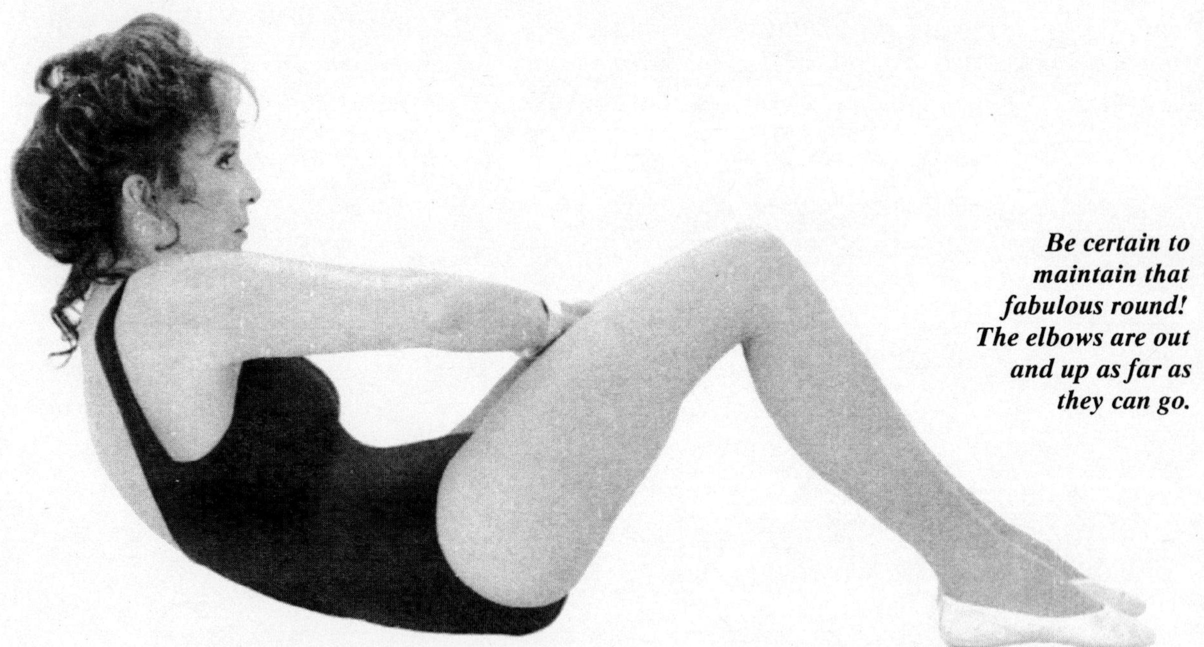

Be certain to maintain that fabulous round! The elbows are out and up as far as they can go.

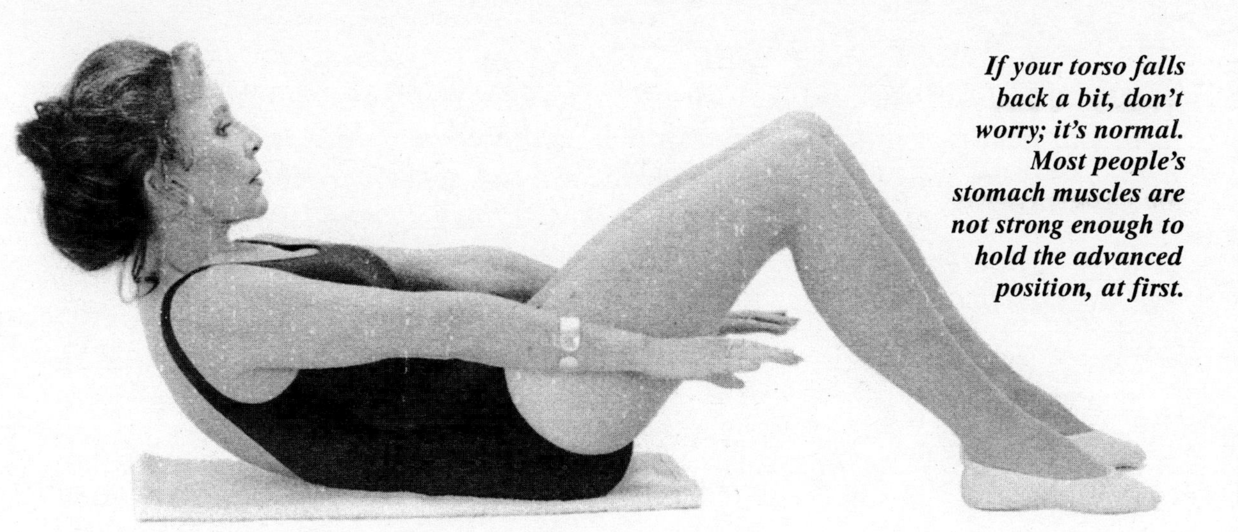

If your torso falls back a bit, don't worry; it's normal. Most people's stomach muscles are not strong enough to hold the advanced position, at first.

❑ Once your torso is rounded as much as possible, gently lower your arms, aiming them straight to the front of you, about 6 to 12 inches off the floor.

❑ Gently, in triple slow motion, do the tiny 1/16- to 1/4-inch motion, back and forth.

IF YOU FEEL THAT YOUR ENTIRE BODY IS MOVING BACK AND FORTH ON THE FLOOR: *Lift your feet 1 to 2 inches up off the floor. Moving back and forth or in a jerking motion is a signal that your back muscles are trying to come in to assist your stomach muscles.*

IF YOU FEEL THAT YOU ARE LOSING CONTROL OF THIS EXERCISE, OR THAT THERE IS A STRAIN ON YOUR LOWER BACK, EITHER: *Move your feet very slightly away from your body;* or, *take your torso down 1/16 inch. If it still feels too difficult, take your torso down another 1/16 inch.*

100 REPS

❑ To come out of this exercise, in triple slow motion, roll your torso down to the floor, one vertebra at a time.

REMEMBER: *Take your breathers when you have to. You may grab your inner thighs with your hands, as in the starting position, and hold your rounded position. Then, before releasing your hands to continue the exercise, take your elbows out and then up, and then round your torso even more. You may also roll down vertebra by vertebra to rest on the floor—but remember to start at Step 1 again when continuing with the exercises.*

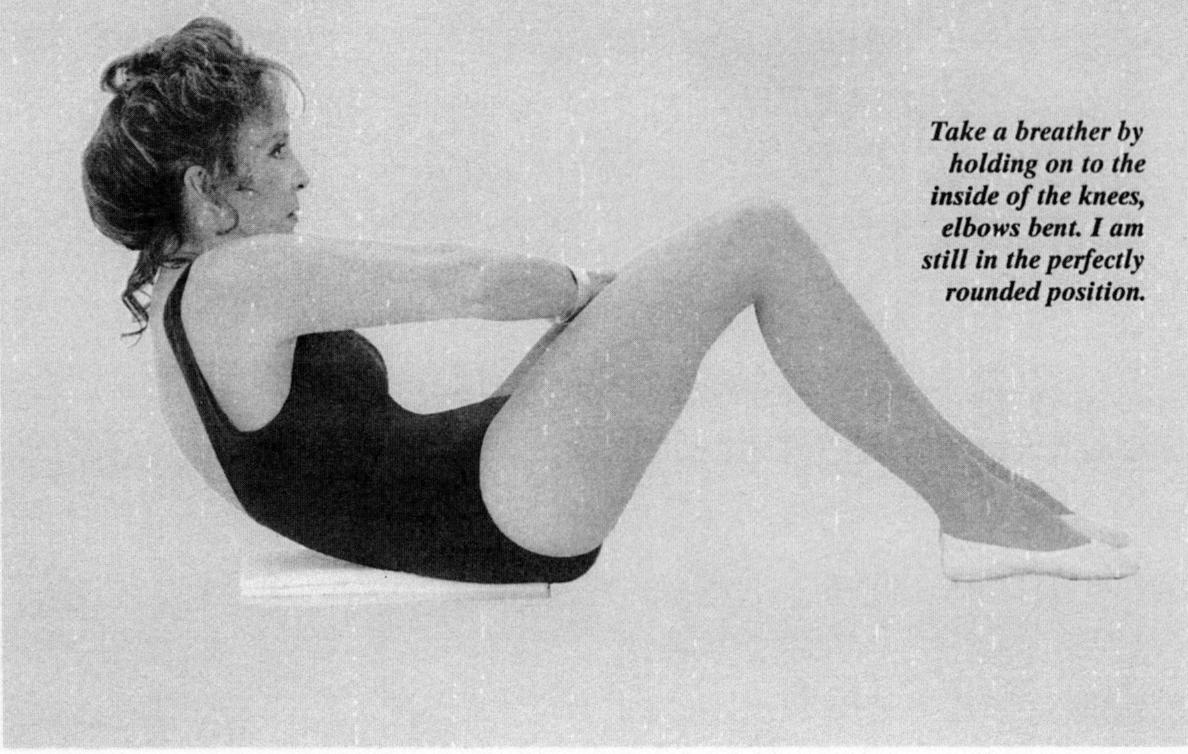

Take a breather by holding on to the inside of the knees, elbows bent. I am still in the perfectly rounded position.

Dos and Don'ts

- ❑ **Do not tighten your stomach muscles. This puts pressure on your lower back. They will certainly be doing enough work!**
- ❑ **Just relax and let your lower back melt into the floor.**
- ❑ **Keep your torso and your shoulders rounded off the floor as much as possible.**
- ❑ **Do not move *just* your arms *or* your shoulders *or* your neck when pulsing. They all move with your upper torso as a unit.**
- ❑ **Relax your buttocks to take pressure off your lower back. They should not move at all.**
- ❑ **Relax your legs.**
- ❑ **Do not tense your neck.**
- ❑ **No jerking or bouncing.**

REMEMBER: *When you are first getting into position, your nose should always be aimed into your chest. Once you have built up tremendous strength in your stomach muscles, you can either continue to keep aiming your nose towards your chest, or, you can raise your head just a tad, aiming your face towards your knees while doing your reps or taking a breather.* Never, *however, aim your face up towards the ceiling. You won't be changing the actual position of your neck—you only should be shifting the position of your head a wee bit. Do whatever is most comfortable for you.*

Single Leg Raise

Most people don't realize that they can actually point their toes without tensing their leg muscles. In the following exercises, as well as in the Leg section, whenever one or both legs are raised, point your toes, but remember to keep your legs perfectly relaxed. This is a wonderful opportunity to start training yourself to relax different parts of your body.

❑ Lying on the floor with your knees still bent, feet a hip-width apart, gently raise your right leg up, toes pointing towards the ceiling, grab the back of your thigh with both hands, below your knee. Both elbows are out as far as they can go, and then aiming up towards the ceiling.

❑ Now, in triple slow motion, round your torso up. At the same time, take your elbows out and then up even more to stretch the upper back. You are aiming your nose towards your rib cage.

❑ When you feel that you can't round any further, take your hands off your legs and extend them, straight out in the direction of your feet, 6 inches to 1 foot off the floor.

❑ Slowly straighten your left leg, raised no more than a foot off the floor.

❑ Now you are in position to gently move your torso, in triple slow motion, 1/16 to 1/4 inch, back and forth.

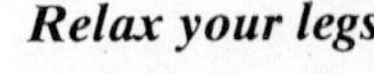

Relax your legs.

100 REPS

❑ When you feel comfortable with this movement, start to lower your upstretched leg 1/2 inch at a time. If you feel your lower back starting to take over—which is the signal that your stomach muscles are not quite strong enough —slowly raise your right leg back towards the ceiling, 1/2 inch at a time, until you feel no strain on your lower back.

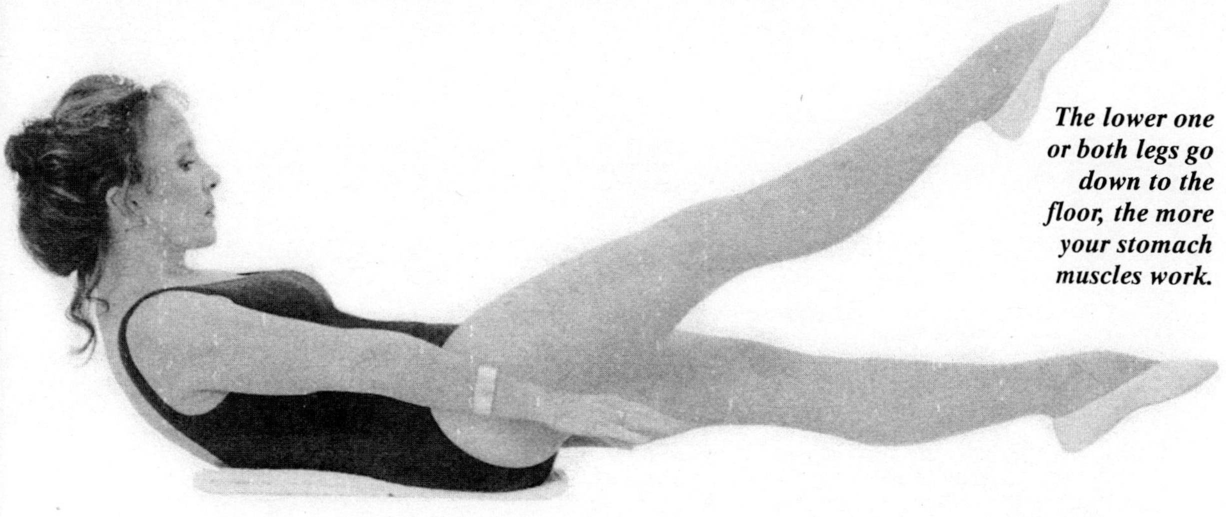

The lower one or both legs go down to the floor, the more your stomach muscles work.

IF YOU STILL FEEL PRESSURE ON YOUR LOWER BACK: *Either gently raise your upstretched leg towards the ceiling, or lower your torso 1/16 inch towards the floor, or rest your outstretched left leg on the floor.*

IF YOU NEED TO TAKE A BREATHER: *Bring your right leg up towards you, to where it feels comfortable, grasp it with both hands below your knee, hold your rounded-torso position with your elbows out, and breathe deeply and naturally. If you need to, rest your left leg on the floor or bend your left knee, resting your left foot on the floor.*

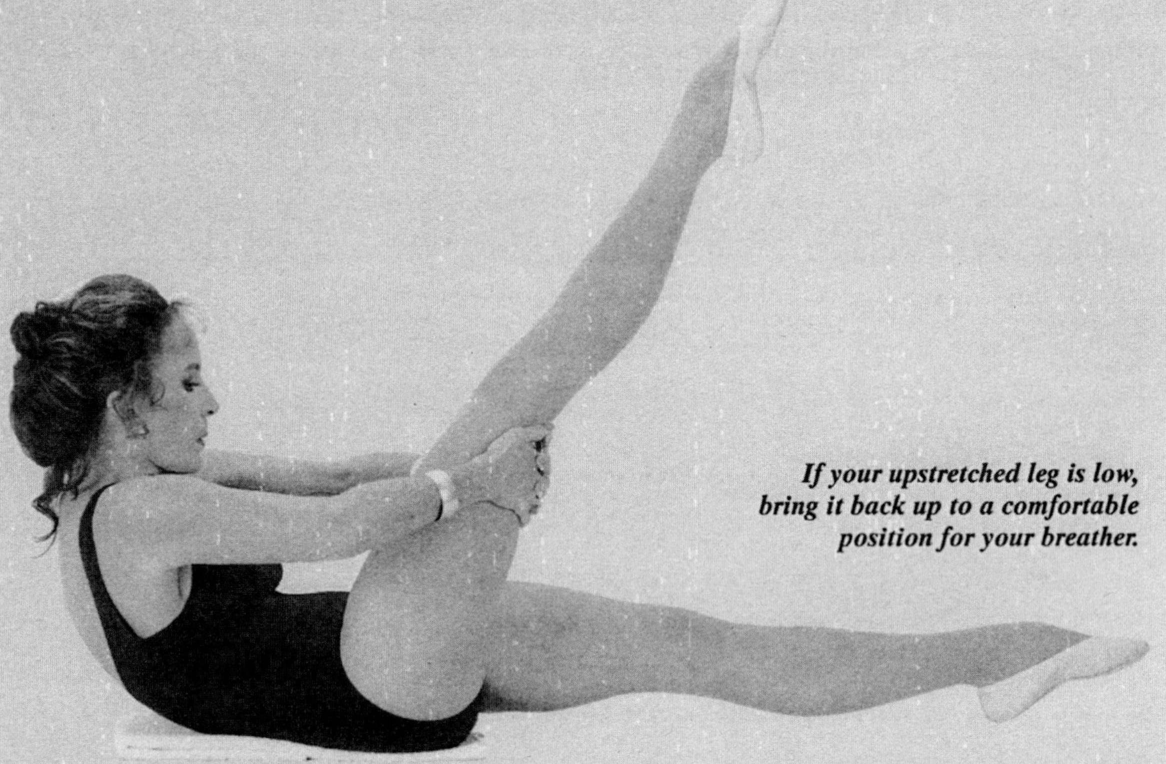

If your upstretched leg is low, bring it back up to a comfortable position for your breather.

When you are ready to start again, still holding on to your leg, round your torso more than you think you can, stretching your elbows out and up towards the ceiling. Let go of your leg, extend your arms out to your sides, then take your right leg down to the position it was in before your breather, and continue to count from wherever you left off. (Don't forget to extend your opposite leg off the floor if you have been resting it on the floor, or if it was bent.)

❑ To come out of this exercise, in triple slow motion—you have no choice!—gently bend your knees, one at a time, so that both feet are resting on the floor, and slowly lower your torso, vertebra by vertebra, until you are resting on the floor.

- ❑ Repeat this exercise on the opposite side.

100 REPS

Dos and Don'ts

- ❑ Your entire body should be relaxed, like a rag doll.
- ❑ Do not let your back take over. Keep it relaxed. How much you can round your upper back depends on how stretched your upper back muscles are, and how strong your stomach muscles have become.
- ❑ If you feel the exercise is getting too difficult, or your back muscles are about to take over, raise your upstretched leg 1/2 inch higher. The lower you can take your raised legs down, the more your abdominal muscles will have to work—but they must be ready for such an *intense* workout.
- ❑ Keep your upper body rounded as much as you can.
- ❑ Keep your legs relaxed.
- ❑ Relax your stomach muscles.
- ❑ Relax your neck.
- ❑ Keep your elbows up and out as high as you possibly can, while getting into position.
- ❑ Do not ever aim your face towards the ceiling; this puts strain on your neck.
- ❑ Do not tighten your buttocks.

Double Leg Raise

❑ Lying on the floor, feet a hip-width apart, bend your knees up to your chest one at a time, and then extend both legs up towards the ceiling. Grab onto your outer thighs, stretch your elbows out then up as high as you can, then round your torso up with your nose pointing into your rib cage.

❑ Once you're rounded and in position, let go of your legs and extend your arms straight out, 6 inches to 1 foot off the floor.

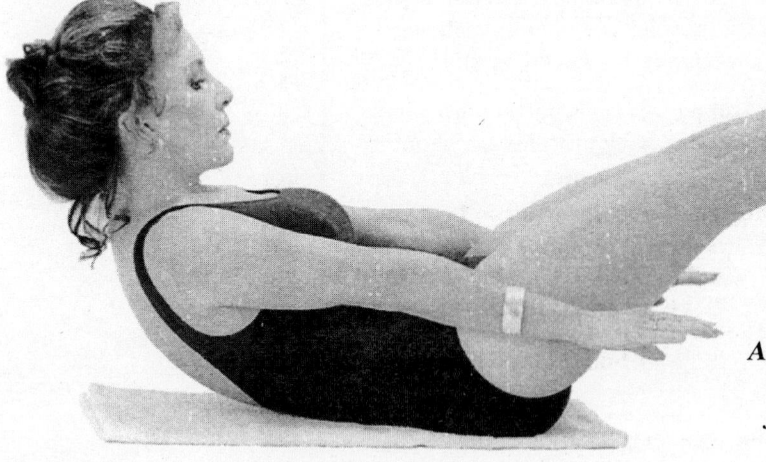

As in the Single Leg Raise, lower your legs only as far as you can without feeling the strain in your lower back. Your legs should feel like feathers.

❑ In triple slow motion, lower your legs as far as is comfortable, then gently move your torso back and forth, 1/16 to 1/4 inch.

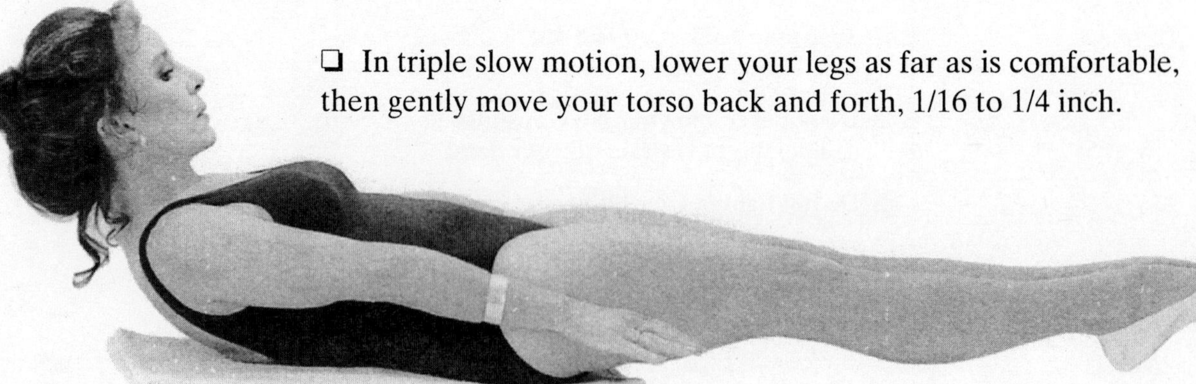

There should be no strain on your body at all—your lower back should always be on the floor, not arched. It takes incredible strength and control to lower your legs this much and still have your body feeling like a rag doll melting into the floor.

❑ If you feel that your lower back muscles are starting to take over, or your lower back is starting to arch, again, this is your signal that your stomach muscles are not yet strong enough to work at this level. Slowly raise your legs back up in 1/2-inch segments until you feel absolutely no pressure on your lower back, or your lower back does not arch, and then continue the exercise at that level.

100 REPS

IF YOU NEED TO TAKE A BREATHER: *Grab onto your outer thighs with both hands, hold your rounded torso position, with your elbows still aimed out to the side, and breathe deeply and naturally. Before letting go to continue the count, round your torso, and bring your elbows up and out more than you think you can.*

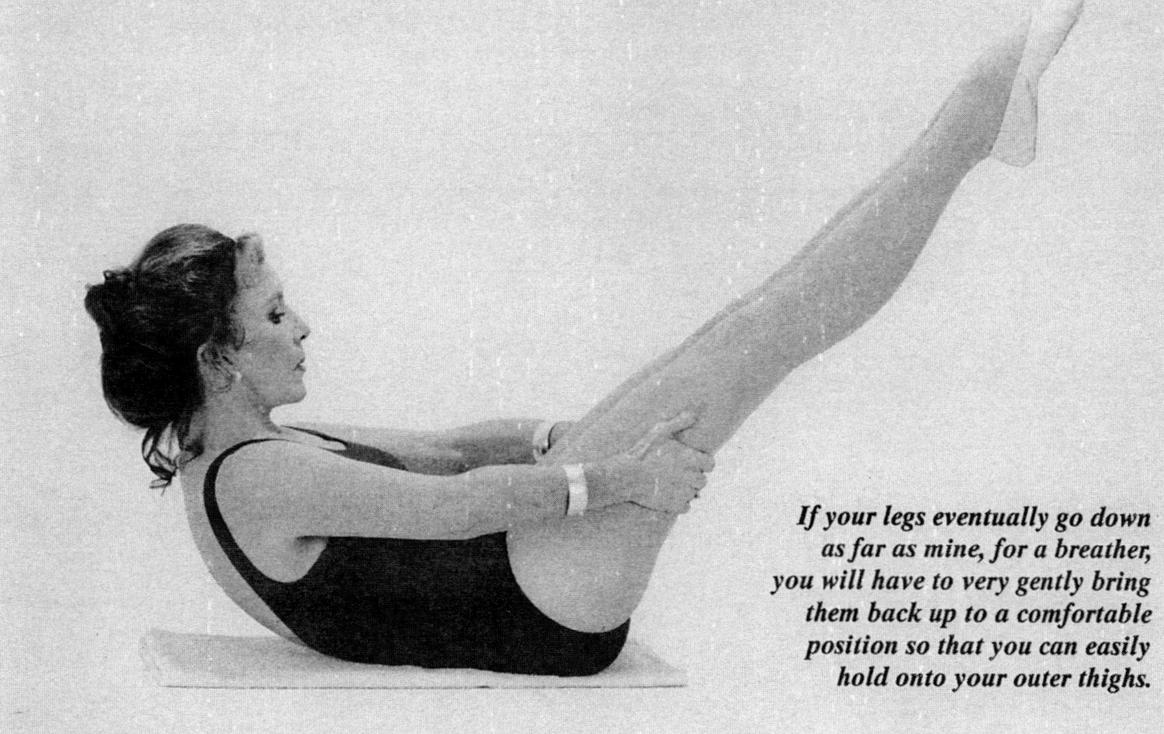

If your legs eventually go down as far as mine, for a breather, you will have to very gently bring them back up to a comfortable position so that you can easily hold onto your outer thighs.

❑ To come out of the double leg raise, in triple slow motion, bend your knees, and lower your feet to the floor, one at a time. Then lower your torso, vertebra by vertebra.

Dos and Don'ts

- ❑ Your elbows must be out and up as far as they can possibly go for the starting position.
- ❑ Keep your shoulders rounded and up off the floor.
- ❑ Keep your entire body relaxed. Especially relax your legs and neck.
- ❑ Relax your stomach muscles.
- ❑ Do not let your lower back arch or come up off the floor. This is another signal that your stomach muscles are not quite strong enough to maintain that position. If so, bring your legs up 1/2 inch. If that's not enough, bring them up another 1/2 inch and continue until you have reached a comfortable position.
- ❑ Let your lower back melt into the floor.
- ❑ Relax your buttocks.

Sit Up and Curl Down

You will be working up to 4 sets of 10 reps each, lowering your torso only by curling up your pelvis. Each set becomes progressively more advanced. You must take a breather between each set.

For this exercise, 1 rep = 1 gentle wave of the arms up and down. Try to do 10 reps for each set.

❑ Sit up with your knees bent, feet a hip-width apart and flat on the floor, your hands clasped just below your knees. Put your head between your knees, with your elbows out to the side. Scoot your buttocks forward until you are not sitting on your tailbone.

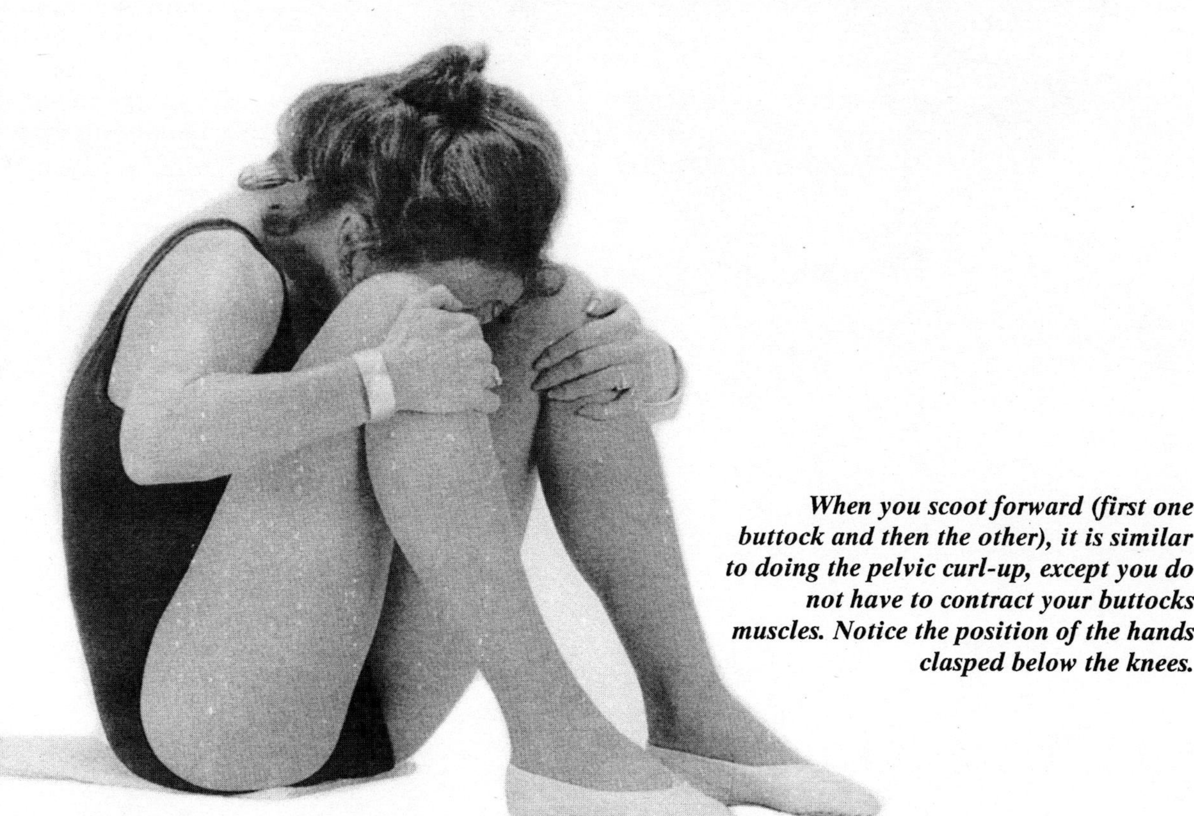

When you scoot forward (first one buttock and then the other), it is similar to doing the pelvic curl-up, except you do not have to contract your buttocks muscles. Notice the position of the hands clasped below the knees.

❑ Tighten your buttocks and curl your pelvis up, which will automatically begin to lower your torso to the floor, vertebra by vertebra. Your back does not do any of the work, and does not move (other than being lowered by the action of your pelvis curling up). Very slowly, keep tightening your buttocks and curling your pelvis up until your curl-up lowers your torso enough so that your arms, which are still holding onto the side of your knees, are now straight. It usually takes 4 to 5 curl-ups to accomplish this.

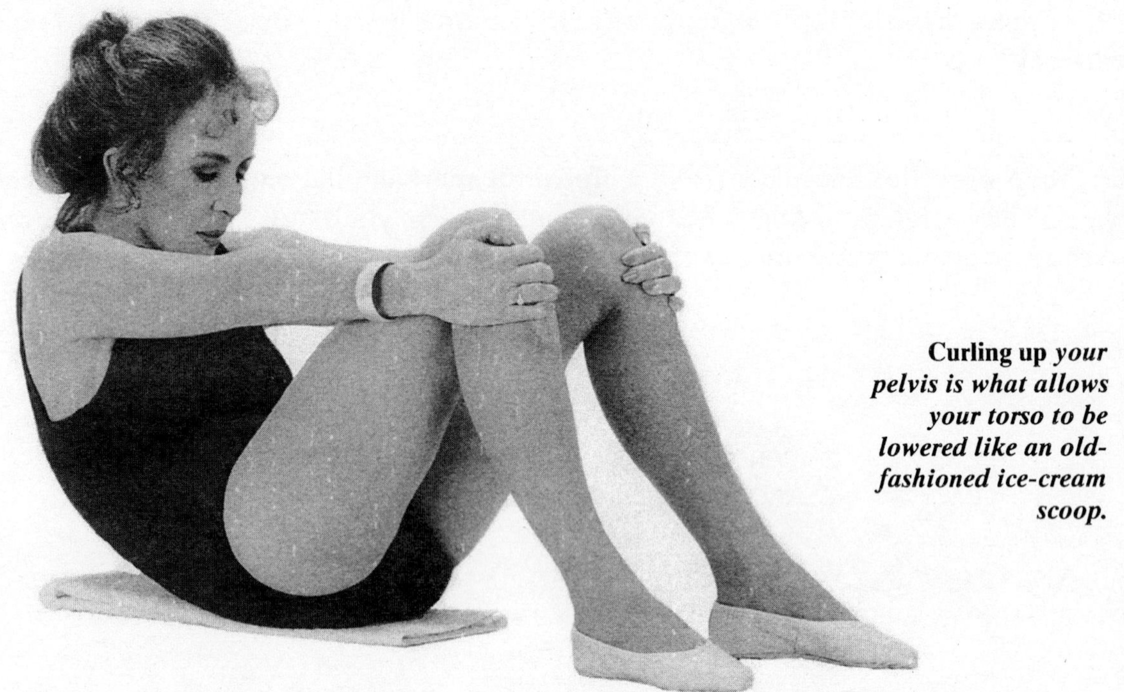

Curling up ***your pelvis is what allows your torso to be lowered like an old-fashioned ice-cream scoop.***

❑ Without moving any other part of your body, let go of your knees. Your torso is still rounded and perfectly relaxed.

❑ With your arms straight, in triple slow motion, take them up as high as you can without forcing, and then back down to the floor in smooth, unbroken waves. Your body is balanced on the strength of your stomach muscles.

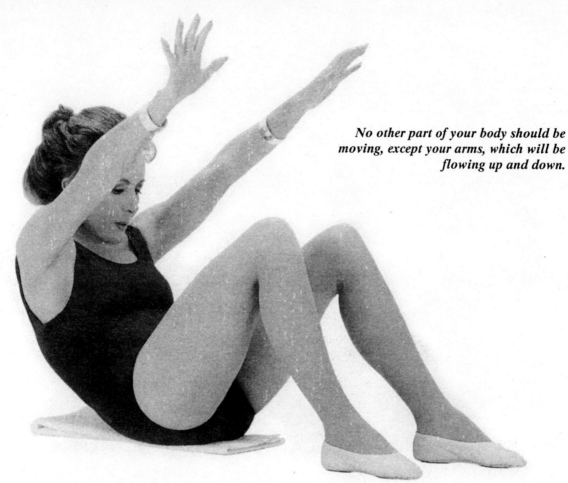

No other part of your body should be moving, except your arms, which will be flowing up and down.

10 REPS OF SLOW, GENTLE ARM WAVES FOR THIS FIRST SET

REMEMBER: *If you feel you are losing your balance, that is your signal that your stomach muscles are not yet strong enough to allow your arms to go as high as you are taking them. Don't take them up as high on the following reps. You can also slide your feet a few inches away from your body or round your torso more towards your knees (or do all three!).*

❑ Slowly clasp your hands up more towards the top of your knees and take a breather. Because your torso is lower now from curling your pelvis up you will need to clasp your hands higher on your knees. Hold your position, taking several deep breaths.

❑ When you are ready to continue, tighten your buttocks and curl your pelvis up even more. These curl-ups will take your torso even lower. Let go of your knees and begin your next set of slow, gentle arm waves.

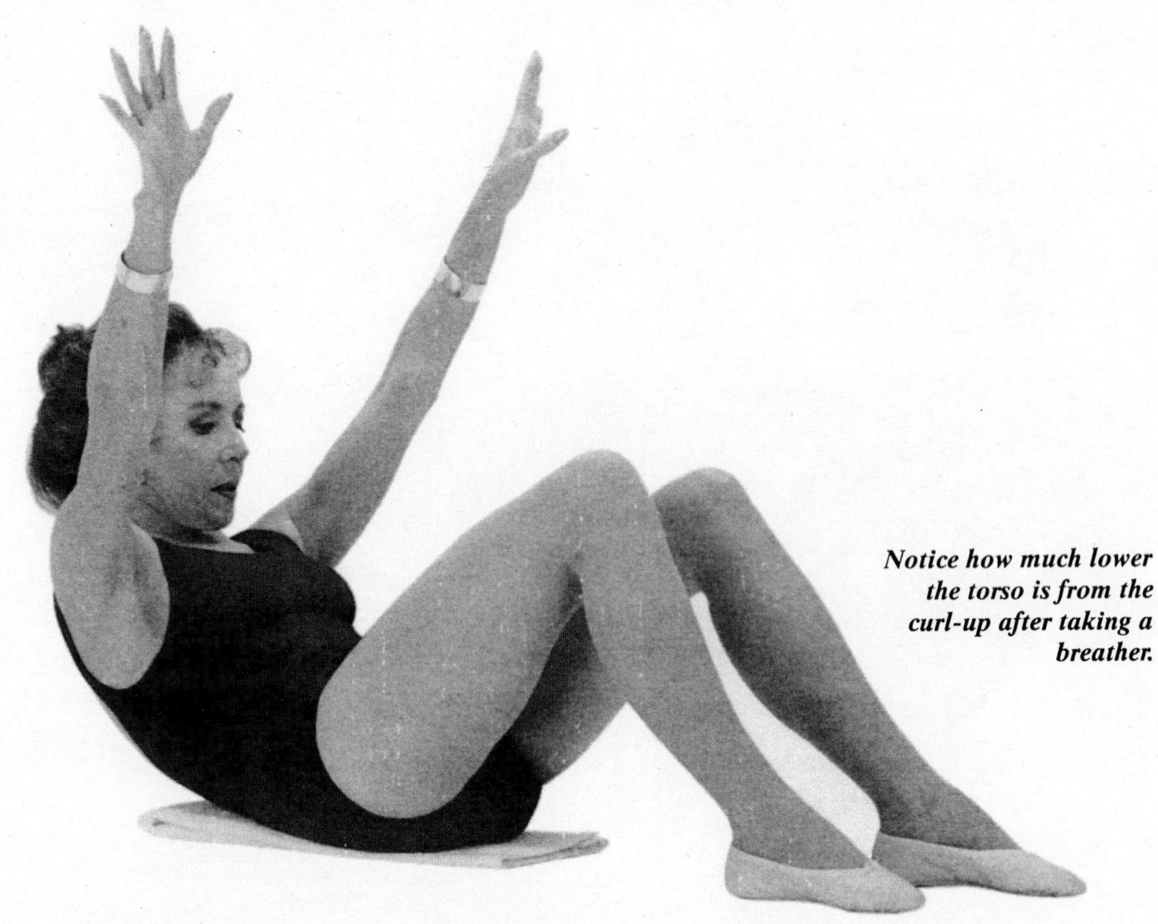

Notice how much lower the torso is from the curl-up after taking a breather.

10 REPS FOR THIS SECOND SET

❑ To come out of your second set and begin your third set, grab the top of your knees, take a lovely breather, curl your pelvis up even more, take your hands off your knees . . . and continue your up-and-down waves with your arms.

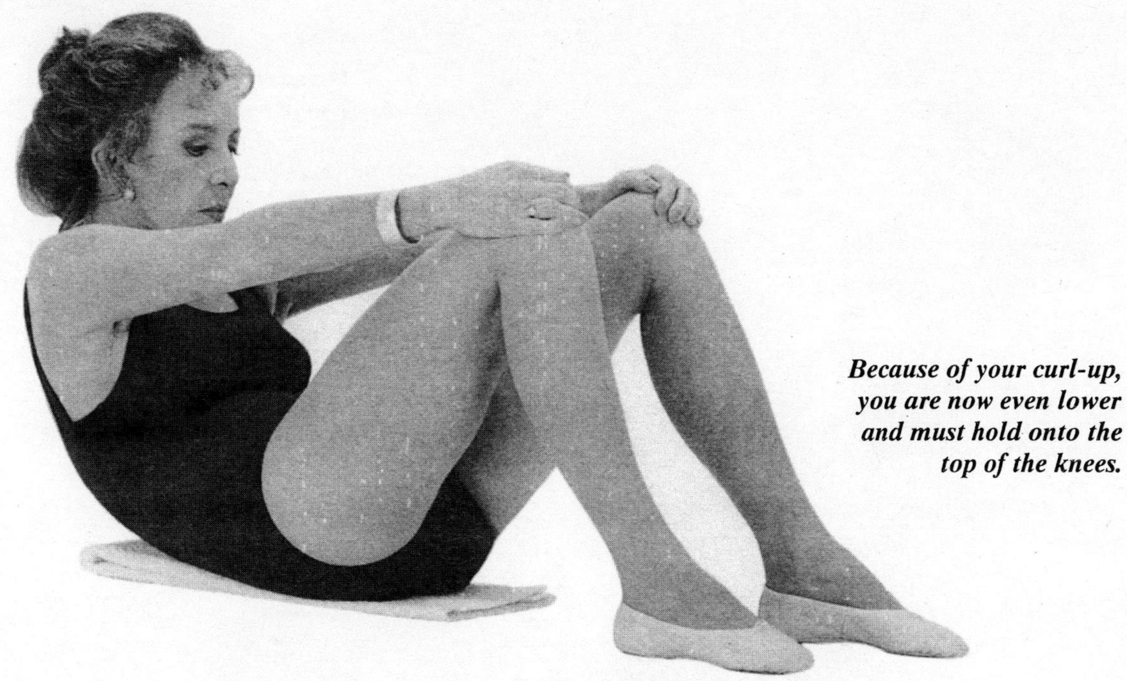

Because of your curl-up, you are now even lower and must hold onto the top of the knees.

10 REPS FOR YOUR THIRD SET

REMEMBER: *At this level, you will probably feel that you won't be able to take your arms up as high. Raise them only as high as is comfortable.*

❑ To come out of your third set and begin your fourth set without moving your body, put your hands above your knees (towards your thigh), take your breather, then continue the routine one more time.

10 REPS FOR YOUR FOURTH SET

❑ To come out of this exercise, slowly lower your torso—even if you are so low that you only have to go down a scant few inches—vertebra by vertebra, tipping your pelvis up more than you think you can as you ease back to the floor.

Dos and Don'ts

- ❑ Keep your back as rounded as possible.

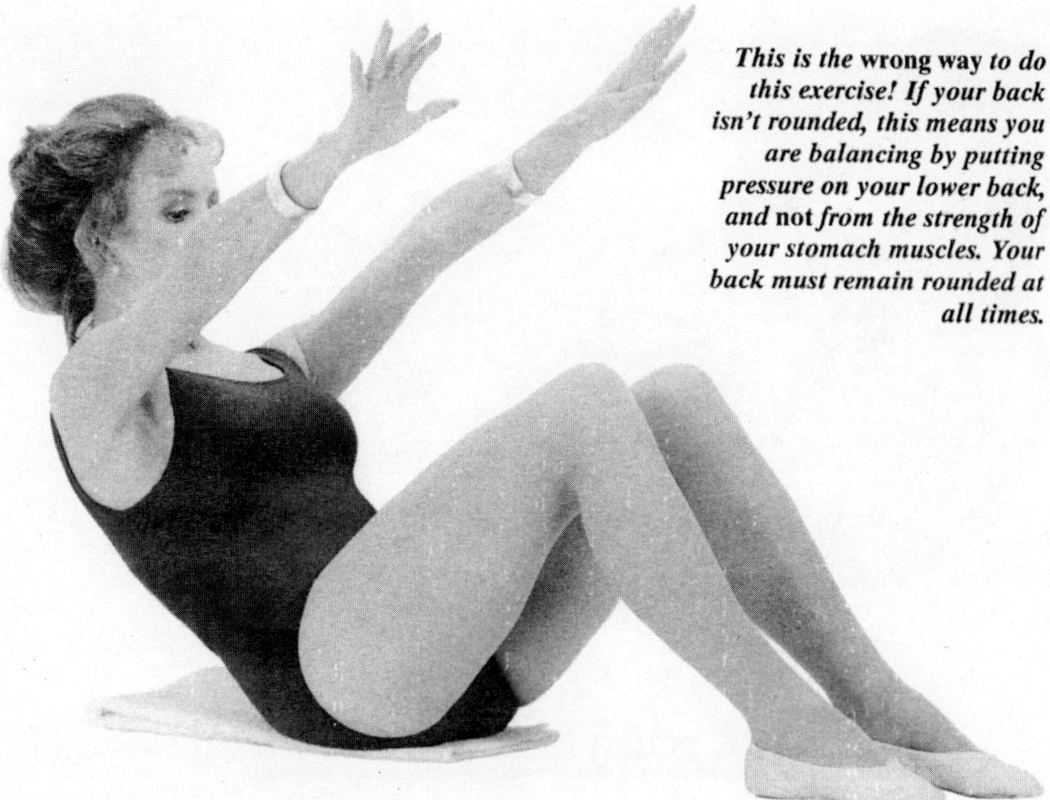

This is the wrong way to do this exercise! If your back isn't rounded, this means you are balancing by putting pressure on your lower back, and not from the strength of your stomach muscles. Your back must remain rounded at all times.

- ❑ Believe it or not, in a short time you will be able to curl your pelvis up so much more than you previously thought humanly possible!
- ❑ Try to bring your arms up as high as you can take them, without forcing. If this exercise is becoming too difficult, don't raise your arms higher than your ears. The more your torso has been lowered to the floor, the less high you will be able to raise up your arms.
- ❑ Concentrate on relaxing. Your arms, gently waving up and down, are the only part of your body that is moving at all.
- ❑ Keep your head down and neck relaxed.
- ❑ Breathe naturally.
- ❑ After each breather, curl your pelvis even more by rolling your pelvis in towards your navel.
- ❑ Do not jerk your pelvis.

Pelvic Ease-Down and Up

❑ Sit erect with your knees bent, feet a hip-width apart and flat on the floor. Scoot up your buttocks as in the previous exercise (Sit Up and Curl Down) so that you are *not* sitting on your tailbone.

❑ Place your head between your knees, and crisscross your hands at the base of your neck.

Notice how rounded the shoulders are in the starting position, and that the hands are crisscrossed at the base of the neck. If that position is too difficult for you at first, you can place your hands behind your head.

❑ Tighten your buttocks, and curl your pelvis up, which will automatically begin lowering your torso towards the floor. Keep your pelvis curled up—never releasing it—as you curl up. Your torso will lower with each curl-up, one vertebra at a time. In triple slow motion, ease yourself down, vertebra by vertebra, until you lie flat on your back. It should take 10 or more curl-ups to accomplish this.

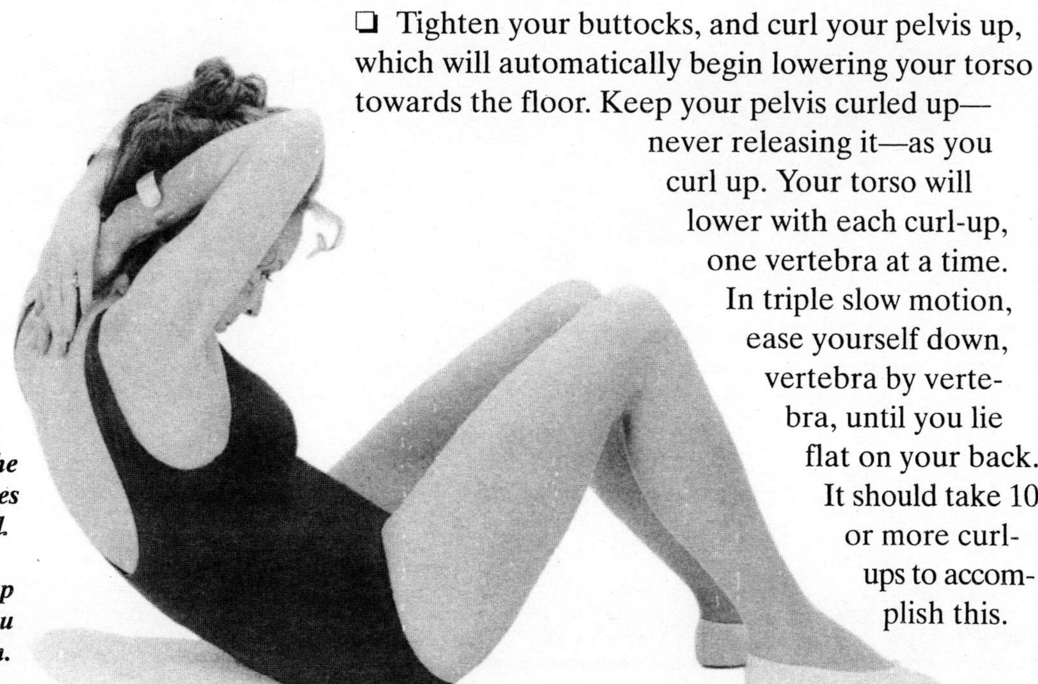

Notice how the torso continues to be rounded. You can always curl up more than you think you can.

❑ Rest on the floor for a few seconds, your arms still crisscrossed at the base of your neck.

REMEMBER: *Many people's stomach muscles will not be strong enough at this point to attempt to ease back up. This is much harder as you must now lift the weight of your torso against gravity to come up. And when you do attempt to ease back up, you will probably laugh—your muscles have to be lethal for you to accomplish this! Don't mentally beat yourself up if you can't do it yet—I don't think even Superman could do this one; it's so powerful! (Well,* maybe *he could if he didn't forget to wear his blue tights!) I must admit even I am shocked when I see men and women in their seventies coming back up with ease.*

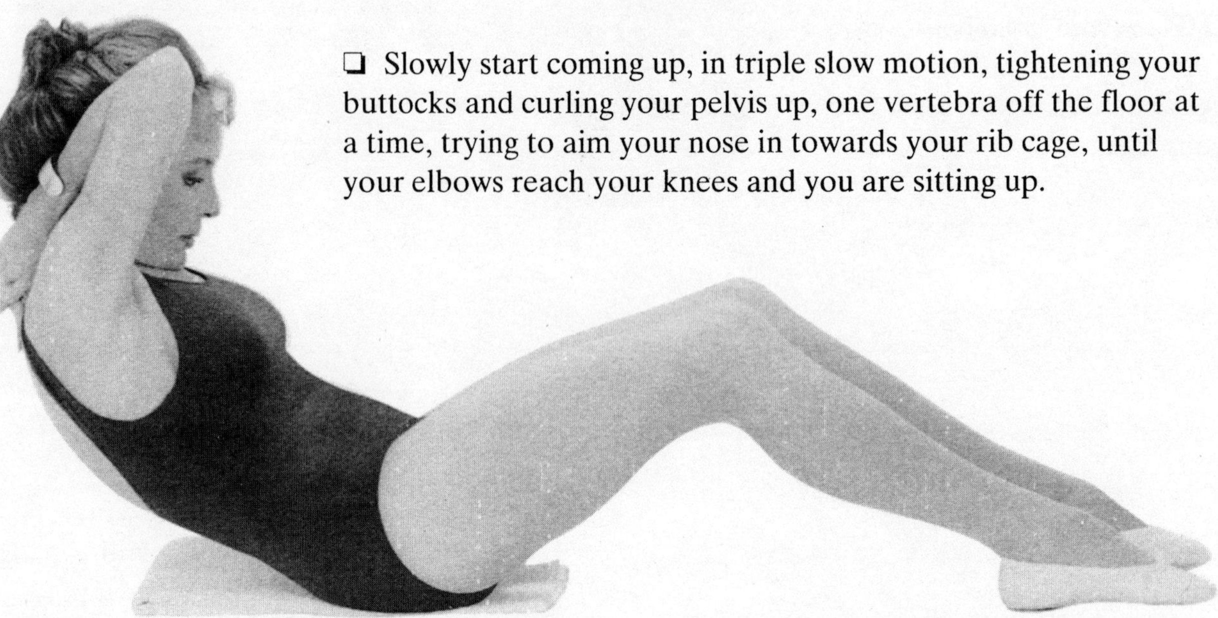

❑ Slowly start coming up, in triple slow motion, tightening your buttocks and curling your pelvis up, one vertebra off the floor at a time, trying to aim your nose in towards your rib cage, until your elbows reach your knees and you are sitting up.

Only attempt this reversal, curling slowly back up, if you are certain your stomach muscles are strong enough to support this position without your lower back taking over. At first, if you feel you are about to lose your balance, you will probably have to move your feet away from your body until your stomach muscles become extremely strong.

This is the total reverse of all the previous steps.

DO 1 REP DOWN AND IF YOU CAN, 1 REP UP, AT YOUR OWN PACE.

Dos and Don'ts

- ❏ You must have incredibly strong stomach muscles to even attempt this exercise—but practice makes perfect.
- ❏ Keep your neck relaxed.
- ❏ You can always curl up more than you think you can.
- ❏ Only by tightening your buttocks and curling your pelvis up will you ease yourself down and up. Do not jerk or thrust your torso, or use your back to lower yourself down—or to bring yourself back up.
- ❏ Breathe normally.
- ❏ Relax your legs—they are like feathers.

Leg Exercises

Pelvic-Wave Leg Strengthener

In this exercise, you will be doing the pelvic wave, slowly down in three stages, and then back up.

By this time, you should be able to appreciate just how incredibly flexible and flowing the pelvis area can be. This is so necessary, as you know, for optimal health and posture.

Your legs should also be strong enough so that you won't ever find yourself holding onto your barre or piece of heavy furniture for dear life again!

One bit of advice, however: Do walk around for a few moments in between the Pelvic-Wave Leg Strengthener and the Plié and Balance exercises. This will give you a breather and help relax your muscles, enabling you to do these exercises more efficiently.

❑ Stand at your barre, or hold onto a piece of furniture, feet a hip-width apart, arms straight but relaxed. Go up on your *toes*—not the balls of your feet—knees bent, and bring your heels together, keeping your back straight and relaxed.

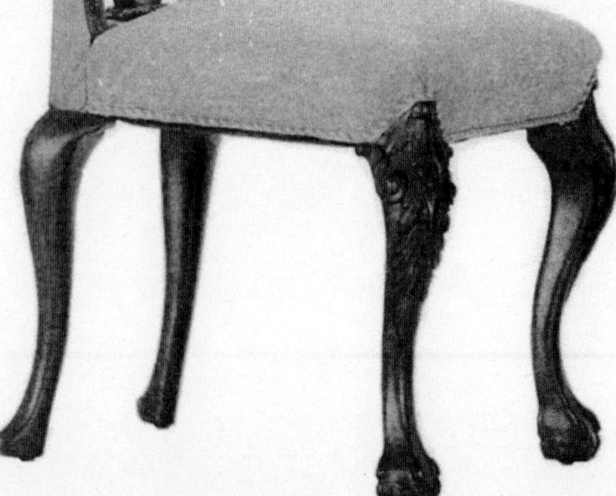

Notice how straight and relaxed the back is. And the knees are not forced out to the sides at all.

❑ In triple slow motion, with your torso erect and your neck stretched towards the ceiling, lower your torso 2 inches straight down towards the floor. Tighten your buttocks and curl your pelvis up. Then curl it up even more than you think you can, and at the same time allow your upper torso to round as much as possible. Hold for a slow count of 3, and then gently release your pelvis without pushing your buttocks back.

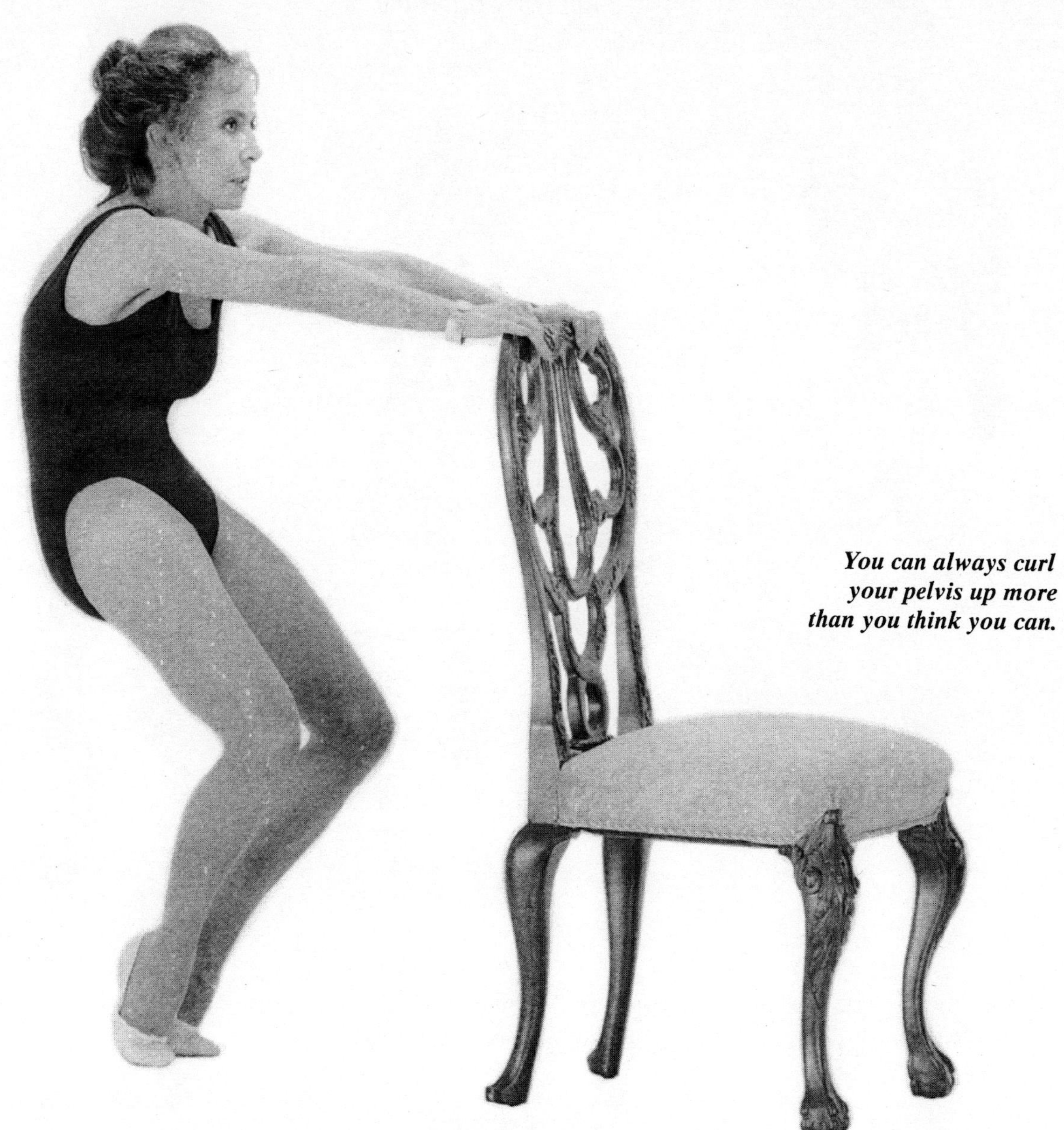

You can always curl your pelvis up more than you think you can.

❏ In triple slow motion, go down 2 more inches, tighten your buttocks, curl your pelvis up even more, hold for a slow count of 3, and gently release.

❏ Go down another 2 inches, tighten your buttocks, curl your pelvis up even more, hold for a slow count of 3, and gently release.

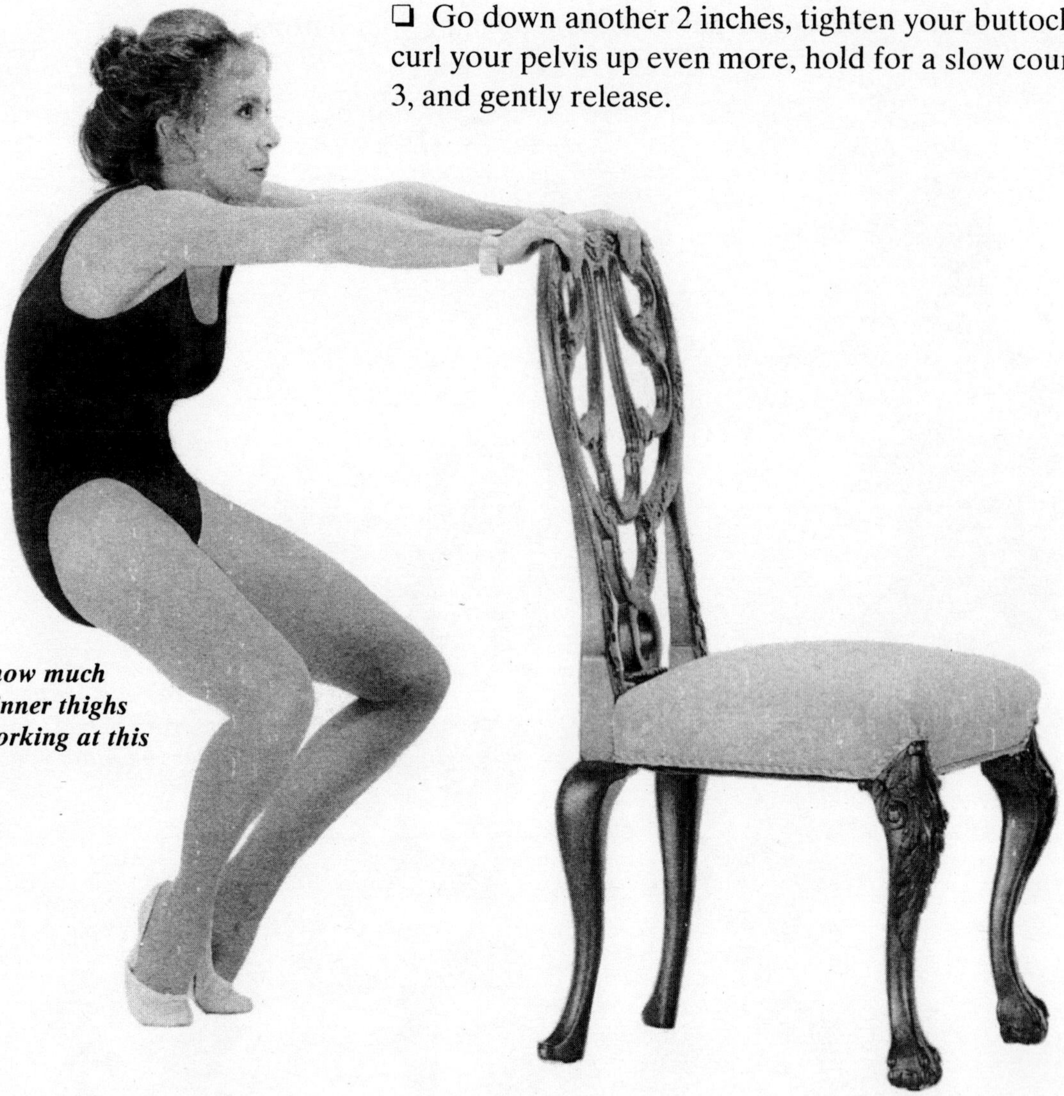

Feel how much your inner thighs are working at this level.

❏ Now reverse the movement, going up 2 inches each time, just as slowly, until you have returned to the original standing position. This equals 1 set.

DO 3 SETS

Dos and Don'ts

- ❑ For the second and third sets, curl your pelvis up even more each time.
- ❑ Your spine is always straight when your pelvis is not curled up. Do not stick out your buttocks when coming out of the pelvic curl.
- ❑ Do not arch your back.
- ❑ Do not try to aim your knees out too far to the side. Let their position be natural.
- ❑ Keep your shoulders relaxed. Your upper back should be as rounded as possible when curling up the pelvis for the most beneficial spine stretch. The more your pelvis is curled up, the more your torso will round, stretching the spine, and the faster your legs will become strong and tight.
- ❑ Keep your balance on your toes.
- ❑ Do not lean your weight on the barre.
- ❑ When lowering your torso, do not allow your buttocks to go below your knees. This puts too much pressure on your knees.

Plié and Balance

❑ Beginning in the same position as the Pelvic-Wave Leg Strengthener, holding your barre or piece of furniture with both hands, your arms straight and loose, stand on your *toes* with your heels together.

❑ In triple slow motion, lower your torso straight down, 10 to 12 inches. Your torso is perfectly erect.

❑ In triple slow motion, raise yourself back up, breathing normally. This exercise is done in one smooth motion.

❑ If you wish, you can take your heels apart and balance even higher on your toes to make this exercise more difficult.

20 REPS

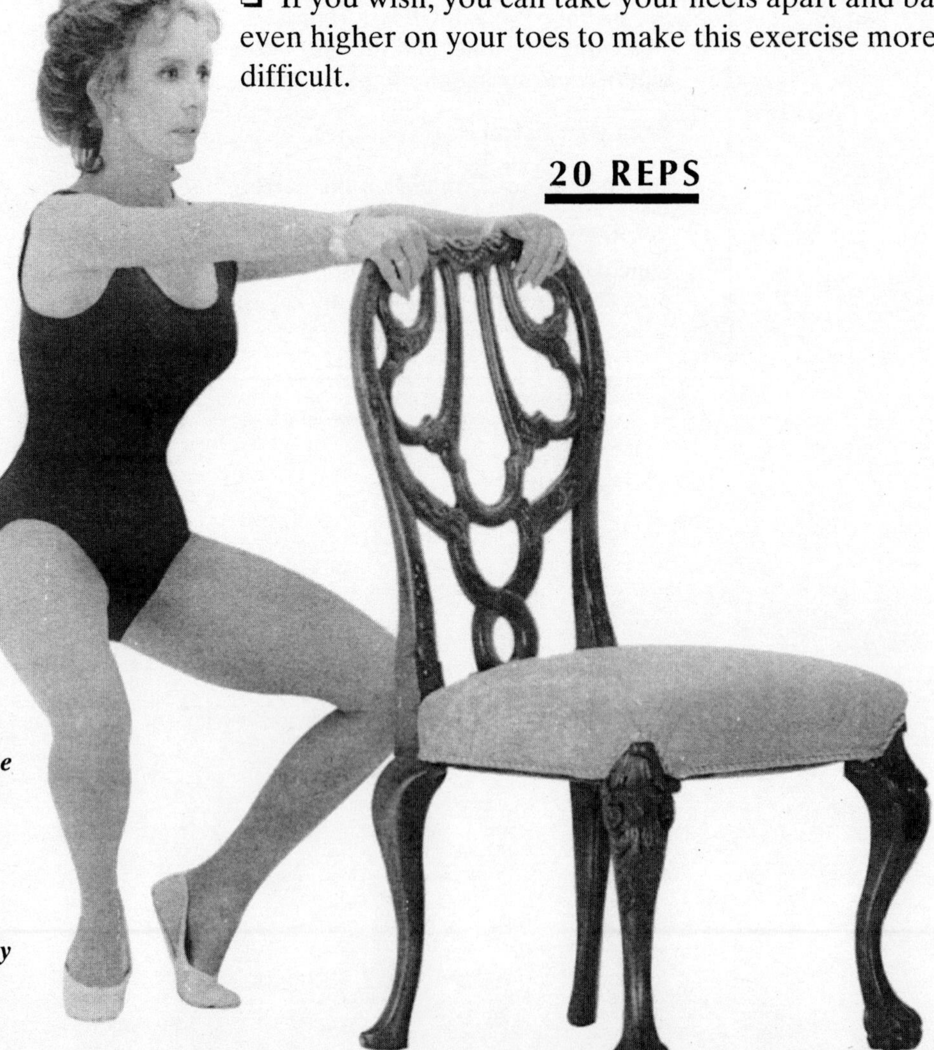

Even though the heels are apart and I am balancing up even higher on the toes, my back is perfectly straight!

IF YOU WANT A MORE INTENSE EXERCISE: *Hold your lowered position for a slow count of 3 to 5 before coming back up.*

DOS AND DON'TS

- ❑ **Do not let your heels drop to the floor when coming up.**
- ❑ **When lowering your torso, do not allow your buttocks to go below your knees. This would mean putting too much pressure on your knees.**
- ❑ **Do not try to aim your knees too far out to the side. Let their position be natural.**
- ❑ **Keep your shoulders relaxed.**
- ❑ **Do not arch your back or stick out your buttocks. Keep your spine straight and your neck stretched.**
- ❑ **If you don't have time to do 20 reps, you can do 10 in even slower motion for the same effect.**
- ❑ **The slower you do this exercise, the stronger your front thigh muscles will become.**
- ❑ **The more erect your torso, the more your thigh muscles are worked.**

HAMSTRING STRETCH #1
Up and Over

While doing the standing hamstring stretches, most people take the foot they're standing on directly out to the side (usually for balance). Try to learn to aim the foot forward (train yourself to do this). It is more gentle on the knees.

(If you have sciatica, always keep your knees bent during this exercise, to relieve pressure on your lower back.)

❑ Standing straight, take your right leg up and rest your heel on your barre or piece of furniture. Your left foot should be turned out slightly for balance, with your left knee straight but relaxed.

❑ Stretch your torso and arms up towards the ceiling. Still stretching up, slowly round your torso over your right leg.

❑ When you're over as far as you can go, crisscross your hands, letting them rest lightly on your right ankle. Take your elbows out to the side and rest your head on your leg. Do not lock your knees.

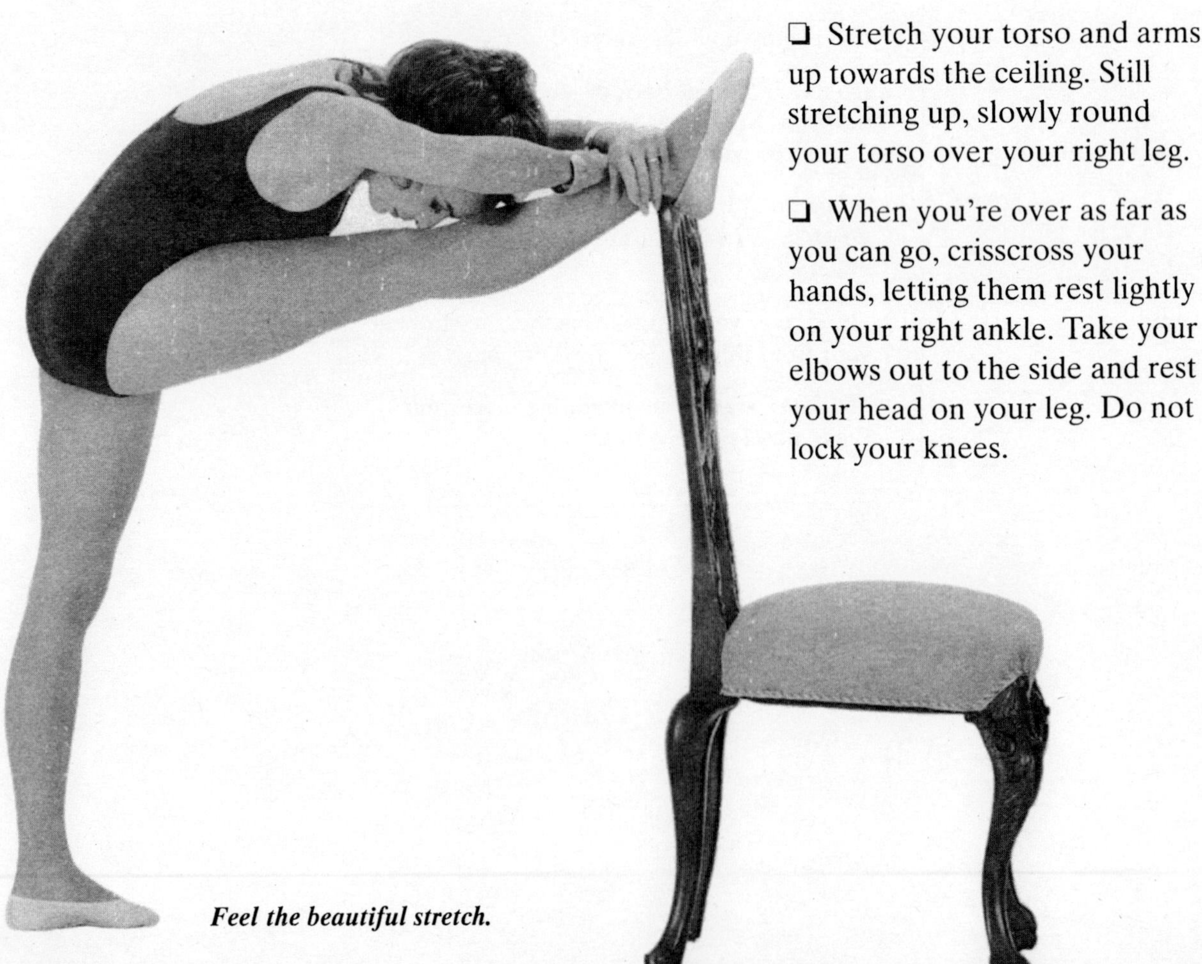

Feel the beautiful stretch.

IF YOU WANT MORE OF A STRETCH: *Once you're in position, try to put your head in between the left side of your right leg and the crook of your arm.*

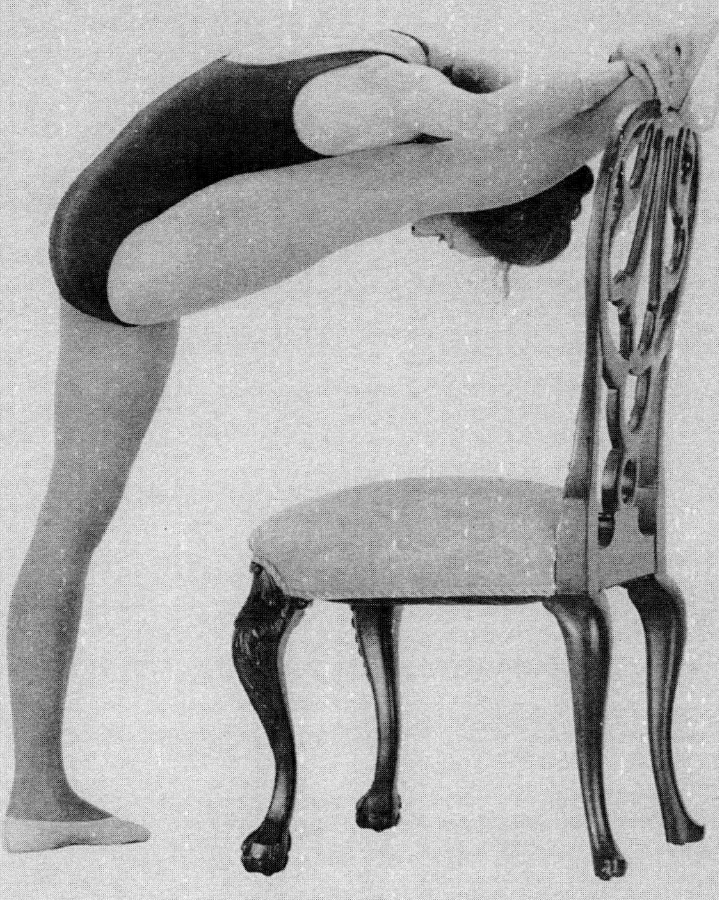

This is a lovely stretch for your neck and spine.

If that's too difficult or you're not quite stretched enough, you can move your hands up a little bit higher on your right leg, and rest your forehead on your leg, wherever it's comfortable (except directly on your kneecap).

❑ Gently move your torso up and down, 1/16 to 1/4 inch, or just hold the position.

50 REPS

- ❑ To come out of this exercise, slowly round your torso up, and gently take your right leg to the floor in *triple slow motion*.
- ❑ Repeat this exercise on the opposite side.

50 REPS

REMEMBER: *A lot of people, especially women, have knees that bulge quite a bit on the inside of their legs. To make this area thinner and smoother, gently turn your raised leg and foot out to the side slightly—your right leg to the right or your left leg to the left.*

Dos and Don'ts

- ❑ It doesn't matter how high your barre is. If you want more of a stretch, gently take your standing leg back, *away* from the barre. (And *never* use a towel rack for a barre! They are not designed to hold your weight! Make sure whatever you use for a barre can support your weight.)
- ❑ If resting your heel on your barre or piece of furniture is uncomfortable, place a facecloth under your ankle.
- ❑ Do not turn the foot you're standing on directly out to the side—unless that is the only way you can keep your balance—and keep that knee relaxed.
- ❑ Keep your hips even.
- ❑ Keep your elbows bent and stretched out.
- ❑ Relax your body.
- ❑ Take advantage of the time you have to relax your neck during this exercise.
- ❑ Do not force your stretch.
- ❑ Do not lock your knees.
- ❑ No bouncing.

Hamstring Stretch #2

Bent Leg

This is a stretch to be respected!

REMEMBER: *If you are standing on a slippery floor and feel that you are about to slip, you can place a suction-cup–type of rubber bath mat under your foot so you don't slide forward under the barre.*

❑ Gently place the arch of your right foot up on your barre or piece of furniture, with your right knee bent. (The back of a sofa or heavy chair is excellent to use as a barre for this exercise.) Place both hands on your barre, each on either side of your foot. Keep the foot you are standing on in whatever position is most comfortable, and bend your left knee slightly. Slowly scoot forward as far as you can on your standing foot, then aim that same foot towards the barre as much as you can.

❑ Crisscross your hands over your right foot, and hold onto the barre.

❑ In triple slow motion, straighten your right leg as far as you can without forcing, which will automatically straighten your left leg. Do not lock your standing knee. Do not force it. Stretch your elbows out to the sides as far as you can, and rest your head on your right leg.

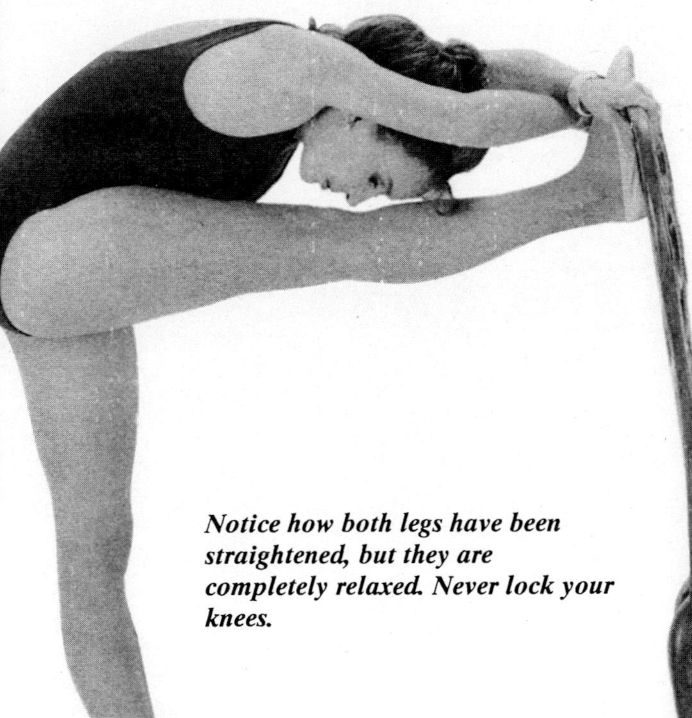

Notice how both legs have been straightened, but they are completely relaxed. Never lock your knees.

HOLD FOR A COUNT OF 50

FOR MORE OF A STRETCH: *Place your head to the right side of your leg.*

You can also bend your left leg and at the same time gently move up and down, just a few inches.

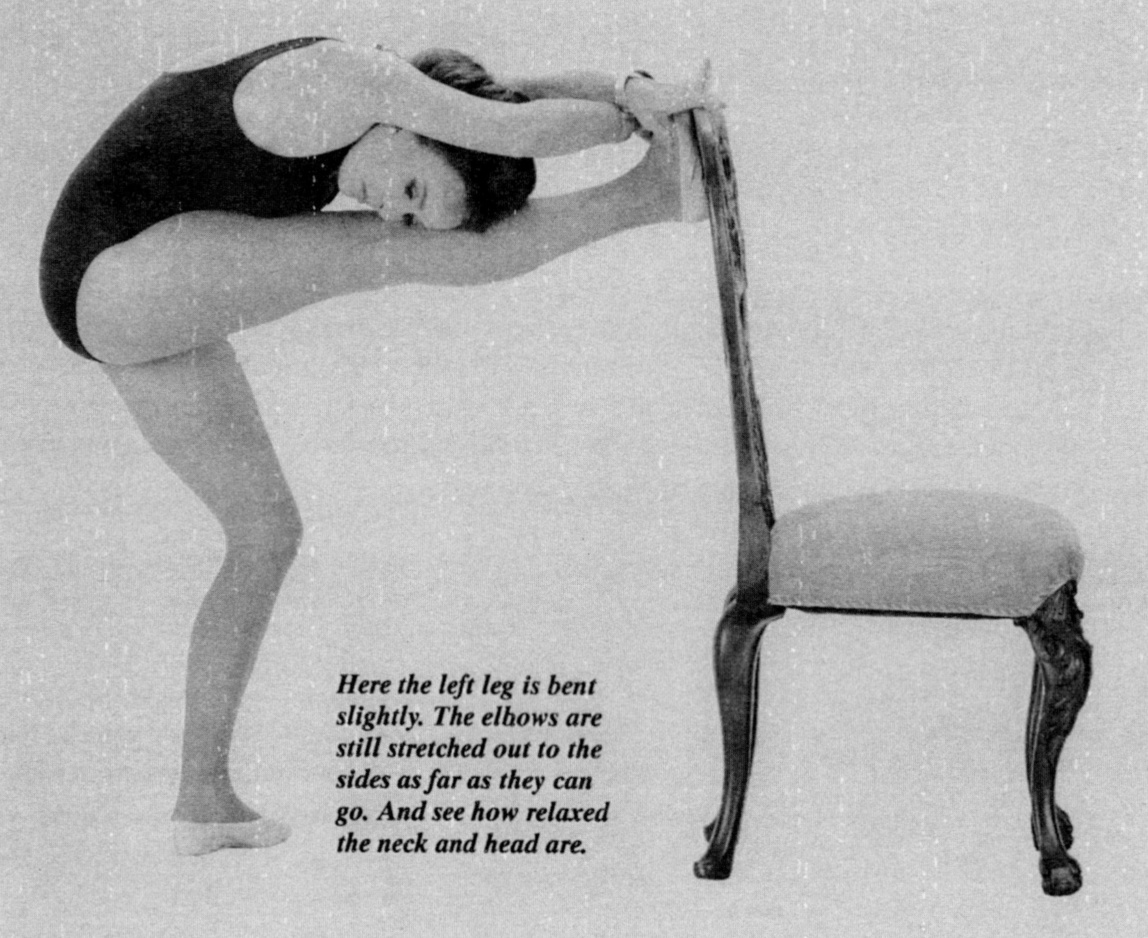

Here the left leg is bent slightly. The elbows are still stretched out to the sides as far as they can go. And see how relaxed the neck and head are.

FOR EVEN MORE OF A STRETCH: *You can place your head to the left side of your leg.*

For an even stronger stretch, gently slide your right foot down slightly so that your heel is underneath the barre.

You can also rotate your left hip out and to the back, while your heel remains underneath the barre. This stretches your buttocks and hip muscles.

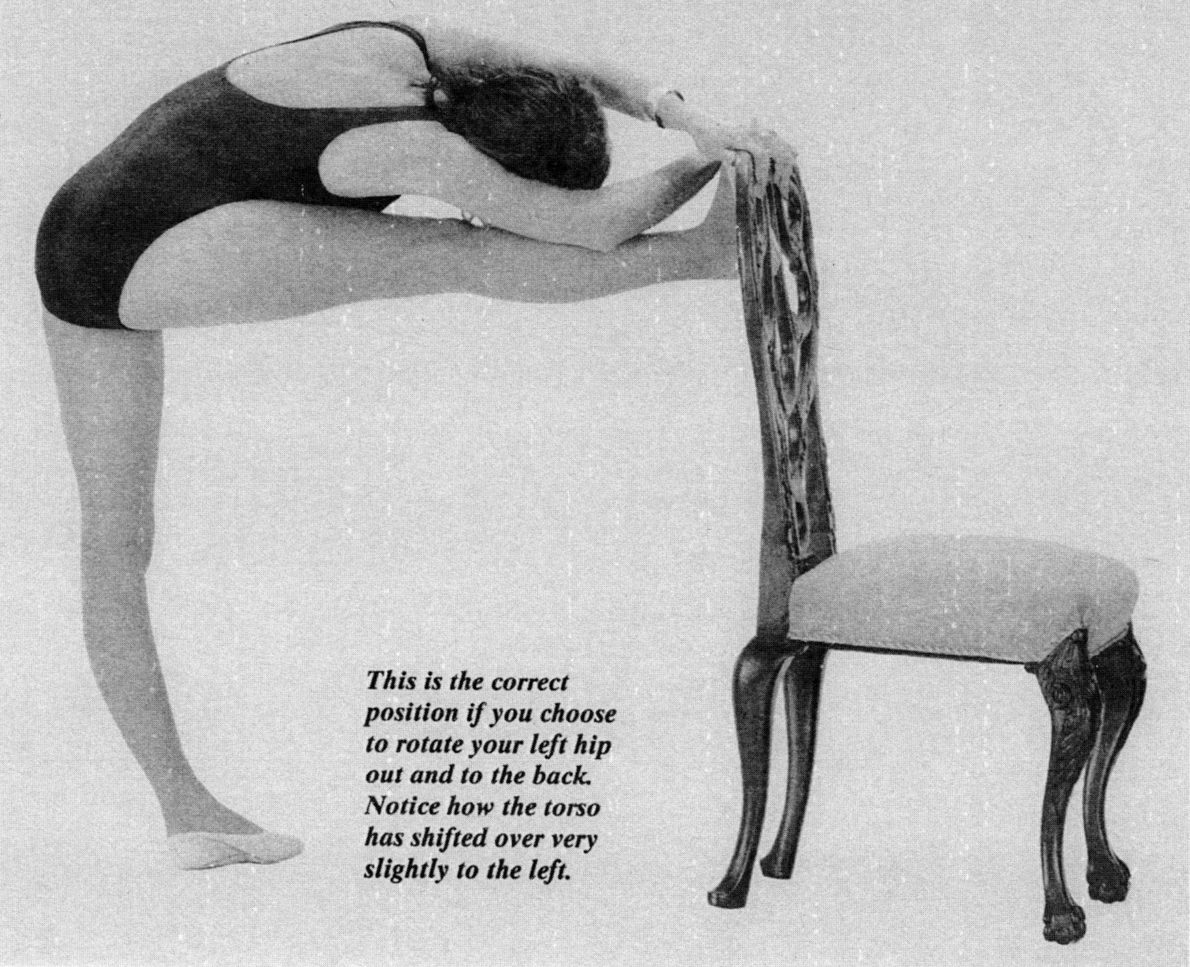

This is the correct position if you choose to rotate your left hip out and to the back. Notice how the torso has shifted over very slightly to the left.

❑ To come out of this exercise, first bend the leg you're standing on and uncross your hands. Then, slowly and gently, take your right leg off your barre or piece of furniture and, in triple slow motion, lower it to the floor.

❑ Repeat this exercise on the opposite side.

HOLD FOR A COUNT OF 50

Dos and Don'ts

- ❑ Never force your leg to straighten more than it comfortably can.
- ❑ Do not overstretch.
- ❑ Keep your body relaxed.
- ❑ Relax the leg you're standing on, even though it's straight. Do not tighten that knee.
- ❑ Do not bounce.
- ❑ Do not tense your arms.
- ❑ Keep your neck relaxed.
- ❑ Think beautiful, soft thoughts.

Leg Strengthener

Knee Bends in the Air

❑ Stand at your barre or piece of furniture, and hold it gently for balance. Bend your right leg out to the side, sliding your right foot up your left leg until your toes are pointing on your left knee. Bend your left knee slightly.

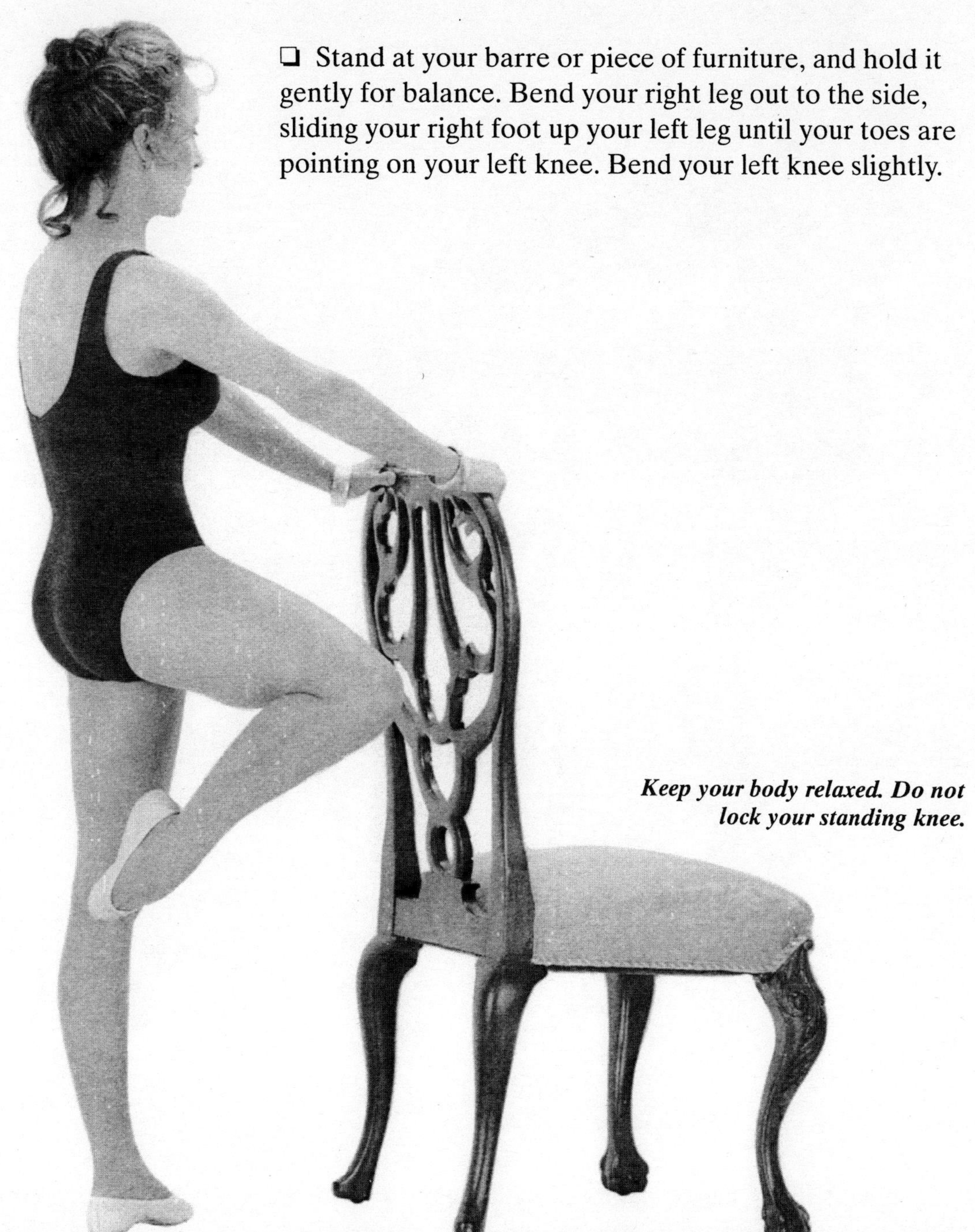

Keep your body relaxed. Do not lock your standing knee.

❑ Straighten your right leg out—halfway between the front and the side of your body—as high as it can go.

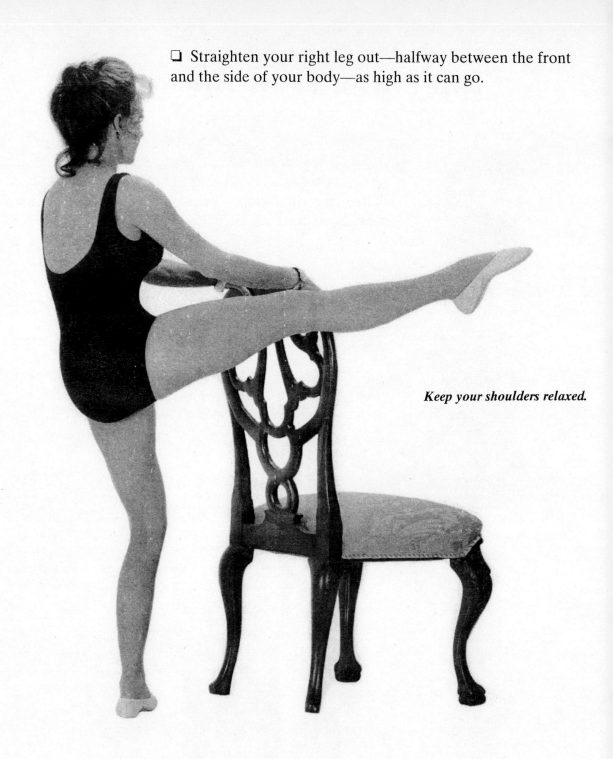

Keep your shoulders relaxed.

❑ Bend your right knee in again taking it higher towards the ceiling and being certain not to let your toes return to your left knee. Your toes are pointed and relaxed. From that position, straighten your leg up even higher.

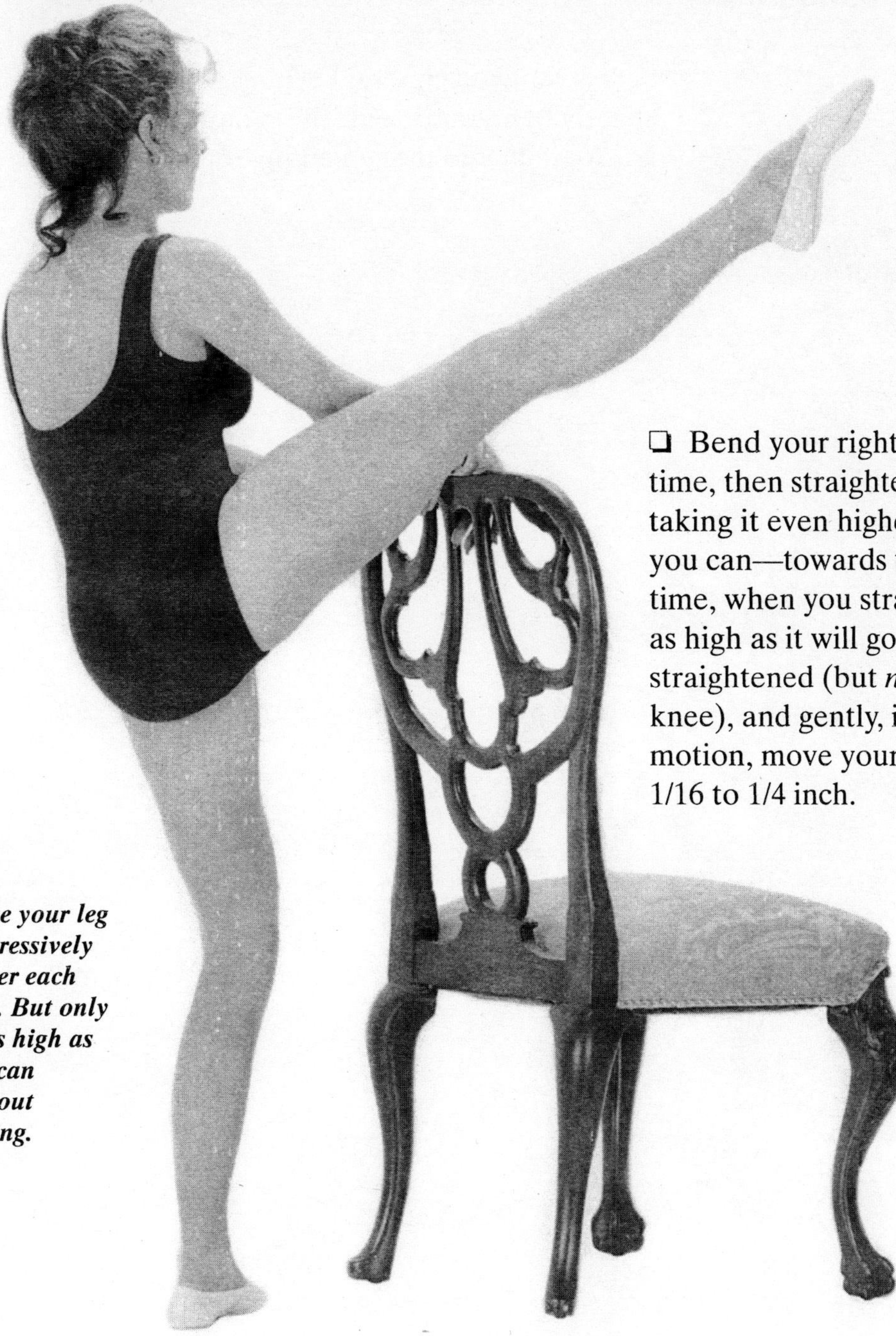

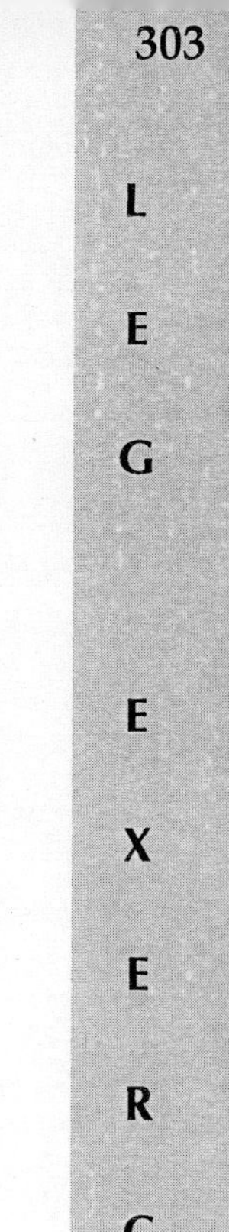

❑ Bend your right knee in a third time, then straighten your leg, taking it even higher—as high as you can—towards the ceiling. This time, when you straighten your leg as high as it will go, *keep* it straightened (but *never* lock your knee), and gently, in triple slow motion, move your leg up and down 1/16 to 1/4 inch.

Raise your leg progressively higher each time. But only go as high as you can without forcing.

5 TO 10 REPS

REMEMBER: *Each time you straighten your right leg, you should try to raise it a little bit higher.*

❑ Then, if you choose, keeping your left knee slightly bent, raise yourself up on the toes of your left foot, and do the remaining reps on your toes.

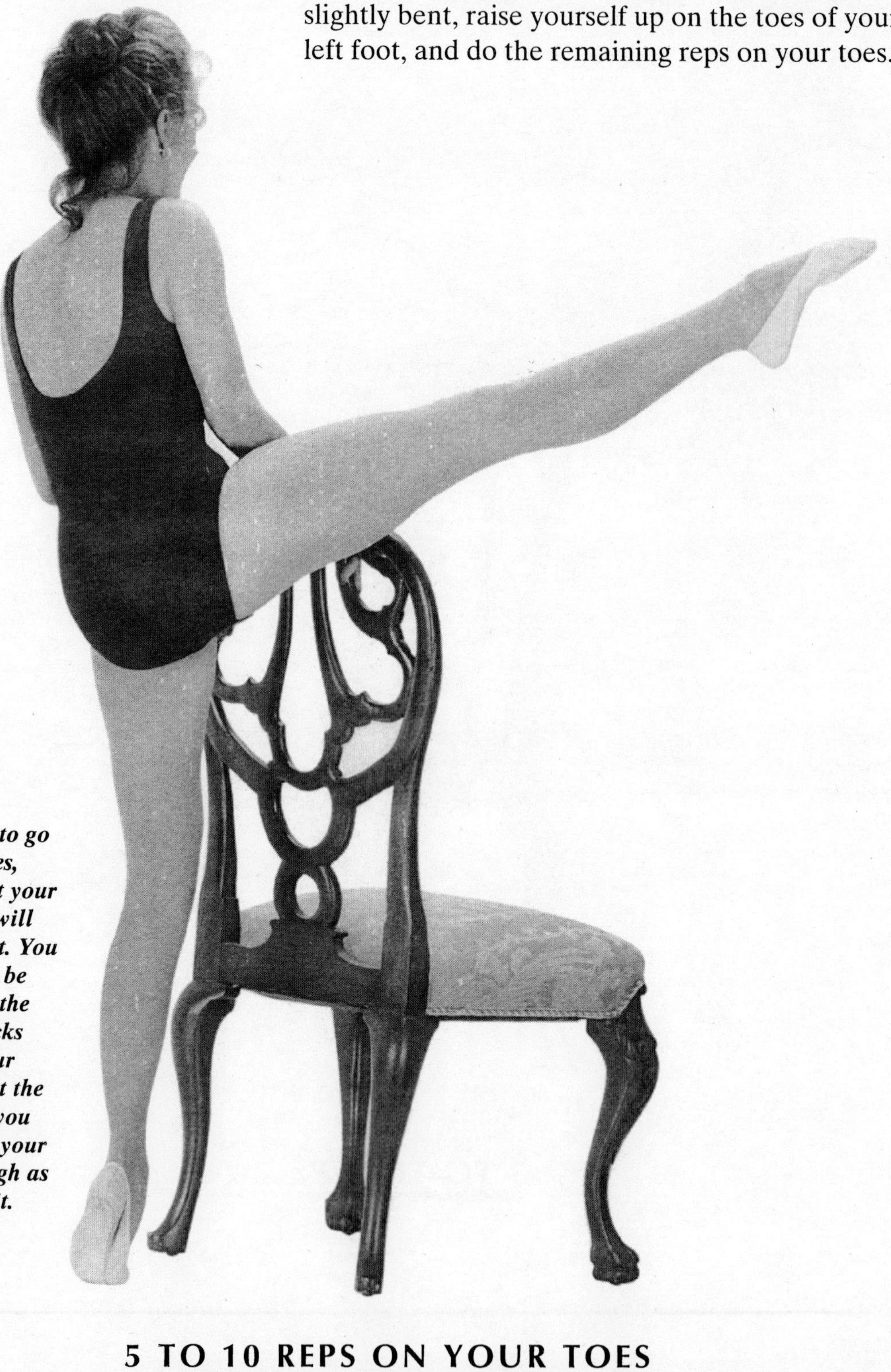

If you choose to go up on your toes, remember that your leg extension will not be as great. You will, however, be strengthening the leg and buttocks muscles of your standing leg at the same time as you are stretching your right leg as high as you can take it.

5 TO 10 REPS ON YOUR TOES

❑ To come out of this exercise, bend your right knee, pointing your toes in towards your left knee. Then, in triple slow motion, lower your right leg to the floor.

❑ Repeat this exercise on the opposite side.

Dos and Don'ts

- ❑ **If you find the amount of reps to be a bit more than you can do at first, start off with 2 to 3 reps with your standing foot flat and 2 to 3 on your toes, gradually working up to 10 reps total. When your legs become stronger, you will be able to do all the reps with your standing leg remaining straight.**
- ❑ **Do not lock your knees.**
- ❑ **Do not lower your leg as you extend it out.**
- ❑ **Do not drop your head.**
- ❑ **Keep your neck and your shoulders relaxed.**
- ❑ **Do not arch your back.**
- ❑ **Keep your torso erect.**
- ❑ **Use your barre only for balance.**
- ❑ **Relax your legs.**

Buttocks–Outer Thighs–Hips

(If you have knee problems, substitute the Sitting or Standing exercises in this section for the Kneeling exercises.)

(If you have a swayback, always round your shoulders as much as you can, or, if you feel it's necessary, you can also let your torso lean over to the opposite side of the leg being used, when doing the exercises in this section. This will stretch the spine even more.)

At this advanced point, you should know how to really curl your pelvis up. The more you curl it up, especially on the Kneeling and Standing exercises of this section, the more your muscles can contract and work, the more your outer thighs will become tight, and the faster you will get those darling round, little peach buttocks!

Also, most of you should be so adept at rolling your hip forward in the starting position that you won't even have to think about using your hand to assist you.

And you should not have to be reminded not to wear shoes for any of the Buttocks—Outer Thighs—Hips exercises. The weight of them is simply too heavy.

REMEMBER: *The more your hip is rolled forward for these first 2 sitting exercises (and the Kneeling Out to the Side exercise), the more you will be working your buttocks muscles.*

Sitting Bringing Up the Rear

This exercise begins in the same starting position as Bringing Up the Rear in *Callanetics Countdown*, or in Behind and Hips in *Callanetics—The One-Hour Program* and *Callanetics for Your Back*—except this time you will be positioning the leg you're resting on further out to the side.

❑ Sitting on the floor or a mat to cushion yourself if necessary, place your hands on whatever you're using as a barre and rest them there lightly. The height does not matter, as long as you are comfortable. Your left knee is bent in front of you. Your right knee is bent and even with your right hip. Your right foot rests on the floor behind you. Still holding onto your barre, move your left knee over to the left 3 to 5 inches, and take your left foot out a little for a balance point.

❑ Making sure that your right hip remains facing the barre, roll it forward as far as you can. As the hip is rolled forward, the torso automatically turns to the left. Your foot will come off the floor.

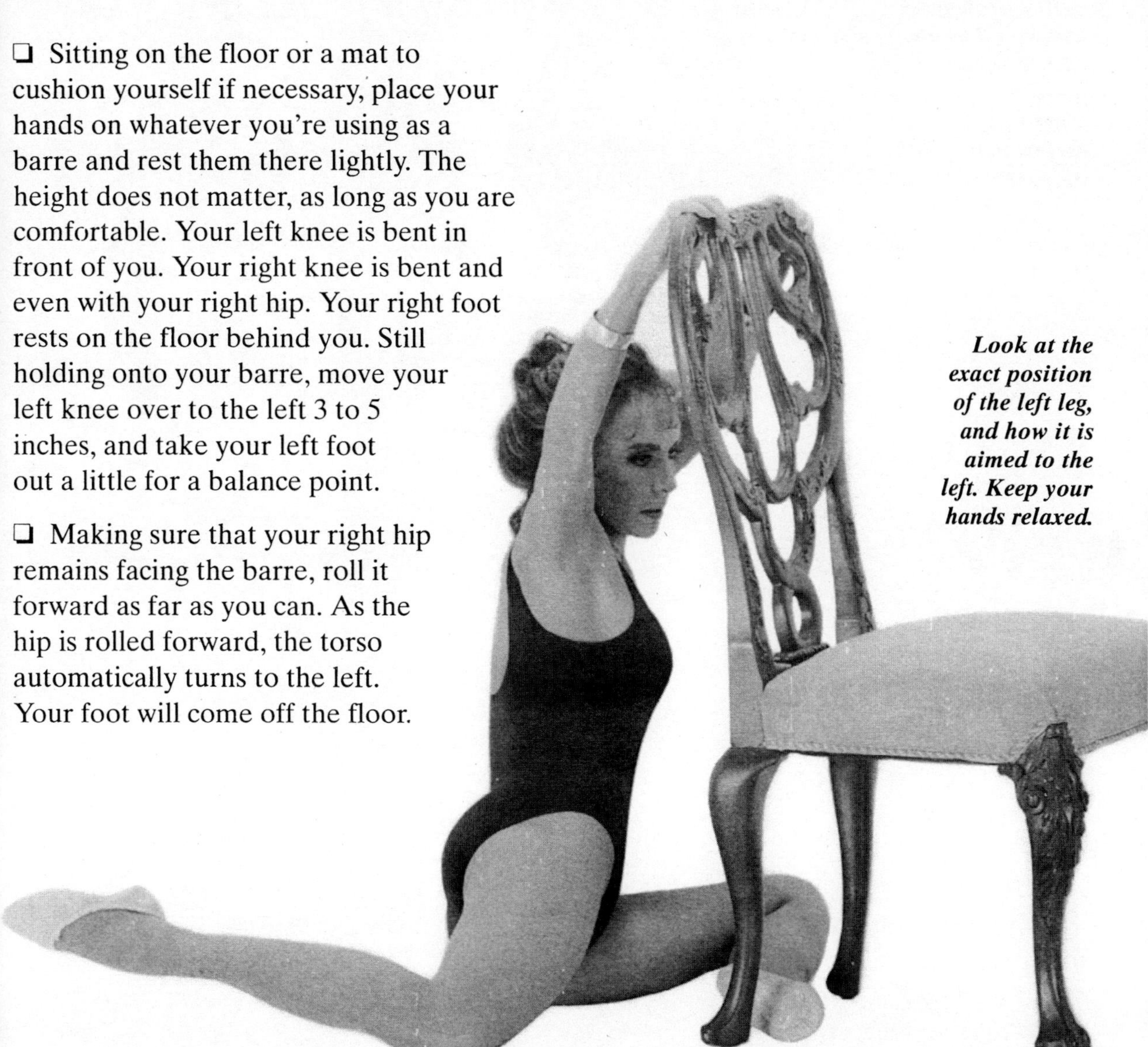

Look at the exact position of the left leg, and how it is aimed to the left. Keep your hands relaxed.

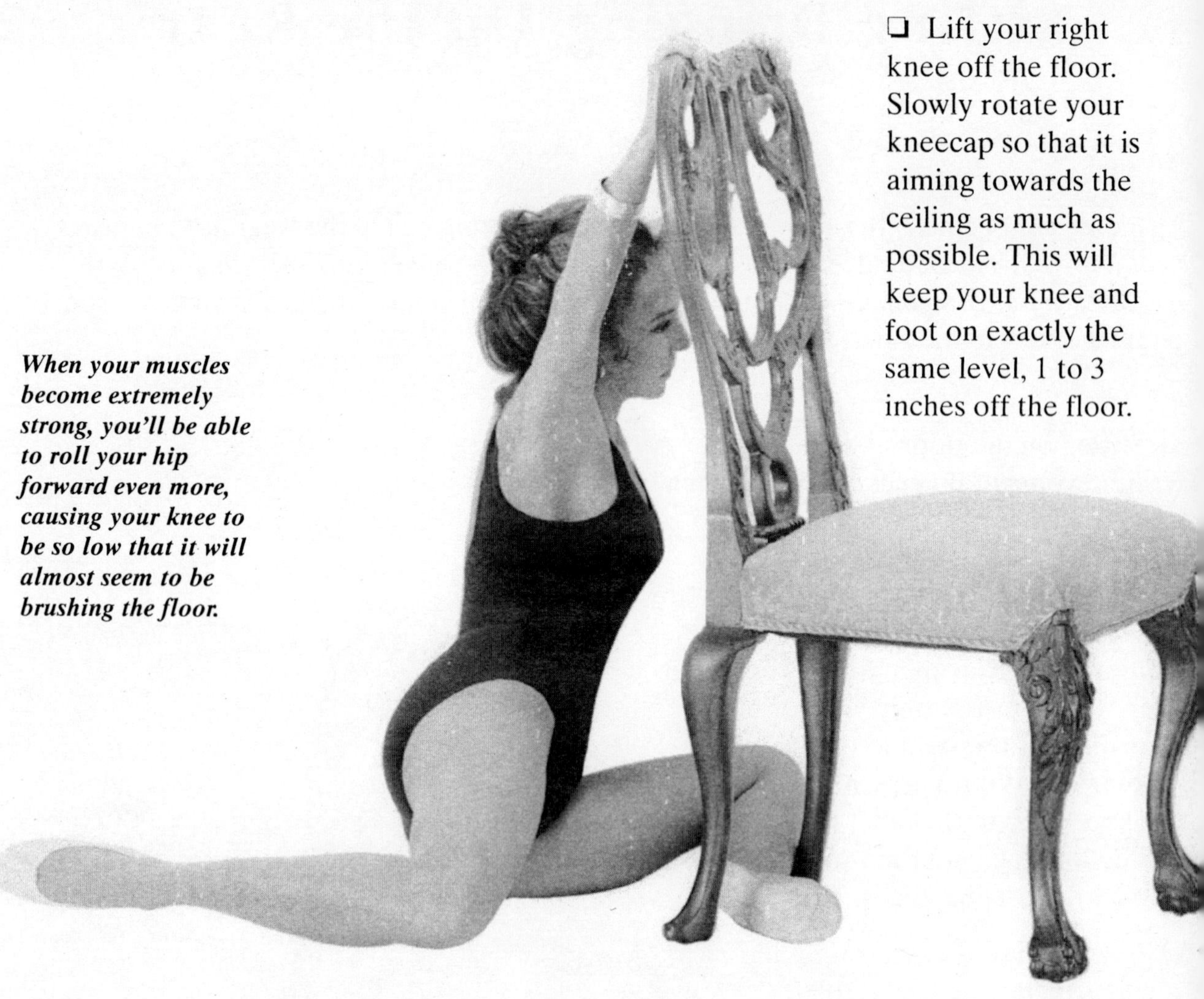

❑ Lift your right knee off the floor. Slowly rotate your kneecap so that it is aiming towards the ceiling as much as possible. This will keep your knee and foot on exactly the same level, 1 to 3 inches off the floor.

When your muscles become extremely strong, you'll be able to roll your hip forward even more, causing your knee to be so low that it will almost seem to be brushing the floor.

❑ Move your knee in triple slow motion back and forth, 1/16 to 1/4 inch.

100 REPS

IF YOU WANT MORE OF A WORKOUT FOR YOUR BUTTOCKS: *Lower your foot a little bit, and aim your kneecap even more towards the ceiling, but do not let your hip rotate to the back.*

For even more of a workout in this same position, you can also lift your knee and foot a wee bit more.

WHEN THIS EXERCISE BECOMES TOO EASY: *Be sure to sit more erect. You can also raise your barre, or place your hands higher up on your piece of furniture. The higher the barre, the more intense this exercise becomes.*

IF YOU FEEL IT'S TOO MUCH, AND YOUR BODY IS BEGINNING TO TENSE UP: *Take a breather, then roll back into position.*

You can also switch sides, but be sure to do a proper count for both sides before continuing this section.

You can also bring your knee forward a wee bit.

❑ Relax your entire body, then repeat this exercise on the opposite side.

100 REPS

Dos and Don'ts

- ❑ Do not arch your lower back.
- ❑ Relax your legs.
- ❑ Relax your neck.
- ❑ The movement back and forth is almost imperceptible.
- ❑ Do not allow the foot of your working leg to rest on the floor. If it starts to feel heavy, take a breather.
- ❑ Do not take the knee of your working leg past your hip when you are returning forward during the little motions.
- ❑ Relax your shoulders. If you feel pressure on your lower back, you have 3 choices:
  - ❑ Round your shoulders more;
  - ❑ Lean over to the opposite side of your working leg just a wee bit, keeping your back straight; or
  - ❑ Tighten your buttocks and curl your pelvis up.

  Some people choose to do all 3 in one go at first.
- ❑ Do not allow your torso to push forward when you are rolling your *hip* forward. This will put pressure on your lower back. Keep your torso erect but relaxed.
- ❑ Keep your hips even.
- ❑ Relax even more!

Sitting Out to the Side

❑ Still seated with your hands up on your barre, bend your left leg out on the floor in front of you. Relax your shoulders.

❑ Move your left knee 3 to 5 inches to the left. Fully extend your right leg out, straight, directly to the side, even with your hip. Then slowly roll your right hip and leg over so that the tops of your toes are aiming into the floor (if possible). Bring your right leg in towards your body. Because your right leg can move in 3 to 4 inches, this will automatically take your hips to the left, causing you to lean slightly to the left.

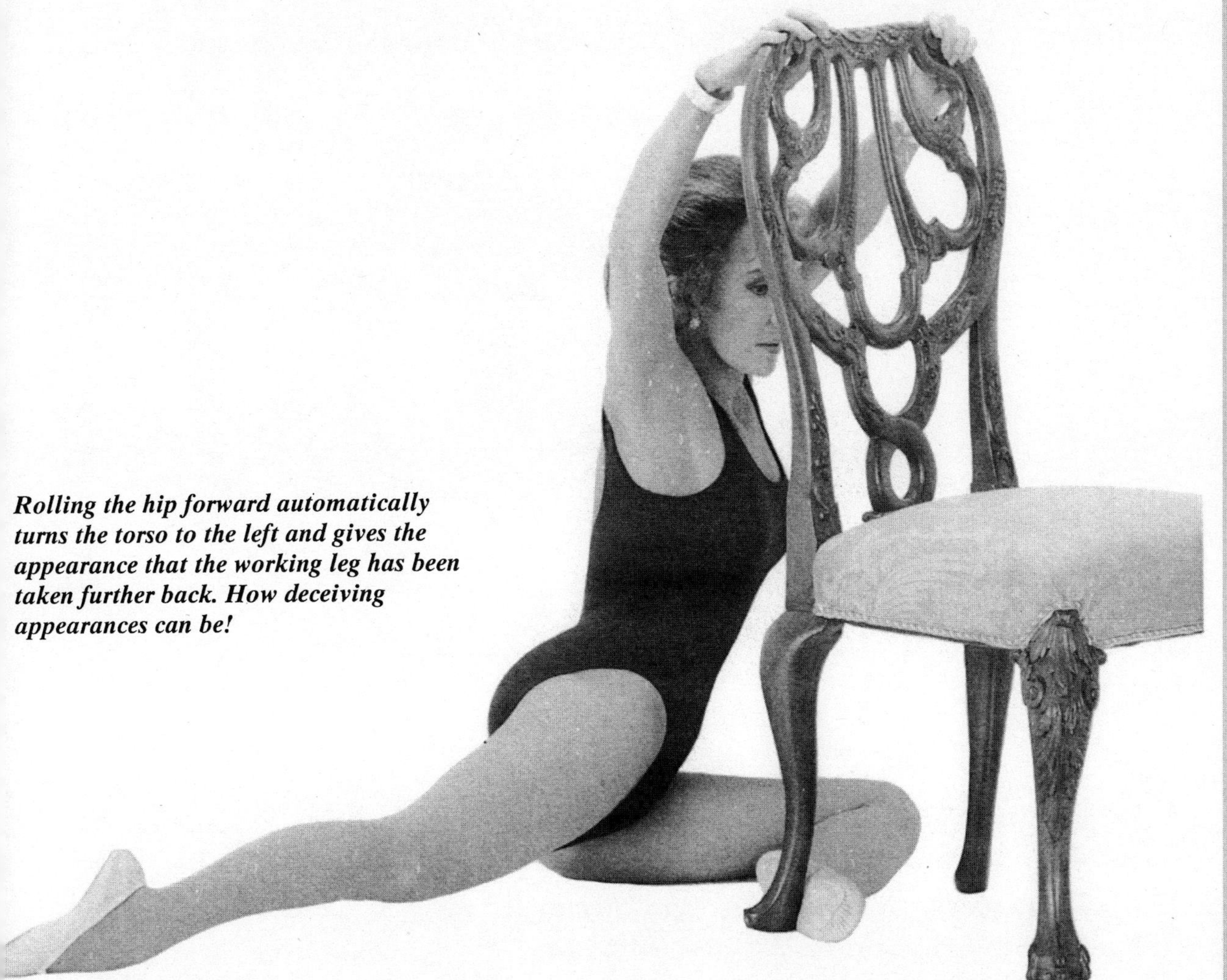

Rolling the hip forward automatically turns the torso to the left and gives the appearance that the working leg has been taken further back. How deceiving appearances can be!

❑ Gently lift your right leg up and down, 1/16 to 1/4 inch.

100 REPS

❑ Repeat this exercise on the opposite side.

100 REPS

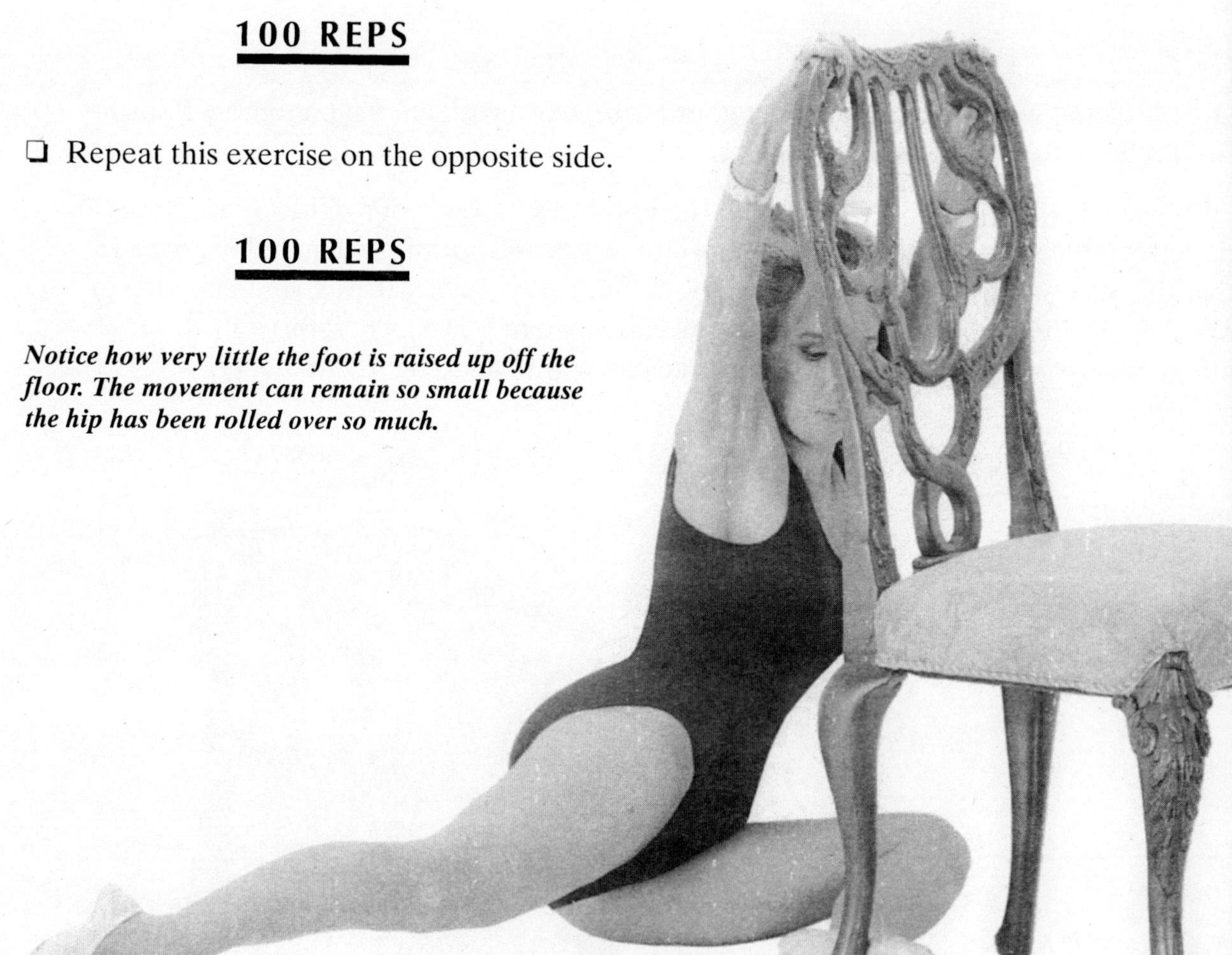

Notice how very little the foot is raised up off the floor. The movement can remain so small because the hip has been rolled over so much.

WHEN THIS EXERCISE BECOMES TOO EASY: *Take your working leg to the back without rotating your hip back. You can also sit more erect.*

IF THIS EXERCISE IS BECOMING TOO DIFFICULT: *Slowly ease your working leg forward a few inches. You can also lean directly over to the opposite side.*

Dos and Don'ts

- ❑ Keep your extended leg very straight, but do not lock your knee.
- ❑ Do not allow your torso to push forward. This will put pressure on your lower back.
- ❑ Keep your working hip rolled forward as much as you can.
- ❑ If you feel pressure on your lower back, you have 3 choices:
  - ❑ Round your torso;
  - ❑ Lean over to the opposite side of your working leg just a wee bit; or
  - ❑ Tighten your buttocks and curl your pelvis up more than you think you can.
- ❑ Never arch your back.
- ❑ If you are in the most advanced position for this exercise, you will only be able to lift your leg 1/16 to 1/4 inch. If you are not yet strong enough for this, you may lean your torso a wee bit to the left and lift your leg higher—but make sure it is no higher than 2 inches off the floor. Otherwise, because you may be tired, you might turn your leg towards the ceiling, and begin working the front thigh muscles instead of the buttocks.

Kneeling Bringing Up the Rear

Even though I know I keep saying 'Round your upper back,' when your muscles become strong enough and you can do the famous pelvic curl-up as second nature, many of you will have noticed that you no longer have to round your upper back during these kneeling exercises.

REMEMBER: *Whenever you tighten your buttocks and curl your pelvis up, your working leg will automatically come forward. Be sure to take your leg back, keeping your knee even with your hip, to get the full benefit of this exercise. The fact that you're taking your knee back does not mean that the hip of that same leg has to move! Be sure, however, that your pelvis stays curled up.*

❑ Kneeling, with knees together and both hands resting loosely on your barre or piece of furniture, arms straight but relaxed, rotate your body, including your legs, to the left. Tighten your buttocks, curl your pelvis up, and round your upper back.

❑ In triple slow motion, take your right knee out to the side and up towards the ceiling as high as it can go without lifting your right foot. When the knee will not go up any further, rotate your kneecap so that it is aiming up towards the ceiling and curl your pelvis up even more than you think you can. Then take your knee up even higher, allowing your foot to lift off the floor as you do so. Because your right knee came forward when you turned your body, now take your knee back as far as you can without moving your right hip or arching your lower back.

❑ Take your left hip towards the left very slightly to distribute your weight off your kneecap.

❑ Tighten your buttocks yet again, and curl your pelvis up even more.

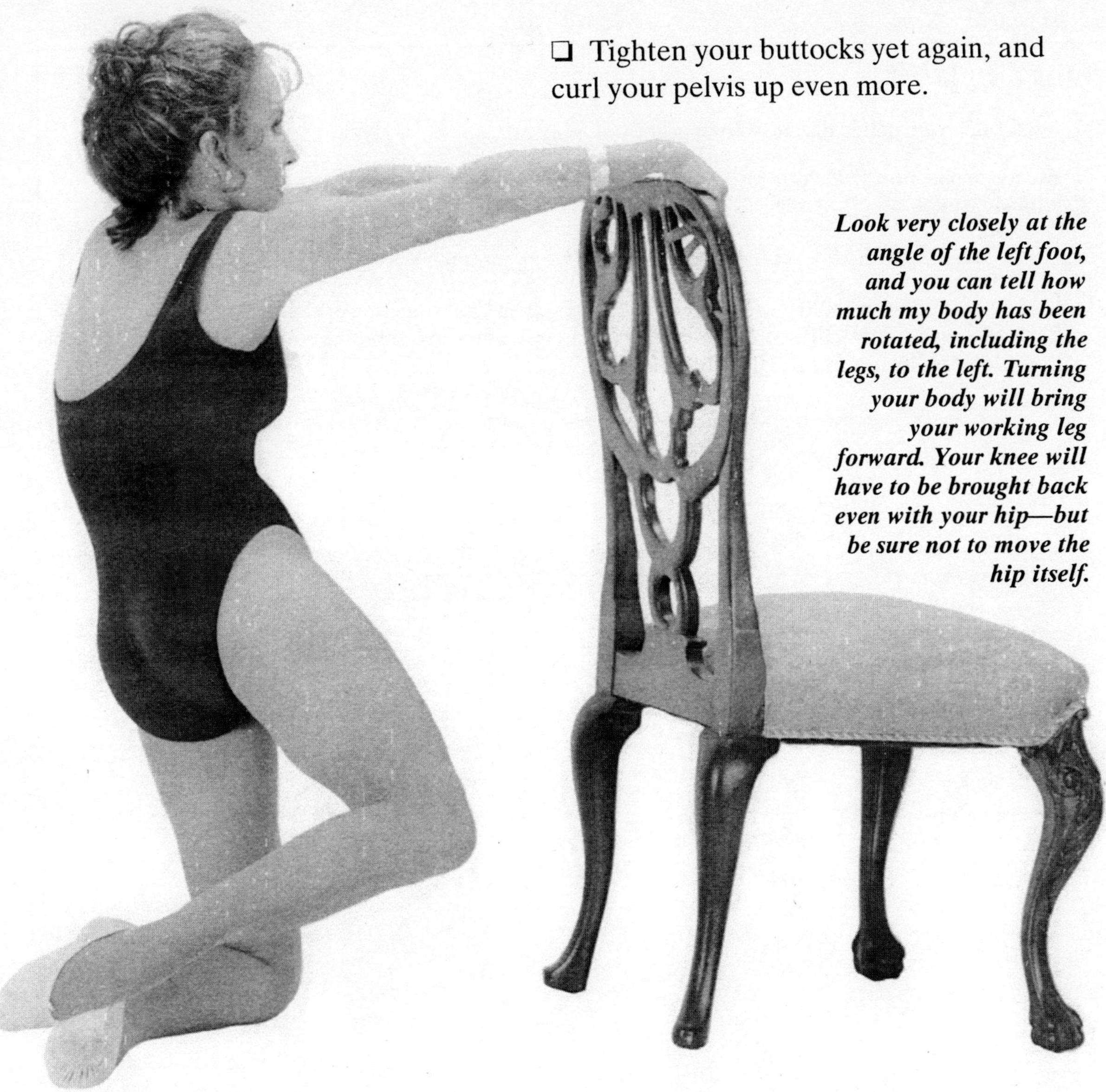

Look very closely at the angle of the left foot, and you can tell how much my body has been rotated, including the legs, to the left. Turning your body will bring your working leg forward. Your knee will have to be brought back even with your hip—but be sure not to move the hip itself.

❑ Gently move your right leg back and forth, no more than 1/16 to 1/4 inch.

100 REPS

❑ Repeat this exercise on the opposite side.

100 REPS

Dos and Don'ts

- ❑ Really tip your pelvis up more than you think you can.
- ❑ Always make sure that your lower back is straight and relaxed, and that your buttocks are not sticking out.
- ❑ If you feel pressure on your lower back, round your shoulders even more.
- ❑ Don't move your hip when taking your working leg back and forth. Aim with your knee, going back and forth in tiny little movements. Try to keep your knee aimed up towards the ceiling, and don't let it go in front of the line of your hip.

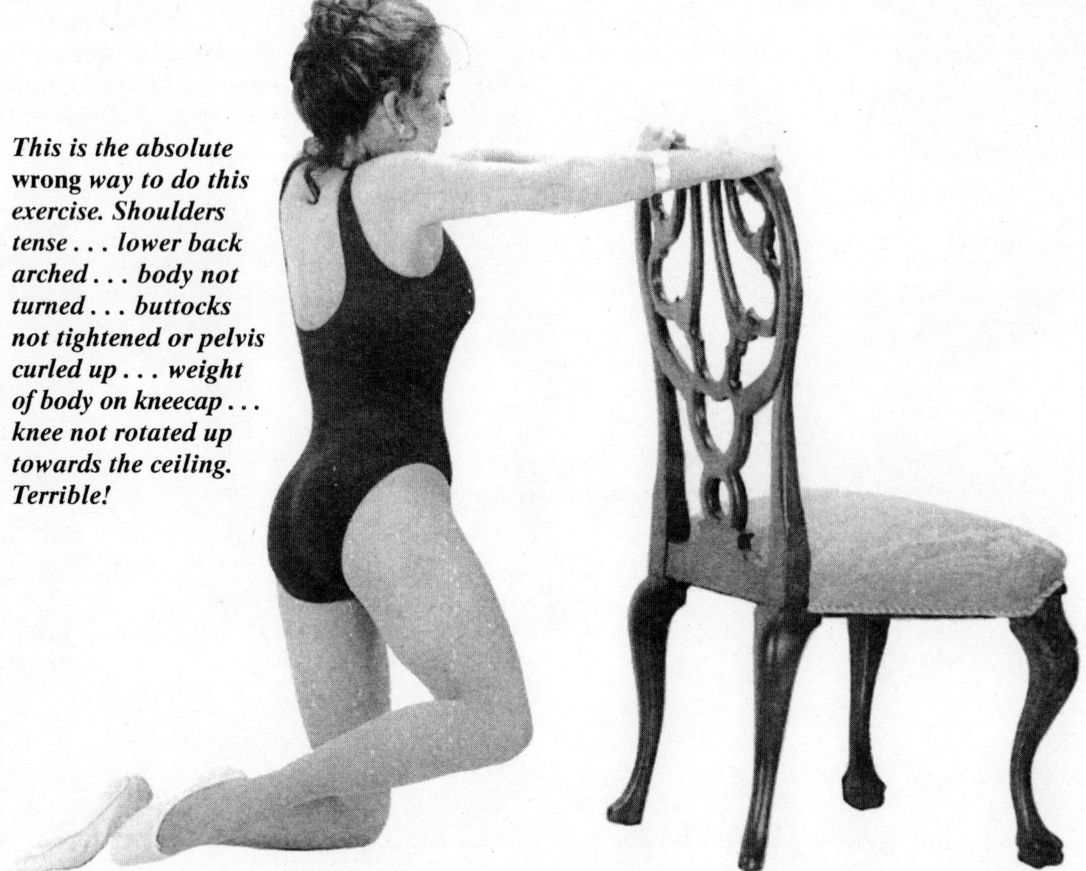

This is the absolute wrong way to do this exercise. Shoulders tense . . . lower back arched . . . body not turned . . . buttocks not tightened or pelvis curled up . . . weight of body on kneecap . . . knee not rotated up towards the ceiling. Terrible!

- ❑ Relax your shoulders, keeping them rounded.
- ❑ Be certain to shift your weight directly off your kneecap. You can place a towel or exercise mat under your knee, if you like.

Kneeling Out to the Side

❏ Kneeling, with both hands on your barre or piece of furniture, stretch your right leg straight out to the side, even with your hip.

❏ Rotate your right leg forward, until the top of your toes rest on the floor, if possible. (This is more of a rotation than in the one-hour Callanetics program.) Allowing your hips to move to the left, bring your right leg in towards your body so that you won't be putting pressure on your kneecap.

❏ Tighten your buttocks, and curl your pelvis up more than you ever thought you could. Round your upper back. Make sure your lower back is straight, not arched, and relaxed.

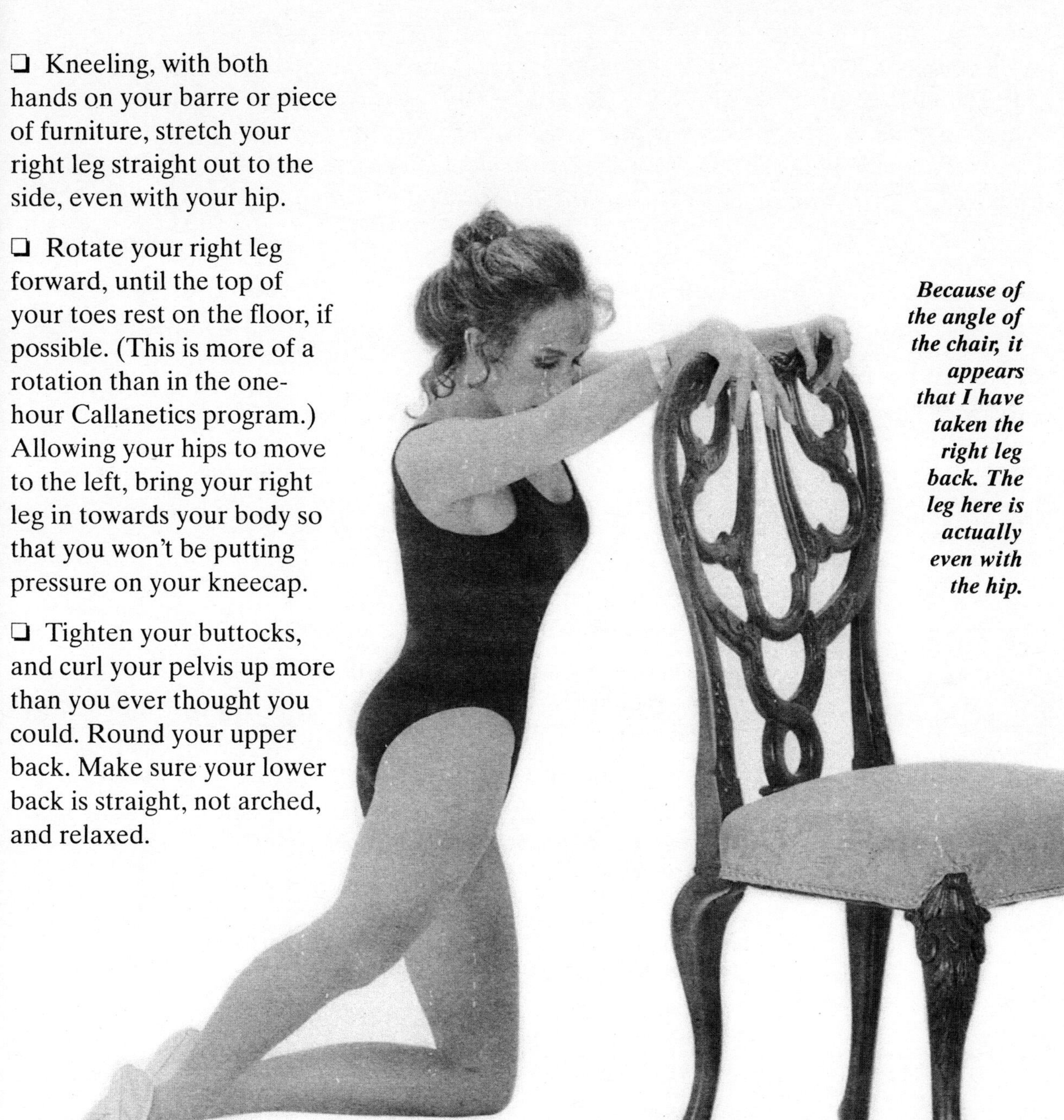

Because of the angle of the chair, it appears that I have taken the right leg back. The leg here is actually even with the hip.

❑ Gently lift your right leg, up and down, in a smooth and tiny motion, 1/16 to 1/4 inch.

100 REPS

IF THIS EXERCISE IS BECOMING TOO DIFFICULT: *Take a breather. If your working leg is starting to feel too heavy, take it a wee bit forward. You can also lean your torso over to the side opposite your working leg. Remember to breathe naturally. If you do take a breather, be sure to get into the original starting position before continuing the exercise.*

❑ Repeat this exercise on the opposite side.

100 REPS

Dos and Don'ts

- ❑ Keep the top of your back rounded, as if you were a cat. Do not arch your lower back; keep it perfectly straight.
- ❑ Keep your pelvis tipped up more than you think you can.
- ❑ Relax your body as much as you can, from head to toe, especially your shoulders and neck.
- ❑ Keep your working leg straight, but your knee remains relaxed. Never lock your knee.
- ❑ Do not ever place your full weight directly on your kneecap. Place a towel or exercise mat under your knee, if you like.
- ❑ Do not stick out your buttocks.

Standing Bringing Up the Rear

THIS EXERCISE WAS DRAWN FROM A POSITION IN CLASSICAL BALLET CALLED AN *attitude*.

❑ Stand at your barre or piece of furniture, your hands resting lightly on it for balance, elbows bent. Your feet are together.

❑ In triple slow motion, lift your right knee and take it up and out to the side as high as you can without moving your right hip up or forward. Keep your right knee even with your right hip. Your right foot will automatically come off the floor when you lift your knee.

❑ Point your foot to the rear, and keep it relaxed. It should always be lower than your knees.

❑ Bend your left knee slightly, the one you're standing on. Tighten your buttocks, and curl your pelvis up. Round your shoulders. Your knee may go forward, so carefully take it back, even with your hip—but don't *move* your hip.

❑ Bend sideways at the waist and aim your right shoulder towards the floor. Relax your shoulders and neck.

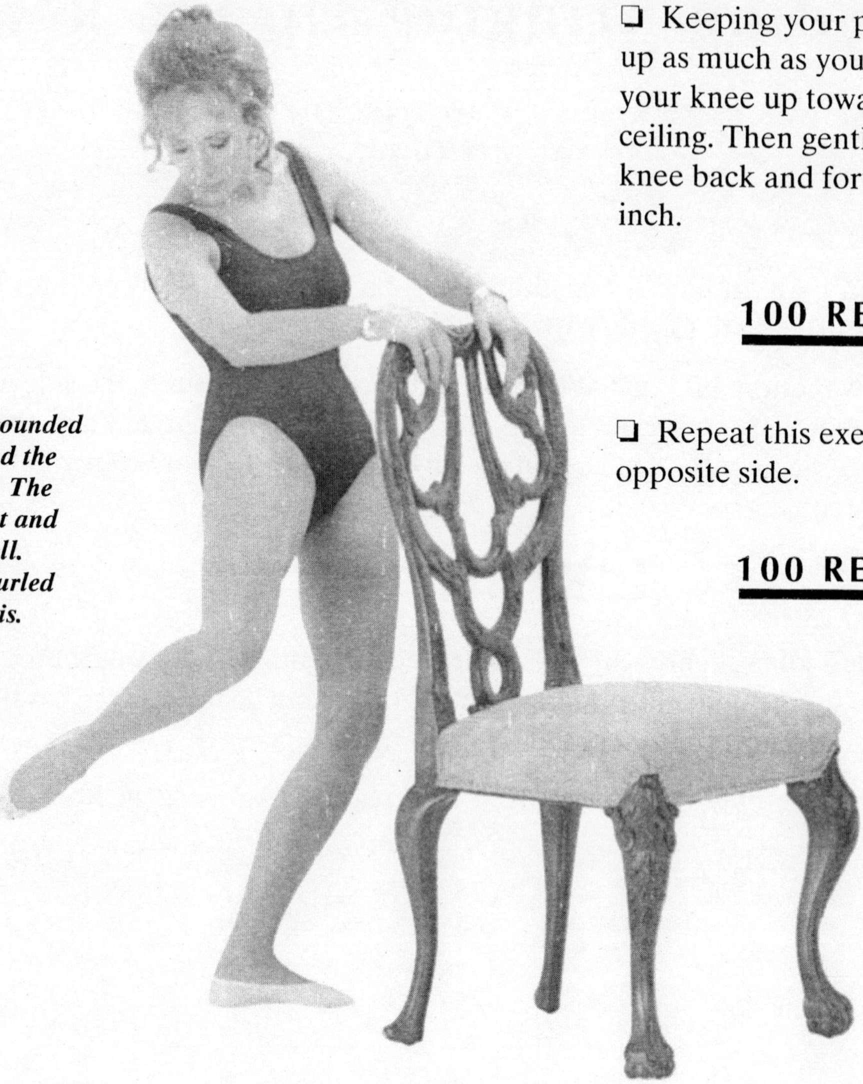

The torso is rounded to the side and the arms relaxed. The left leg is bent and relaxed as well. Notice how curled up the pelvis is.

❑ Keeping your pelvis curled up as much as you can, rotate your knee up towards the ceiling. Then gently move your knee back and forth 1/16 to 1/4 inch.

100 REPS

❑ Repeat this exercise on the opposite side.

100 REPS

DOS AND DON'TS

❑ Make sure your lower back is stretched. Do not arch your back at all.

❑ Keep your hips even.

❑ Relax your shoulders and your neck.

❑ Do not lock your knees.

❑ Make sure the leg you're standing on is slightly bent.

❑ Relax your entire body—and stay relaxed!

Standing Out to the Side

THIS EXERCISE WAS ALSO DRAWN FROM A POSITION IN CLASSICAL BALLET CALLED AN *arabesque.*

❑ Stand at your barre or piece of furniture, your hands resting lightly on it for balance. Your feet are together.

❑ Take your right leg directly out to the side, even with your hip, pointing your toes like a ballet dancer's but keeping them relaxed. They should be aiming forward. Your leg is straight, but your knee remains relaxed. Bend your left knee slightly.

This is one exercise I definitely take advantage of while standing having a conversation with someone. When you become stronger, you will not have to hold onto anything! The movement is so ridiculously tiny that no one ever knows I'm even doing it. At that level, you should keep your torso straight and relaxed.

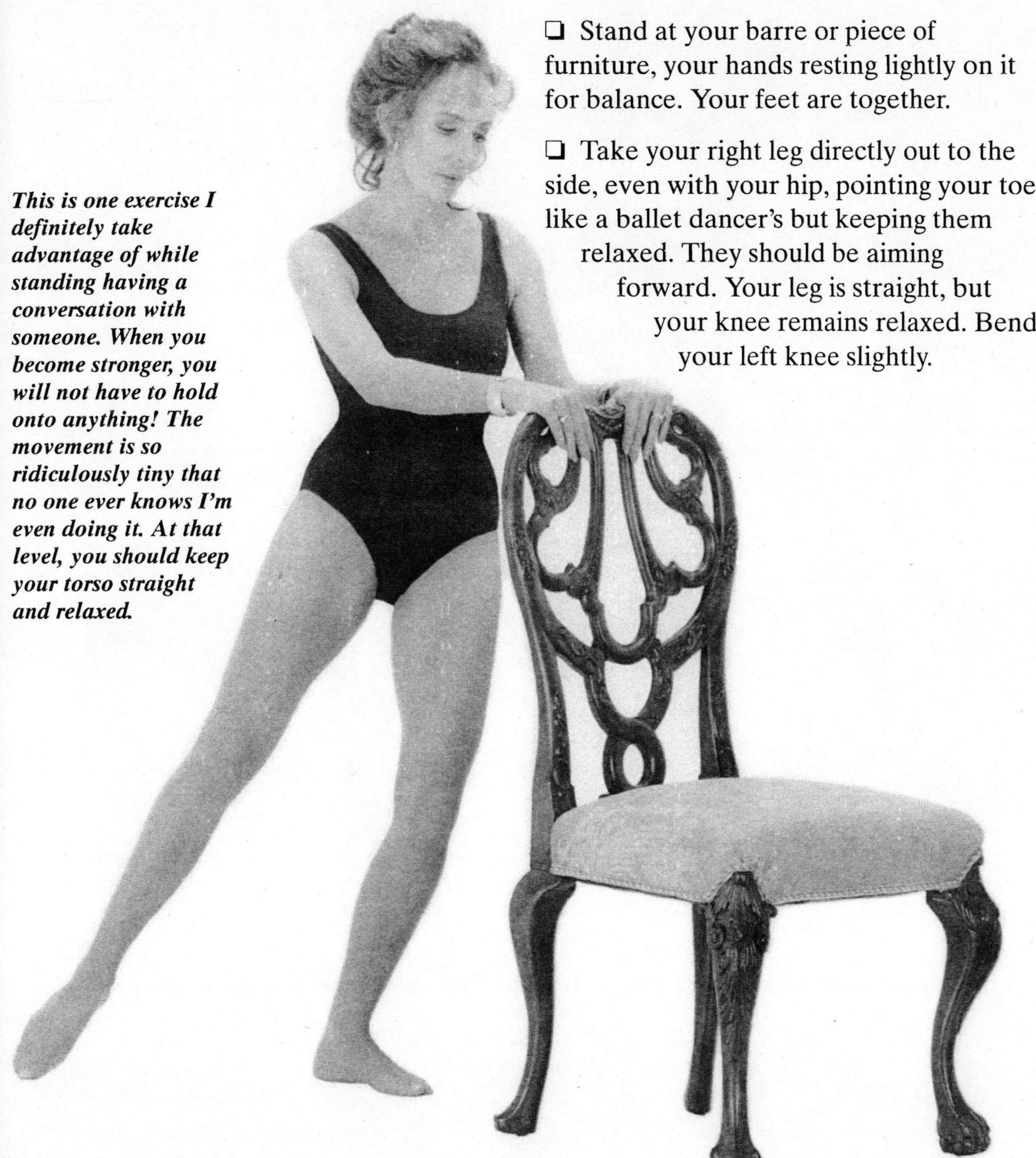

❑ Allowing your hips to move to the left, bring your right leg in towards your body. It can usually come in about 4 to 6 inches.

❑ Tighten your buttocks and curl your pelvis up.

❑ Bend at the waist and aim your right shoulder towards the floor.

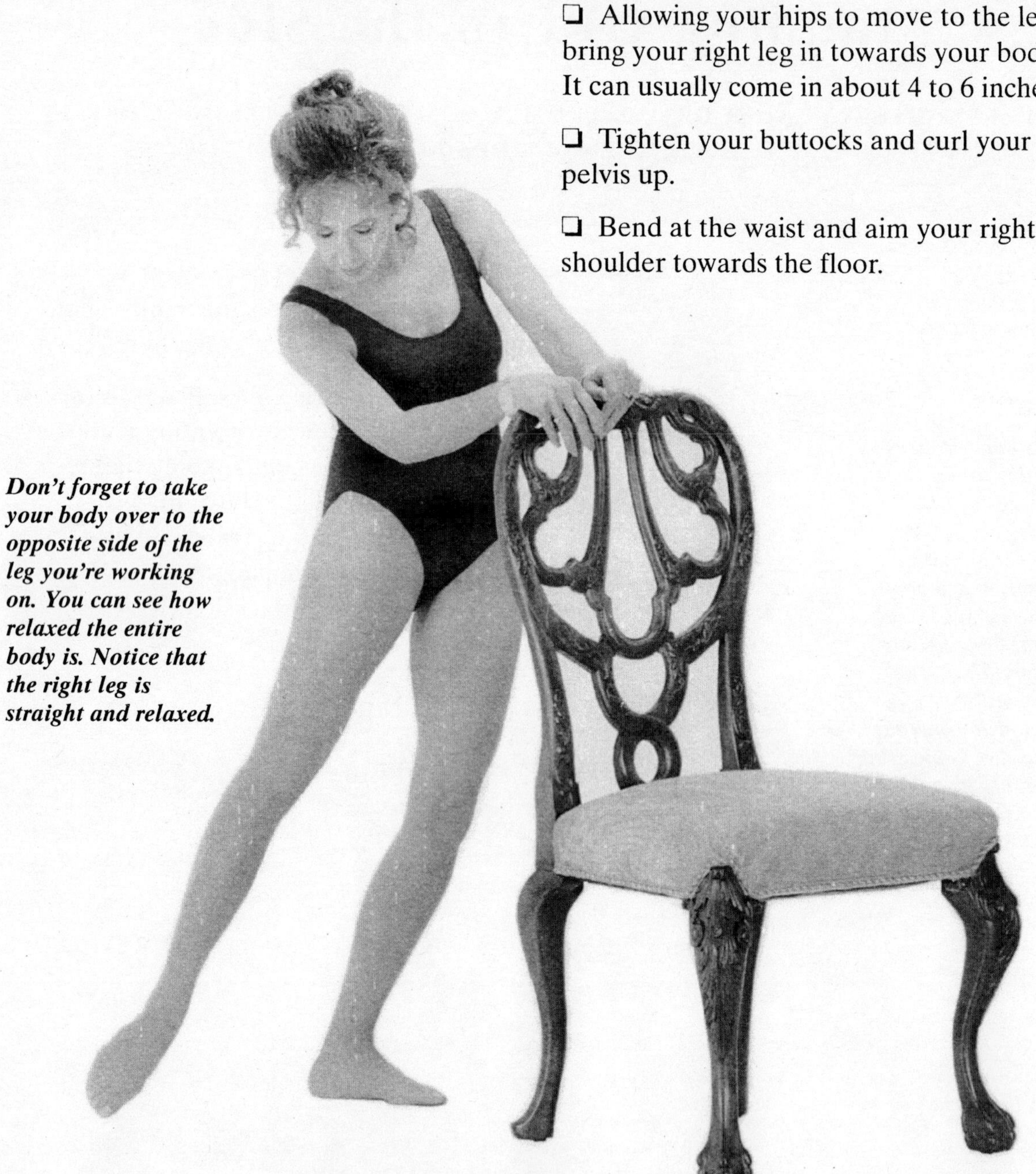

Don't forget to take your body over to the opposite side of the leg you're working on. You can see how relaxed the entire body is. Notice that the right leg is straight and relaxed.

❑ Tighten your buttocks and curl your pelvis up even more than you think you can.

❑ Gently start moving your leg up and down, 1/16 to 1/4 inch.

100 REPS

❑ Repeat this exercise on the opposite side.

100 REPS

DOS AND DON'TS

❑ **Keep your shoulders relaxed; they should be doing absolutely nothing.**

❑ **Keep your hips even. They should not be moving at all.**

❑ **Do not arch your back.**

❑ **Always keep the pelvis tipped up more than you think you can.**

❑ **If you feel you're losing your position and your arms are taking over, take a breather. Or you can take the working leg forward a wee bit.**

❑ **Do not lock your knees.**

❑ **Keep your working leg straight, but do not lock its knee.**

The Entire Body

Open and Close

This exercise builds up incredible strength throughout the entire body. In ballet school, before classes, some students and I would do Open and Close for stamina, leg strength, and for a higher extension of the leg. At the beginning, the more you do, the lower your legs will go. Expect this—don't think you're not doing this exercise correctly if it happens! Believe it or not, there are some people in their seventies who can do fifty Open and Closes effortlessly, without breathers, and their legs remain at the same height.

But as with so much of Super Callanetics, this is an exercise that must be respected. Most people with back problems have found that Open and Close has helped their backs tremendously—because they knew their own limitations and did not force the exercise. This means they *stopped* when they felt that the lower back was about to take over, and only did what they felt they could do *properly* at that particular time.

And as you should be aware from the one-hour program, even though this is basically a leg exercise, it requires tremendous use of the stomach muscles as well. This is why, if your abdominals are not particularly strong, your lower back will inevitably take over—which is not what you want! Build yourself up slowly, and you'll soon find that another wonderful benefit of this exercise is that your stomach muscles also become stronger.

REMEMBER: *If you feel you're losing strength, or your lower back is about to take over, lower your legs a few inches, or bend your knees as you open and close. Or take a breather. If you find that you're still feeling pressure on your lower back, you must discontinue this exercise until you have built up more strength in your stomach and leg muscles.*

REMEMBER: *Height does not matter. Work at your own level. All of the Green Beret and Special Forces that I taught in Berlin discovered in horror that they couldn't even lift their legs off the floor! They had to drag them back and forth across the floor (no comment!).*

BUT DON'T FORGET: *Open and Close must be treated with the respect it deserves!*

❑ Sit on a mat with your upper back against a sofa or counter, and hold onto it as if there is a barre above your head. (Some people use a chest of drawers with one drawer open in place of a barre.) If you have a barre, sit under it with your hands or wrists draped lightly atop it. (By this time, you shouldn't find yourself holding onto it for dear life!)

❑ Bend your knees and take them up towards your chest. Point your toes. Scoot your buttocks forward a few inches so that you are not sitting on your tailbone. Gently drop your chin. This will help stretch your spine more.

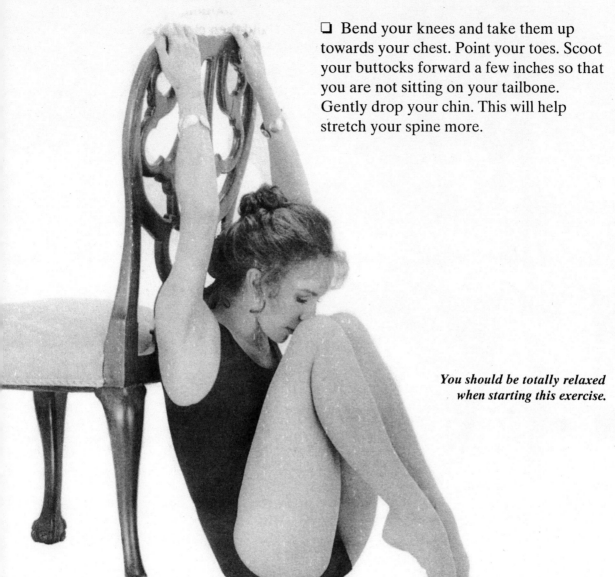

You should be totally relaxed when starting this exercise.

❑ Slowly, straighten your legs, without locking your knees, pointing your toes up towards the ceiling as high as you can without forcing. You are sitting in a jackknife position.

❑ In triple slow motion, open your legs as wide as you can, and then close them.

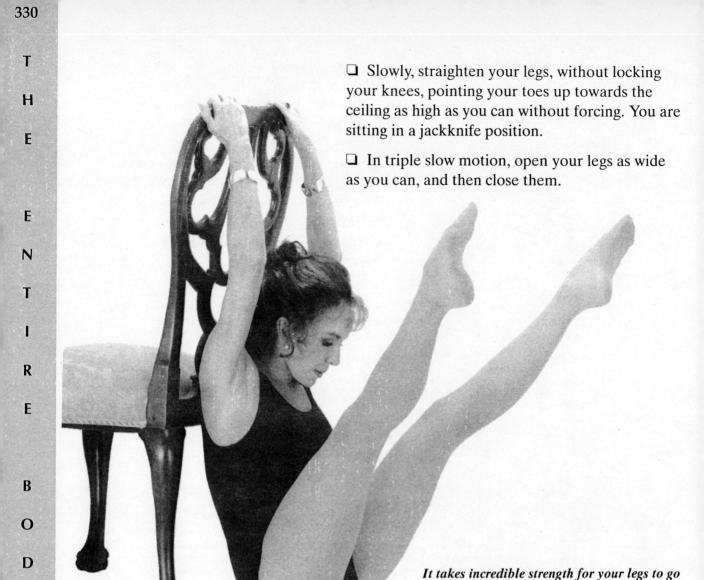

It takes incredible strength for your legs to go this high with ease. Work at your own pace.

DO 5 SETS OF 10, 2 SETS OF 25, OR 50 REPS

❑ To come out of this exercise, gently bend your knees in the closed position, bringing your legs in close to your body, and lower them to the floor.

REMEMBER: *At this point in Super Callanetics, you should already be able to do 50 continuous reps. If, however, you need to break them into 2 sets to avoid putting pressure on your lower back, please do so.*

Some people do Open and Close in sets of 10.

Dos and Don'ts

- ❑ If your muscles are not particularly strong, stop and take breathers, and gradually work up to a set of 25, increasing slowly as your muscles tighten and strengthen.
- ❑ The closer you can place your buttocks up against a wall or piece of furniture, the more difficult this exercise. It is much harder to raise your legs when you are sitting that way—just try one and you'll understand—and as you know, the higher you can raise your legs, the harder Open and Close becomes.
- ❑ Take as many breathers as you wish.
- ❑ Your body must stay relaxed. Do not tighten your grip on the barre or furniture.
- ❑ Always make sure that the object you're holding onto is sturdy enough to hold your weight (without your having to worry about it!).
- ❑ Relax your legs, especially the knees; eventually they will be light as feathers.
- ❑ Keep your chin down.
- ❑ Although your toes are pointed, keep your feet relaxed.
- ❑ Never force your legs to move more than they can.

Stretches

(If you have sciatic pain, always keep your knees bent during all of these stretches. This will help relieve the pressure. If that is not helpful, discontinue these stretches until it is better.)

Sitting Inner-Thigh Stretch

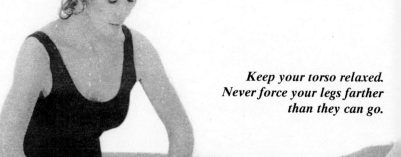

❑ Sitting on the floor, stretch your legs out so they are spread as far apart as they can be without forcing. Place your hands either in front or in back of you—whichever you prefer—and gently push your pelvis into the floor.

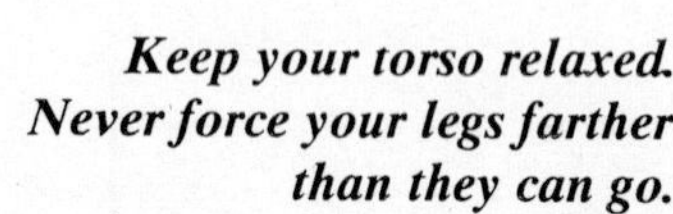

Keep your torso relaxed. Never force your legs farther than they can go.

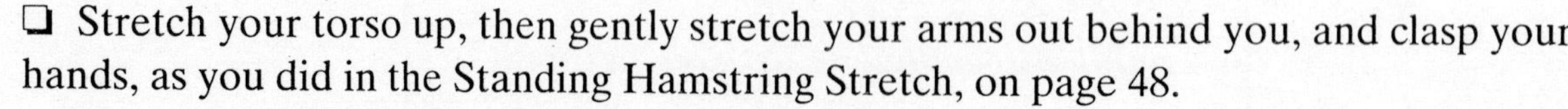

❑ Stretch your torso up, then gently stretch your arms out behind you, and clasp your hands, as you did in the Standing Hamstring Stretch, on page 48.

❑ In triple slow motion, round your upper back forward until your head and shoulders are down as far as they can go without straining. (If you are very stretched, you should be able to touch the floor with either your face, your nose, or your upper torso.)

❑ Gently let your arms move even higher behind your back; try to stretch your torso so that your arms are aiming directly up towards the ceiling.

Move your arms up as high as you can without forcing.

❑ Relax your body, and feel the stretch in your lower back and inner thighs. If you are stretched enough to be resting on the floor, however, simply take advantage of this time to let your body melt into the floor, especially your neck. (This stretch can be so relaxing—careful that you don't fall asleep!)

HOLD FOR A COUNT OF 50

❑ Or, if you are *not* resting on the floor, gently move your torso 1/16 to 1/4 inch, up and down.

50 REPS TO THE CENTER

❑ Next you will be going over to your right leg. Unclasp your hands and slowly take your torso over to your right leg, bringing your arms over at the same time. (Or, if you prefer, you may walk your hands over in front of you on the floor.)

❑ Lower your hands lightly and crisscross them on your ankle, taking your elbows out and forward to stretch your waist. (It's the opposite arm going forward that stretches your waist.) Let your head rest on your leg.

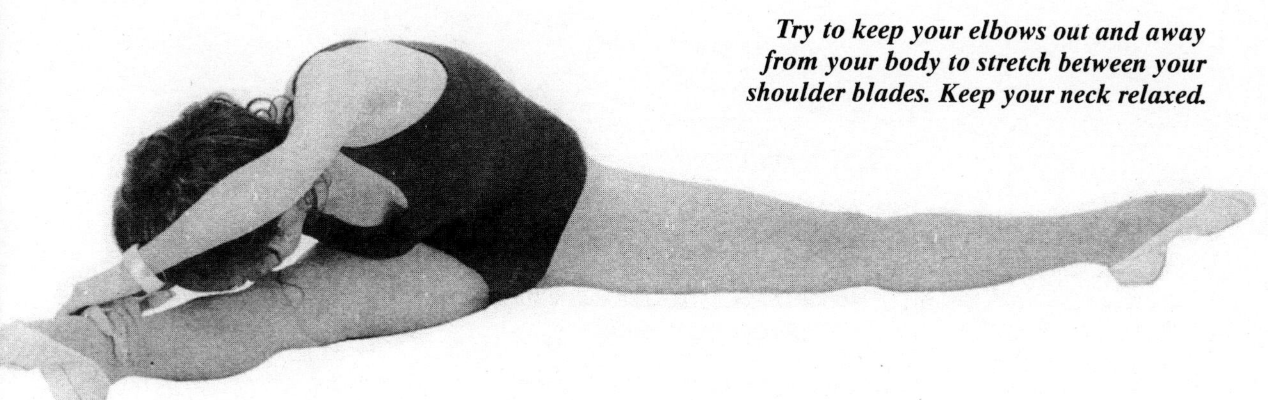

Try to keep your elbows out and away from your body to stretch between your shoulder blades. Keep your neck relaxed.

❑ In an almost imperceptible motion, gently move your head and torso towards your feet or the floor, 1/16 to 1/4 inch, and then back.

50 REPS TO THE RIGHT

❑ Gently walk your hands over to your outstretched left leg, and again crisscross them to rest on your ankle. Let your head rest on your leg.

❑ Delicately move back and forth, 1/16 to 1/4 inch.

50 REPS TO THE LEFT

❑ To come out of this exercise, in triple slow motion, gently walk your hands up your leg (do not touch your knee) or place your hands on either side of your leg and walk your hands up as you roll your torso back up to the starting position, vertebra by vertebra.

FOR MORE OF A STRETCH ON EACH SIDE: *Keep your elbows out away from your body. The more you aim your elbows forward, the more you will be stretching your waist. You can also rest your head on either side of your leg, then move gently back and forth towards your foot.*

DOS AND DON'TS

❑ **Do not force your body down.**

❑ **Do feel the stretch in your lower back and inner thighs—*feel* the waist stretch when you're over to the side.**

❑ **Do not bounce.**

❑ **Do not pull forward with your neck.**

❑ **Relax your toes and your legs.**

❑ **Relax your entire body, especially your neck.**

Sitting Hamstring Stretch

(If you have sciatica, always keep your knees bent during this exercise.)

This is the stretch I do when I feel like my neck is becoming like a brick (not even crumbling!) from stress. It should be able to help you as well.

This is basically the same movement forward as the Sitting Inner-Thigh Stretch, done with your legs together.

❑ Sitting up on the floor, close your legs so that your feet are together in front of you, pointed but relaxed.

FOR MORE OF A STRETCH: *Especially for your calves, turn your feet up so they are flexed.*

❑ Stretch your arms out behind you, and clasp your hands. Now gently raise them up as high as you can take them.

❑ Stretch your torso up, then slowly round your upper torso forward until your head and shoulders are down as far as they can go without forcing. Feel the stretch in your lower back as you go down. Try to rest your head on your legs.

❑ Let your arms move up gently even higher behind your back; try to stretch your torso so that your arms are aiming directly up towards the ceiling.

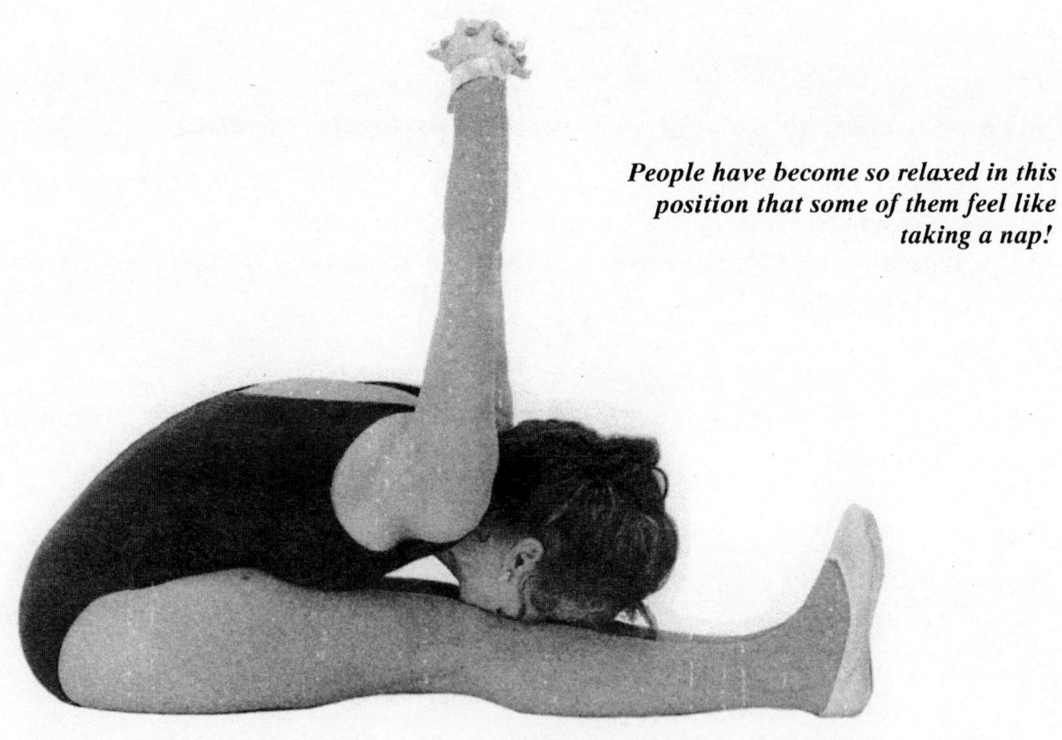

People have become so relaxed in this position that some of them feel like taking a nap!

❑ Relax your body, and feel the stretch in your lower back and hamstrings.

❑ Gently move your torso 1/16 to 1/4 inch, up and down, if you are not resting your head on your legs. If you are stretched enough to be resting on your legs, however, simply take advantage of this time to let your body melt into your legs, especially your neck. Or, if you prefer, you can gently move your head towards your feet, forward and back, 1/16 to 1/4 inch.

HOLD FOR A COUNT OF 50

❑ To come out of this stretch, bring your arms down in triple slow motion, unclasp your hands, and rest them on the floor.

❑ Slowly bring your body up, rounding your torso, one vertebra at a time.

Dos and Don'ts

- ❑ Your torso is rounded—not straight—when you're going down. Otherwise you'll be putting pressure on your lower back.
- ❑ Relax your legs, especially your knees.
- ❑ Relax your neck and shoulders. Allow your neck to melt into the floor.
- ❑ Do not force your body down.
- ❑ Do feel this stretch in your lower back.

Lying-Down Hamstring and Calf Stretch

(If you have sciatica, always keep your knees bent during this exercise, to relieve pressure on your lower back.)

❑ Lie on your back and bend your knees. Keep your feet flat on the floor.

❑ Bend your right knee up into your chest, and then straighten that leg.

❑ Clasp your hands around your calf or ankle with your elbows up and out, and, in triple slow motion, bring your leg as close to your body as you can.

❑ Gently straighten your left leg on the floor, without locking your knee, and rest your left heel on the floor.

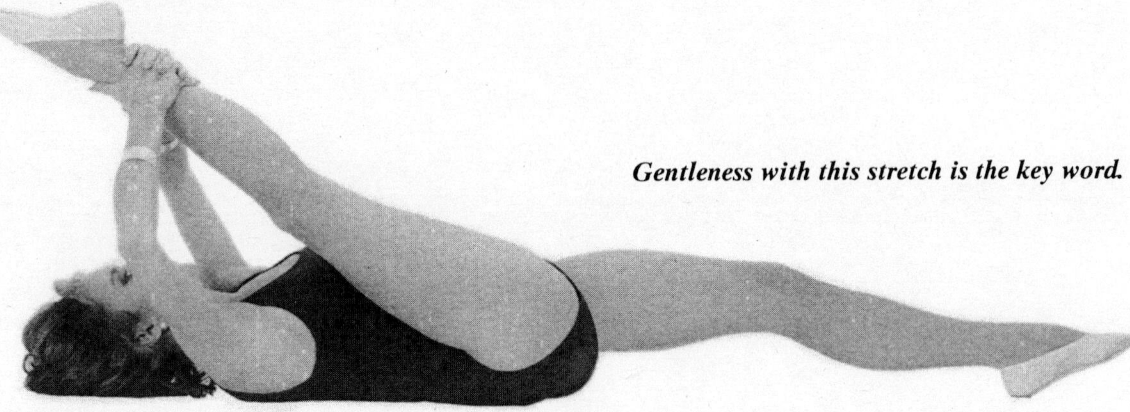

Gentleness with this stretch is the key word.

❑ With an almost imperceptible motion, move your right leg towards your body, 1/16 to 1/4 inch.

50 REPS

FOR MORE OF A STRETCH, OR TO STRETCH YOUR CALVES: *Flex your feet towards you. Do not point them up towards the ceiling.*

❑ To come out of this stretch, bend both your knees in a smooth, gentle motion, and place your feet flat on the floor. Bring your arms down as well, and rest them by your side.

❑ Repeat this exercise on the opposite side.

50 REPS

DOS AND DON'TS

❑ Do not force your leg up higher than it can go.

❑ Do not lock your knees.

❑ Keep the leg that is resting on the floor as straight and as low as possible, as long as your knee remains relaxed.

❑ Keep the foot of your raised leg pointed but relaxed.

❑ Do not tighten your grasp on your calf or ankle.

❑ Keep your neck and shoulders very relaxed. Take advantage of this time to relax your neck and entire body.

Spine Stretch

Remember in the one-hour Callanetics program I explained that this was a gentle adaptation of a chiropractic manipulation—and that after doing the Spine Stretch, my hips became even for the first time in my life? Well, nearly twenty years later, my hips are *still* even . . . but of course I always take advantage of this spine stretch as much as I can.

❑ Still lying on the floor with your knees bent and feet resting flat, bring your arms up to your shoulders.

❑ Bending from the elbow, place your forearms at a right angle to the side of your head, resting them lightly with your palms facing upward. Your elbows must remain on the floor.

❑ In triple slow motion, lift your right knee, bent, up to your chest. Let your left leg gently ease down until it rests on the floor. Take your bent right knee over to your left side, away from your body as much as you can, trying to rest your foot and knee on the floor.

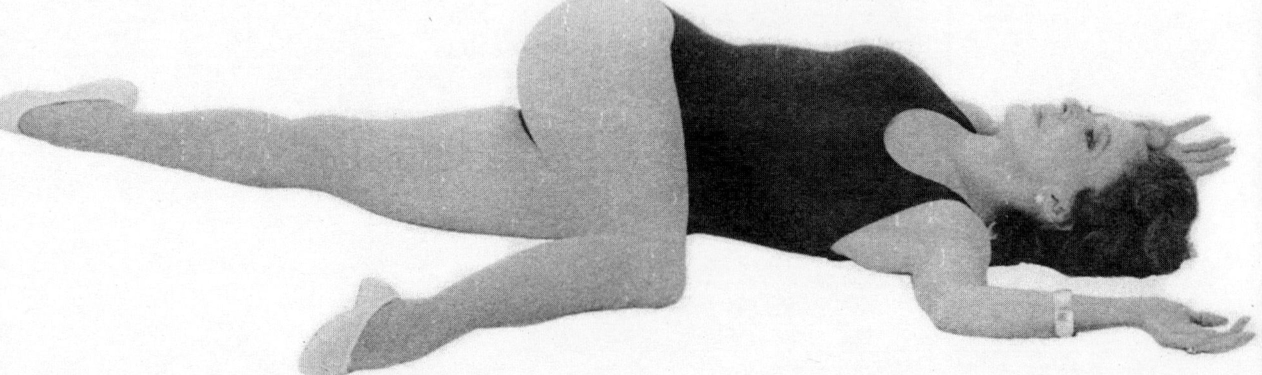

Notice the position of the left leg, resting on the floor—and how far back it has been taken for even more of a stretch. Both knees are very relaxed.

FOR MORE OF A STRETCH: *Gently move your right knee up to your left elbow.*

FOR EVEN MORE OF A STRETCH: *Ease your straight leg to the back of you, as shown in the photo above.*

HOLD FOR A COUNT OF 50 TO 100

❑ To come out of this stretch and go over to the other side, in triple slow motion, keeping your right knee bent, bring it back to your chest and then place your right foot on the floor, with your knee bent.

❑ Bend your left knee to your chest, and then slide your right foot down to the floor. This is all done in one smooth, continuous motion.

❑ Repeat this stretch on the opposite side.

HOLD FOR A COUNT OF 50 TO 100

❑ To come out of this stretch, in triple slow motion, keeping your left knee bent, bring it back to your chest, and then place your left foot on the floor. Bend your right knee, and place that foot flat on the floor. Then ease yourself up to a standing position in the same manner as you did after the stomach exercises **or** if you are able to, or if you choose to, you can go directly into the Leg Splits.

Dos and Don'ts

- ❑ **Do not force your bent leg down to the floor.**
- ❑ **Do not lift your shoulders or elbows off the floor.**
- ❑ **Do keep your body completely relaxed.**
- ❑ **Do take advantage of this time to relax your neck.**
- ❑ **Remember, gravity is doing the work, not you!**
- ❑ **Think beautiful, happy thoughts!**

Leg Splits

❑ Moving directly from the end position of the Spine Stretch, roll over and ease yourself up into a sitting position. Extend your right leg in front of you, with your hands resting on the floor to the sides of your right leg.

❑ Extend your left leg as straight behind you as you can.

Do not attempt this until you feel you are very stretched. And then be very careful.

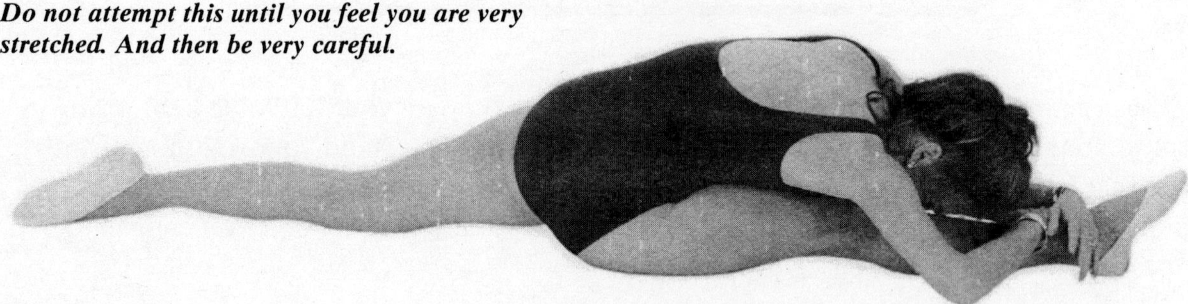

FOR MORE OF A STRETCH: *Bring your torso down to your outstretched right leg, allowing your head to rest on your leg. Keep your elbows out and your arms relaxed, or crisscross your hands over your ankle.*

HOLD FOR A COUNT OF 25

❑ To come out of the split, raise your torso slightly by walking your hands either up your leg or on the floor to the sides of your leg. Bend your right knee and slide it in towards your body. Bend your left leg as well and slide it forward.

❑ Gently ease yourself up by putting your hands on the floor and then gently returning to a standing position, vertebra by vertebra.

Dos and Don'ts

- ❏ Do only as much of a split as you can.
- ❏ Do not ever try to force your body down further than it can go. If you can only do a partial split, that's perfectly all right.
- ❏ Keep your upper body relaxed.
- ❏ If you are not able to rest both legs straight on the floor, don't worry! You can use your hands to support your body by resting them by your sides, gently on the floor. Be sure, however, not to push into the floor (this is a stretch, not a push-up!).

Pelvis– Front and Inner Thighs

Pelvic Rotation

(If you have knee problems, you can do the Pelvic Rotation in a standing position, with your knees bent. You will not see results as quickly, but as you already know, your health and safety are far more important!)

As most of you already will have experienced from the one-hour program, the reason the Pelvic Rotation is such a challenge is because it helps you gather strength from your entire body (including your toes!). As one student commented in class, 'It's excitingly frightening how much your pelvis can curl up!'

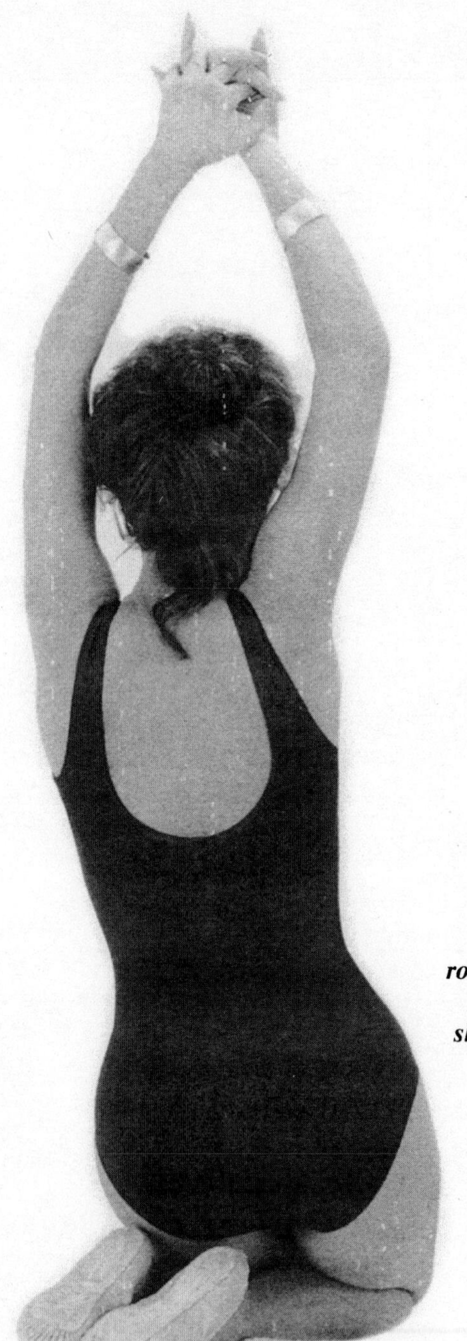

The entire routine is one continuous slow motion.

❑ On a mat, sit comfortably on your heels. Your knees are together and your legs relaxed.

❑ Stretch your arms up over your head and clasp your hands together. Keep your torso erect, and feel the stretch in your back.

❑ Lift your torso 2 to 3 inches up off your heels.

❑ Take your right hip over to the right side as far as you can. Roll your pelvis forward, to the front, at the same time curling it up and aiming it into your navel. Move your left hip over to the left side as far as you can. Then move your buttocks to the back, completing a circle.

The motion is a smooth, flowing circle—hip—pelvis—hip—behind. Only your pelvis moves in an unbroken circle.

20 REPS OF A CIRCLE, STARTING WITH YOUR RIGHT HIP OVER TO THE SIDE

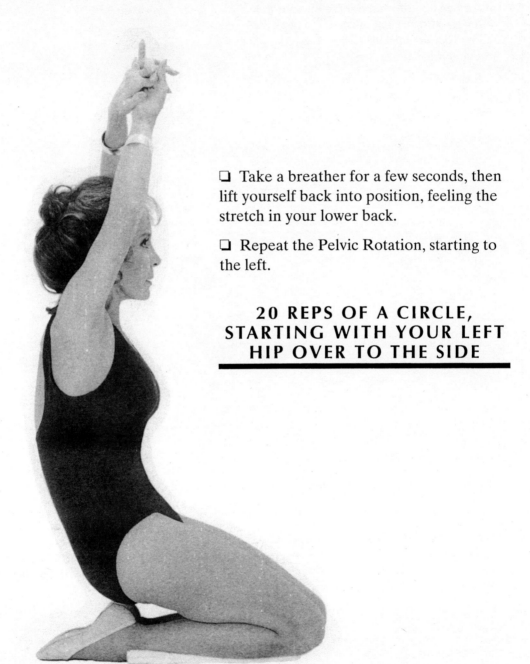

❑ Take a breather for a few seconds, then lift yourself back into position, feeling the stretch in your lower back.

❑ Repeat the Pelvic Rotation, starting to the left.

20 REPS OF A CIRCLE, STARTING WITH YOUR LEFT HIP OVER TO THE SIDE

Your pelvis can curl up more than you think it can.

Dos and Don'ts

- ❑ Whichever Callanetics you have been doing, at this point you should be able to make a larger, more flowing circle. The Super Callanetics Pelvic Rotation allows you to aim your buttocks back, because you should have more flexibility in that area by now, and can complete a full circle without difficulty. This is not an up-and-down motion with your pelvis but a smooth circular motion. Do not ever allow your movements to become jerky—they should always flow.

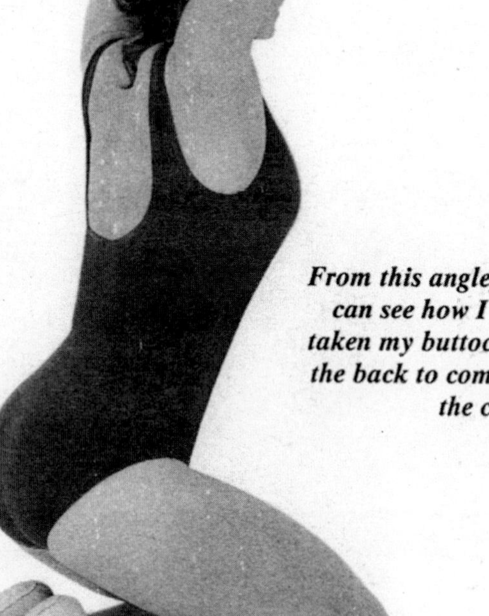

From this angle, you can see how I have taken my buttocks to the back to complete the circle.

- ❑ Do keep your entire body relaxed.
- ❑ The more you can curl your pelvis up into your navel, the more effective this exercise.
- ❑ Take breathers whenever you feel it necessary.
- ❑ Most men find it difficult to sit directly on the bottom of their feet. They can either turn both ankles out towards the floor—this creates a nice little hollow space for their buttocks to rest in. Or they can place the bottom of their toes on the floor and sit on their heels, which would then be facing up towards the ceiling.

Pelvic Rotation—Figure 8

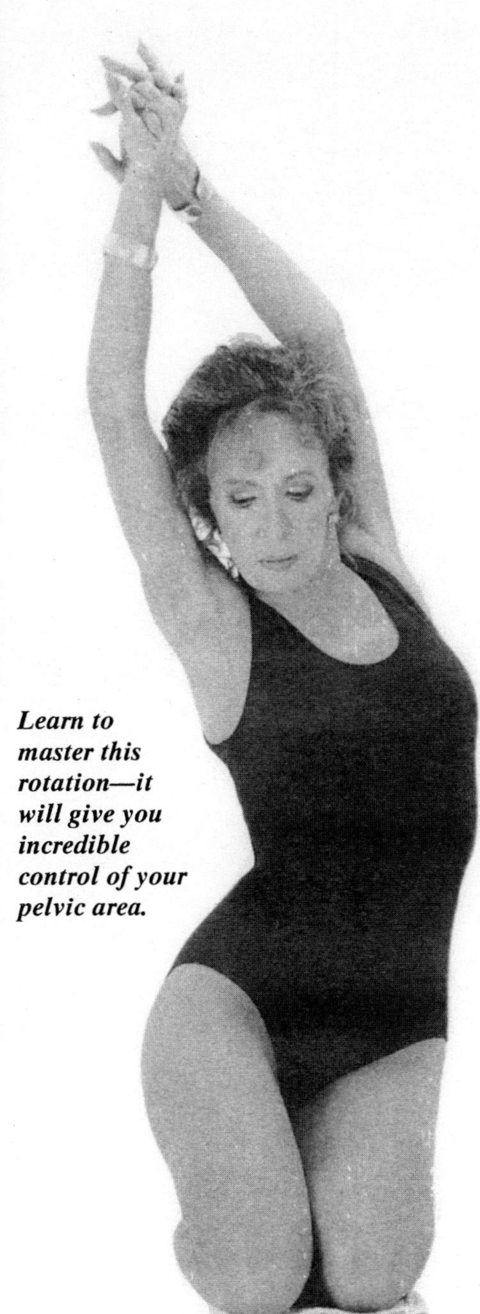

Learn to master this rotation—it will give you incredible control of your pelvic area.

This exercise is done in exactly the same manner as the Pelvic Rotation.

❑ Sit on your heels, knees together, your legs relaxed.

❑ Lift your arms up over your head and clasp your hands together. Feel the stretch in your lower back, and keep your torso erect.

❑ Lift your torso 2 to 3 inches up off your heels.

❑ Take your right hip out to the side, as far as you can. Then roll your right hip forward, aiming it up. As you do this, your left hip will autoı5atically lower a few inches, and be aimed more towards your back.

❑ Then, take your left buttock back as far as it will go. When your left buttock can't go back any further, gently start rounding your left hip forward in a half-circle to the point where your left hip is up and forward as far as it can go. Your right hip is now back.

DO AS MANY AS YOU CAN

The motion is a smooth figure 8—one hip up—the opposite buttock down and back—one hip up—the opposite buttock down and back.
Only your pelvis moves.

Dos and Don'ts

- ❑ You must be terribly strong in your inner thighs to attempt this figure 8.
- ❑ Do not arch your back or stick out your buttocks.
- ❑ Do keep your body relaxed.

Pelvic Scoop

❑ Kneel on a mat, knees together, with your feet outstretched behind you and your legs relaxed.

❑ Lift your arms up over your head and clasp your hands together. Feel the stretch in your lower back.

❑ Lower your arms in front about a foot. Round your torso a wee bit forward. Now, keeping your spine straight, aim your buttocks down towards your heels. *Do not arch your back.*

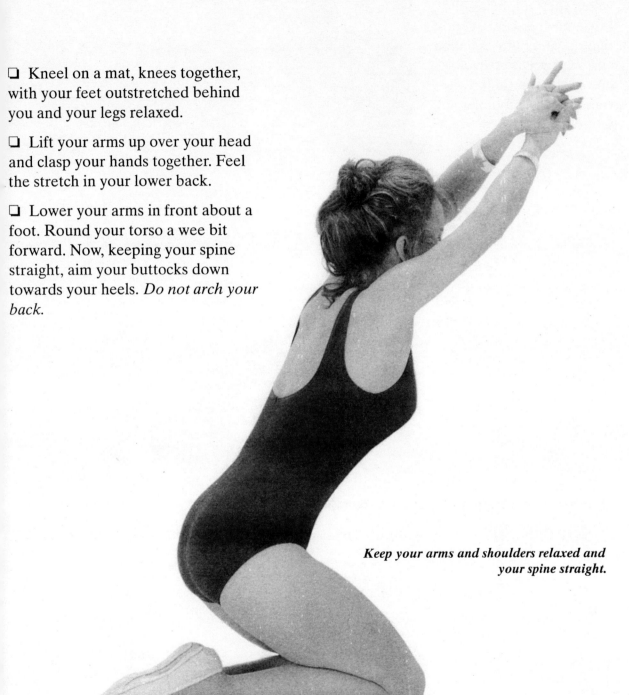

Keep your arms and shoulders relaxed and your spine straight.

❑ When you have stretched your buttocks to the point where they are delicately brushing your heels, gently tighten your buttocks, then curl your pelvis up even more than you think you can, in a slow scooping motion.

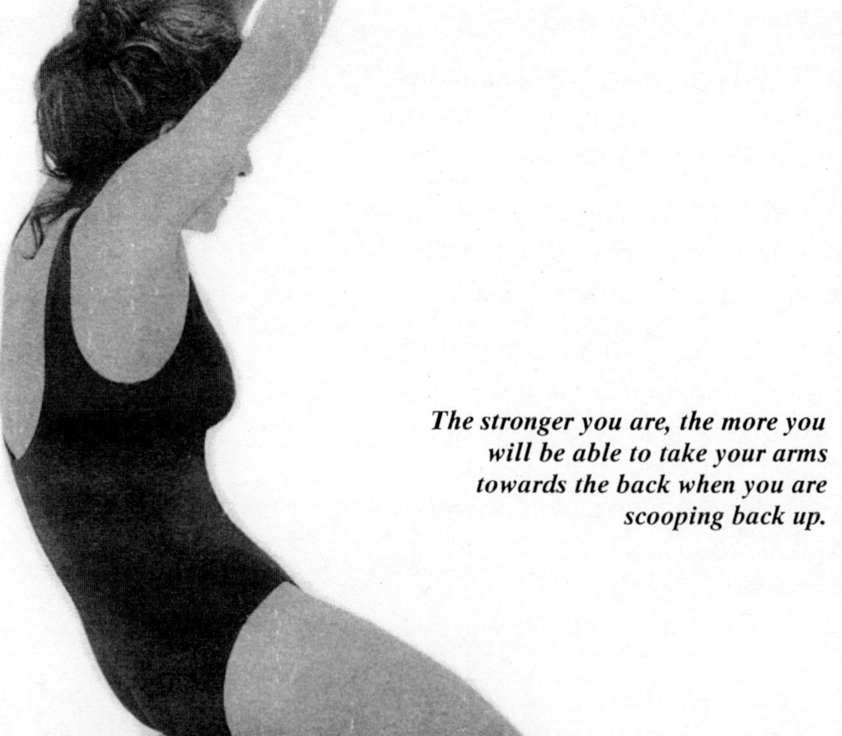

The stronger you are, the more you will be able to take your arms towards the back when you are scooping back up.

❑ Raise your arms back up till your hands are above your head in the starting position.

❑ Keep curling your pelvis up until you have returned to the original kneeling position.

REMEMBER: *The more you can take your arms and torso back when you are returning to the original kneeling position with your curl-up, the faster your thigh muscles will strengthen. This is, however, quite a challenge.*

And the higher you can curl your pelvis, the more you will be strengthening your inner thighs.

10 TO 20 REPS

FOR MORE OF A CHALLENGE: *Push your knees together when you are returning to the starting position.*

Dos and Don'ts

- ❑ **Do keep your entire body relaxed.**
- ❑ **Do keep your arms and shoulders relaxed. Do not strain your arms forward.**
- ❑ **Keep your pelvis curled up when you are returning to your original position.**
- ❑ **Do not arch your back.**
- ❑ **Keep your buttocks tightened when you are returning to the kneeling position.**
- ❑ **If you find yourself needing a breather, take one. Relax your body and breathe naturally. Then resume the original position and continue.**
- ❑ **If you feel a strain in your calves when you are returning to the starting position, bend your arms and torso forward.**

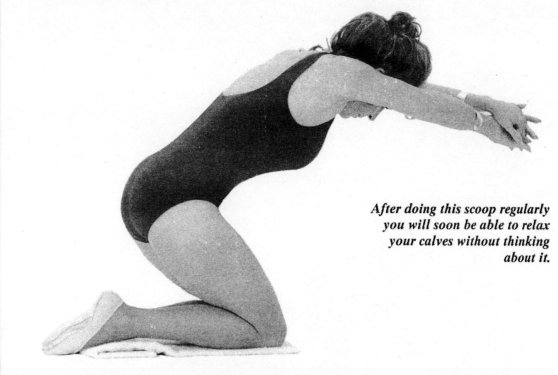

After doing this scoop regularly you will soon be able to relax your calves without thinking about it.

Front-Thigh Stretch

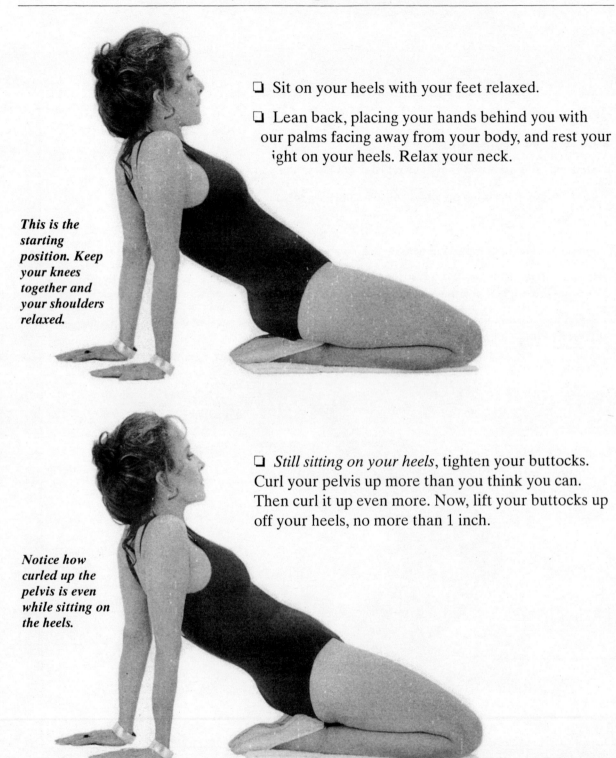

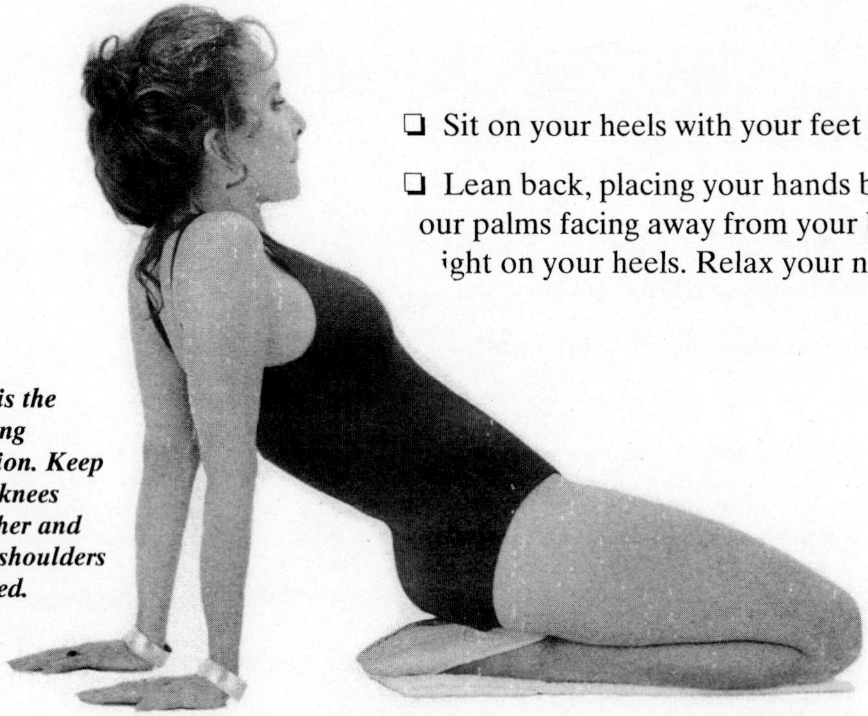

❑ Sit on your heels with your feet relaxed.

❑ Lean back, placing your hands behind you with our palms facing away from your body, and rest your ight on your heels. Relax your neck.

This is the starting position. Keep your knees together and your shoulders relaxed.

❑ *Still sitting on your heels*, tighten your buttocks. Curl your pelvis up more than you think you can. Then curl it up even more. Now, lift your buttocks up off your heels, no more than 1 inch.

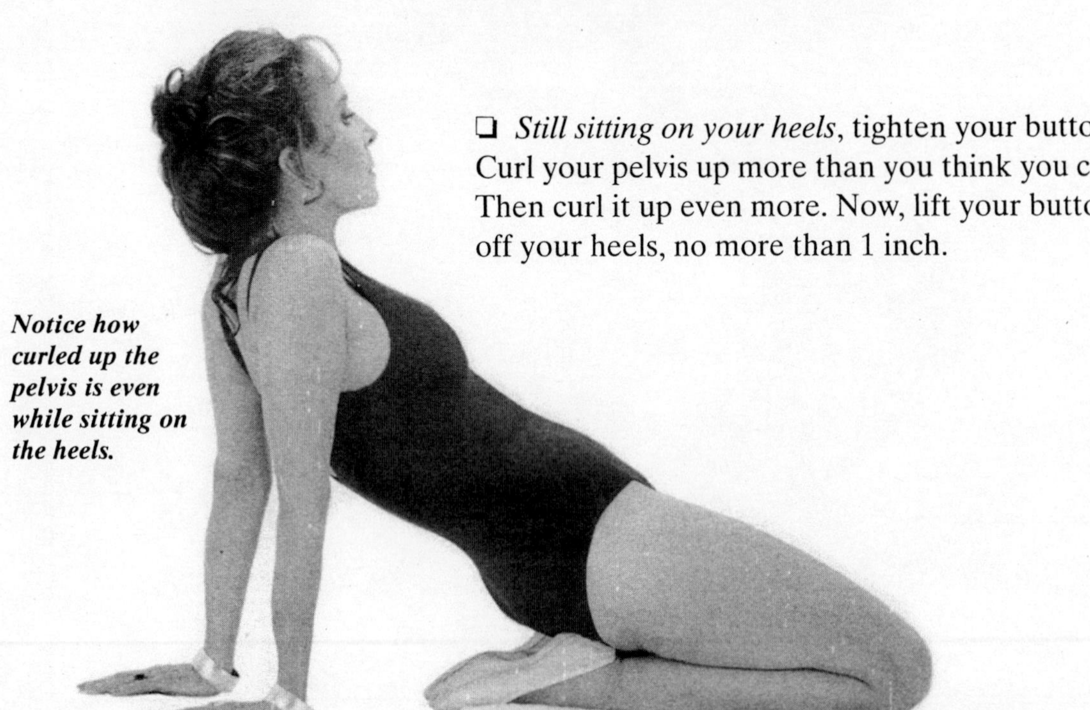

Notice how curled up the pelvis is even while sitting on the heels.

❑ Curl your pelvis up even higher.

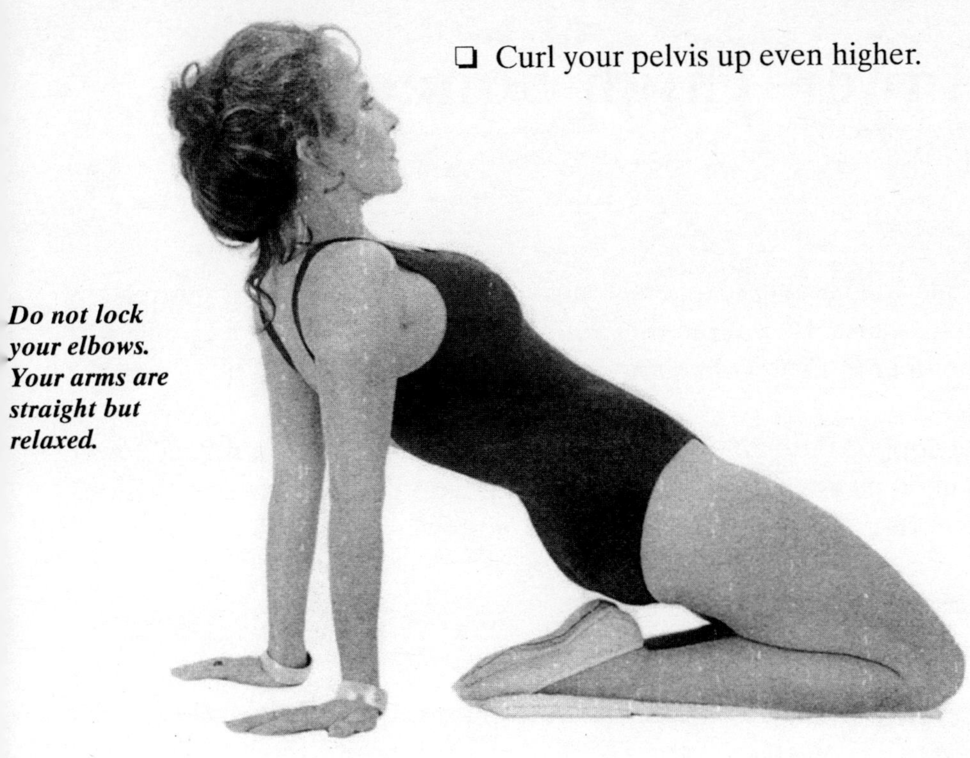

Do not lock your elbows. Your arms are straight but relaxed.

❑ Move gently up and down no more than 1/16 to 1/4 inch.

20 REPS

Dos and Don'ts

- ❑ Do not arch your back. Keep your spine straight.
- ❑ Keep your neck relaxed.
- ❑ Do not move your head up or down.
- ❑ The more you curl your pelvis up, the more your thighs will stretch.
- ❑ Do not put too much pressure on your hands.
- ❑ Relax your entire body.

Inner-Thigh Squeeze

By now, most people will be able to sit erect during this exercise, without putting pressure on their lower backs. If you find that your lower back is still assisting during the Thigh Squeeze, remember to keep your shoulders rounded. You can also take breathers if you need to.

This is also a lovely opportunity to be able to stretch your neck. Let your head lower forward slightly, taking it down in a delicate, slow motion, until your chin is resting on your chest. Or, if you prefer, gently stretch your neck up towards the ceiling.

❑ Facing a chair or legs of a table, sit on the floor, your back straight. Your arms are at your sides, resting lightly on the floor.

❑ Place the arch of each foot on the chair or table legs, up as high as you can keep them without feeling any strain in your lower back. Relax your shoulders.

❑ Keeping your toes pointed and relaxed, squeeze as if trying to bring the legs of your piece of furniture together.

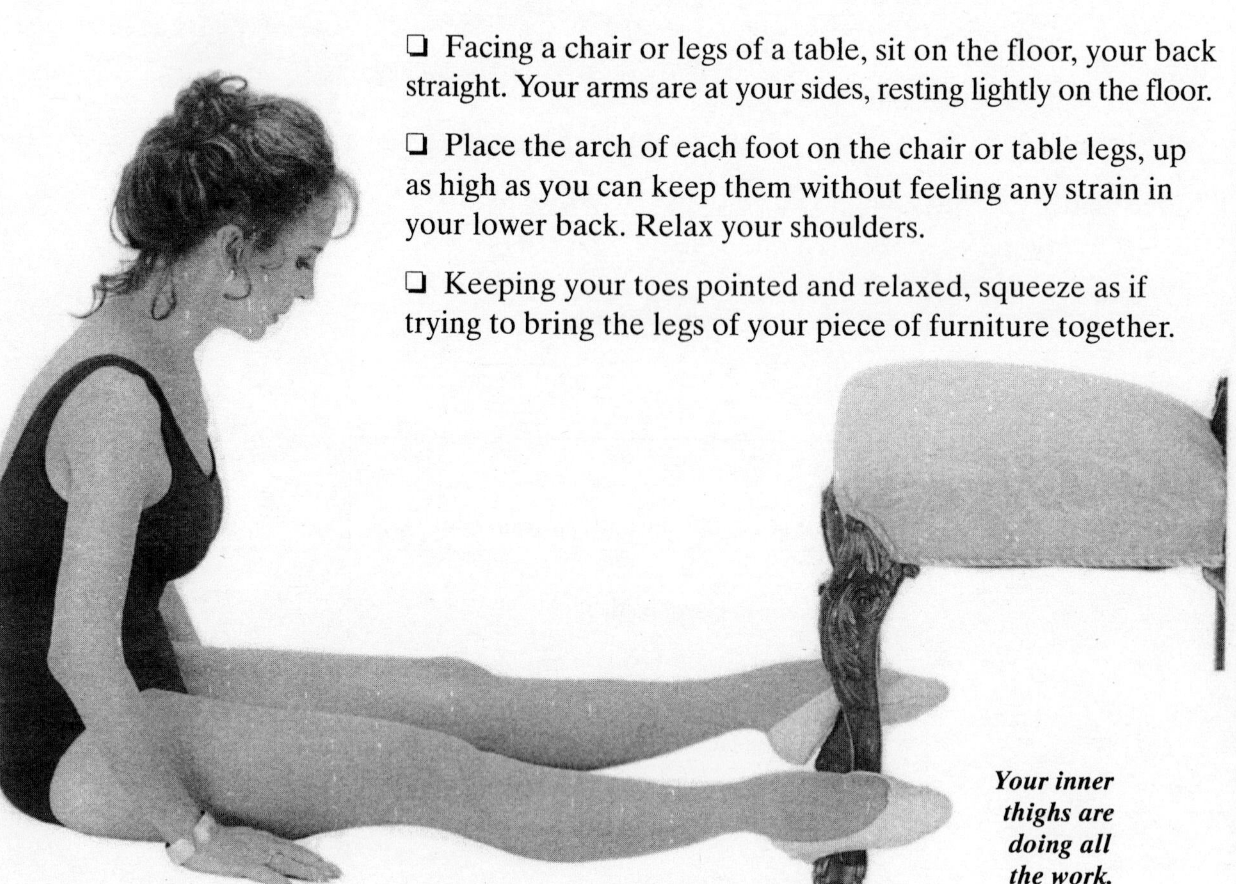

Your inner thighs are doing all the work.

100 REPS • WORK UP TO 300

FOR MORE OF A CHALLENGE: *Place the arches of your feet higher on the outside of the chair or table legs and squeeze.*

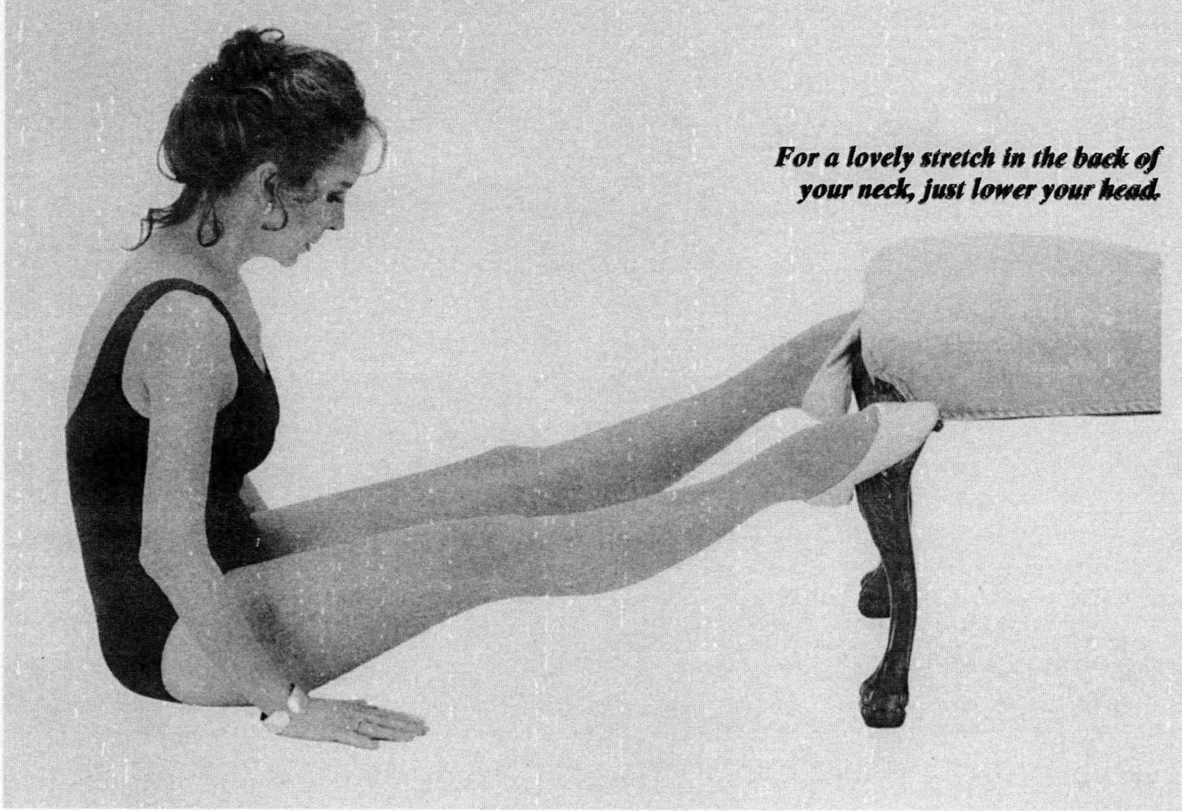

For a lovely stretch in the back of your neck, just lower your head.

FOR EVEN MORE OF A CHALLENGE: *With your legs resting on the floor, place the inside of your heels on the outside of the chair or table legs. Point your toes away from the chair or table legs, and squeeze with your heels.*

DOS AND DON'TS

- ❑ Keep your shoulders relaxed.
- ❑ Keep your legs relaxed.
- ❑ Do not lock your knees.
- ❑ Relax your lower back.
- ❑ Keep your hands and arms relaxed and comfortable.

The Twenty-Minute Super Callanetics Routine

The Twenty-Minute Super Callanetics Routine

When I am very rushed and don't have time to do the entire Super Callanetics routine, I still allow myself twenty minutes to do some of the exercises. These will still give me strength, stamina, and flexibility throughout my body. (I would be so horrified if my muscles and skin started to sag—anywhere!)

These exercises are what I choose to do in twenty minutes, but *remember,* my muscles are extremely strong, so I can breeze through this routine. At first, you may not be able to do all of these exercises in twenty minutes. Don't worry about that! Simply choose several of them, and as your strength increases, you will be able to add on until you have mastered these as well.

I must stress, however, that a twenty-minute routine is no substitute for the regular Super Callanetics one-hour regimen. These are only designed to be substitutes when you are severely pressed for time.

WARM-UPS

1. The Waist-Away Stretch • 100 REPS EACH SIDE
2. Underarm Tightener • 100 REPS

STOMACH

3. Sit Up and Curl Down • FOLLOW DIRECTIONS CAREFULLY!

LEGS

4. Pelvic-Wave Leg Strengthener • 3 SETS
5. Hamstring Stretch #2—Bent Leg • HOLD FOR A COUNT OF 50

   Try to do this with your heel underneath your barre.

BUTTOCKS—OUTER THIGHS—HIPS

6. Standing Out to the Side • 100 REPS

THE ENTIRE BODY

7. Open and Close • 50 REPS

STRETCHES

8. Spine Stretch • HOLD FOR A COUNT OF 100 ON EACH SIDE

PELVIS—FRONT and INNER THIGHS

9. Pelvic Rotation • 20 REPS OF A FULL CIRCLE TO THE RIGHT, AND THEN 20 REPS OF A FULL CIRCLE TO THE LEFT

10. Inner-Thigh Squeeze • 100 REPS

The one exercise I always do whenever I can, even while standing and talking to someone, is the Standing Out to the Side. Most people don't have a clue I'm doing it. If you do attempt this exercise, make sure you do an equal amount on each side, for this exercise works so fast, your buttocks will become lopsided if you favour one side over the other. How embarrassing this would be in a tight dress or tight trousers!

If it's appropriate, I'll also try to do the The Waist-Away Stretch and the Underarm Tightener when other people are around. They usually join in with enthusiasm! Play around with these—you will soon be quite surprised what you can accomplish (and where!). Your balance will soon improve so drastically that you won't have to worry about holding onto anything for support.

A Final Message

Not long ago an elderly man who does Super Callanetics regularly said to me, 'Callan, don't use up your energy trying to explain to people what the difference is between Super Callanetics and other exercises. There's simply no way they will understand until they've done Super Callanetics themselves. Just tell them it's like the difference between the postman and a fax machine. Both of them will deliver a letter, but you can get that letter so much faster with a fax. And there's no damage to it.'

I like that analogy. Super Callanetics has offered so many people an incredible opportunity to take their body strength beyond what they would have classified as their limitations, without stress or strain—no damage to it. It is such a wonderful feeling to know that your very own body can accomplish incredible feats that you never even thought possible.

And so I will continue to take advantage of all that Super Callanetics has to offer, along with the thousands of other people who have used it to transform their bodies. And the reason I can do so with complete confidence is because I have a guarantee that every time I do Super Callanetics, I know that not only will I have a tighter body when I have completed the routine, but I will not ever have to worry about injuring myself. Super Callanetics is a more efficient way to maintain—in less time—the incredible results you already will have obtained from mastering the one-hour program. And Super Callanetics provides an incredible challenge for those of you who have trained your muscles so well. Even more important than your physical transformation will be your *mental* transformation—the glowing look that accompanies self-confidence and an improved self-image.